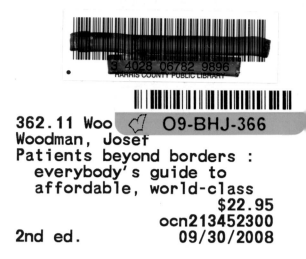

"A useful new book on this topic. . . ."

—*Savvy Senior*

"I am considering elective surgery and this was a great compendium of information scattered all over the Internet."

—Amy Tupper (Sanford, NC)

"I spent a lot of time on the Internet trying to research this topic on my own and looking for certain procedures (mainly dental and cosmetic surgery). I wound up getting dental work done in Mexico at a facility reviewed in this book and am happy with my experience. I recommend this book to anyone even remotely considering foreign medical travel."

—K. Williamson (Los Lunas, NM)

"Woodman's father is not alone in looking abroad for a medical overhaul. After all, if the American healthcare system is not completely broken, it is certainly dysfunctional: 47 million people have no health coverage, and 130 million have no dental insurance. As baby boomers age into more medical problems with spotty coverage and would prefer not to deplete their retirement savings, they are looking at all available options."

—*Financial Times*

". . . a must-read for those considering medical tourism . . ."

—*ABC News*

"A practical guide to planning a medical trip . . ."

—*The Washington Post*

Patients Beyond Borders
Second Edition

Patients Beyond Borders

Everybody's Guide to Affordable, World-Class Medical Travel

Second Edition

Josef Woodman

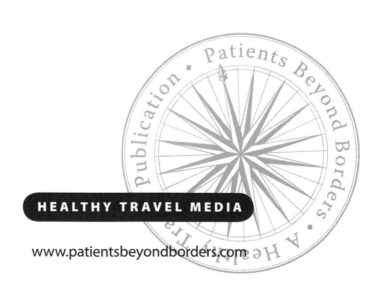

HEALTHY TRAVEL MEDIA

www.patientsbeyondborders.com

PATIENTS BEYOND BORDERS:
Everybody's Guide to Affordable, World-Class Medical Travel
Second Edition

Copyright © 2008 by Josef Woodman

ISBN 13: 978-0-9791079-2-4

Cover art and page design: Anne Winslow
Developmental Editing, First Edition: Yvette Bozzini
Developmental Editing, Second Edition: Faith Brynie
Copy Editing: Kate Johnson
Proofreading: Barbara Resch
Index: Madge Walls
Typesetting and Production: Copperline Book Services
POD Printing: Catawba Publishing, LLC;
Offset Printing: Bethany Press

Printed in the USA and Hong Kong

Healthy Travel Media
P.O. Box 17057
Chapel Hill NC 27516
919 370 7380
info@healthtraveler.net
www.patientsbeyondborders.com

To Angelmine

ACKNOWLEDGMENTS

NEARLY FOUR YEARS and the collaboration of hundreds of patients, practitioners, providers, and institutions went into the creation of what is now the Second Edition of *Patients Beyond Borders.*

I would like to thank literary agent Peter Beren, whose tireless energy and encouragement breathed early life into the manuscript. Gerald and Kathleen Hill contributed greatly to the early research.

I have so much gratitude to the dozens of gracious professionals at Apollo Hospitals in Delhi and Chennai, who helped me gain an early understanding of the important health considerations behind any medical journey. Special thanks to Anil Maini, Sunita Reddy, and the consummate surgeon Vijay Bose. Also to Doug and Anne Stoda, whose courageous medical trip helped me to locate the true voice and audience for the First Edition.

For their many insights and observations during research for the Second Edition, my appreciation goes to Jason Yap of Singapore Medicine; Dan Snyder of Parkway in Singapore; Vishal Bali of Wockhardt; Curtis Schroeder and Mack Banner of Bumrungrad in Thailand; Dr. Mingyen Wu of the Taiwan Task Force in Medical Travel; James Bae of Council for Korea Medicine Overseas Promotion in South Korea; and Dr. Steven Tucker of the West Excellence Clinic in Singapore.

Health travel planners and concierges, already pre-disposed toward empathy and assistance, offered so much potentially competitive information, which greatly enhanced the offerings in Part Two. Special thanks to Jag and Dipa Jethwa of Taj Medical Group; Julie Munro of Cosmetic Surgery Travel; Suresh Ponnudurai of Malaysian Healthcare Networks; Rich Feldman of Medical Tourism of Costa Rica; Rudy Rupak of Planet Hospital; Pat Marsek of MedRetreat; and Stephanie Sulger of Medical Tours International for indulging my relentless queries.

Deep thanks also to David Boucher, Avery Comarow, Sharon Kleefield, and Karen Timmons for their pearls of wisdom, which led to new paths of research.

Finally, a heartfelt note of appreciation to the editors, copywriters, proofreaders, and indexers who reshaped the First Edition, distilling heaps of new data into an accessible and engaging work. Special thanks to our Editorial Director, Faith Brynie, who collected a vast amount of information from around the world and organized it into a readable, coherent form; and to copyeditor Kate Johnson, who hammered and polished these pages and did them proud.

Josef Woodman
Chapel Hill, NC
May 2008

Contents

PART THREE: RESOURCES AND REFERENCES

Foreword

LITTLE MORE THAN a year has passed since the First Edition of *Patients Beyond Borders* was printed. In that brief time, medical "tourism" — better termed medical travel — has continued to grow and to transform the way we all perceive — and receive — medical care. As an American physician practicing oncology in Singapore since 2006, I've been fortunate to have witnessed this medical revolution from the front lines.

Prior to my journey to Asia, I worked as a clinical oncologist specializing in prostate cancer in Los Angeles. Around the year 2000, I started treating more and more traveling patients, not just from across the US, but from all around the world. Patients would come to LA from as near as San Francisco, St. Louis, or Boston and as far away as London, Berlin, and Delhi. Honestly, it never struck me as unusual that, in today's increasingly international climate, patients were willing to travel for high-quality medical care. However, I was shocked when I learned they also wanted to visit me monthly—even weekly—for chemotherapy if needed. Often the cost of travel exceeded the cost of the medications. Nonetheless, I always tried to get these patients involved with doctors in their hometown or home country with whom I could work as a team.

Some patients were leery of the team approach at first, but with adequate planning, evaluations before and after travel, electronic records, email, Skype, and digital imaging, it soon became common for me to see my patients quarterly and let them work closely with their local physicians the rest of the time. Over a few years I built a reliable network of specialists who could care for my cancer patients across the world. I learned that I could obtain any medicine, procedure, or test for my patients anywhere on the globe if I armed them with a well-reasoned letter or rationale. And I discovered that my patients could go to centers of excellence closer to them than LA; we just needed to network with the right people.

Fast-forward to 2006, when I was offered a chance to develop a US-style cancer center in Singapore. I was approached for the task because my peers knew that 30 percent of my practice came from outside the US and another 40 percent from outside California. Healthcare leaders in Singapore could see that the cracks in the US healthcare system might grow wider, and they saw medical travel as a potential safeguard against spiraling costs. My experience in global networking made me an ideal candidate for the post.

It was only after settling into my position that I realized I had been facilitating medical travel for years! In Los Angeles, 70 percent of my patients came from outside of California. In Singapore, 70 percent of my patients come from outside of Singapore, many seeking high-quality care not available in developing countries. In LA, I often worked with a Spanish translator. In Singapore, I work with a Chinese translator. In Singapore, I see a large number of new Asian patients, but I also see my follow-up US patients along with Australians and Europeans who were already traveling to Singapore for healthcare before I arrived. The reality is that I did not turn patients into medical travelers; they had done that for themselves years before.

The US and the rest of the world are now filled with medical travelers, but the phenomenon, in fact, is not new. For thousands of years, people have been willing to travel great distances to obtain the best healthcare at any price. The industry can cite as many historic pilgrimages to ancient physicians, such as Hippocrates and Galen, as it can modern journeys to hospitals in India, Thailand, or the US. Seeking the best in medicine for our families is no different from seeking education or employment. What is different today is that with so many centers of healthcare excellence, the disparity in cost is glaringly obvious — and patients are learning they can do something about it. The huge numbers of Asian patients who travel to obtain high-quality care are being joined in the waiting room by a small, but increasingly Westernized, crowd seeking not only high quality but also lower costs.

With this Second Edition of *Patients Beyond Borders*, Josef Woodman and his team will again help tens of thousands of patients safely cross borders for medical care. As the globalization of healthcare services and delivery matures, it's my deepest personal and professional desire that we all come together to offer the highest quality of care to more and more patients. For our children as much as for our parents, I envision a world filled with expanding healthcare choices, even greater safety, and financial transparency for medical services.

Steven Tucker, MD, FACP
President, International Medical Travel Association
May 2008

Introduction

When the First Edition of *Patients Beyond Borders* was released in 2007, I was immediately and unexpectedly overwhelmed with responses — from the media, from industry leaders, and from patients. The *Washington Post* called. National Public Radio and Fox News called. AARP and the AMA called. The phone never stopped ringing, and all my callers had the same questions: Why are people traveling outside their home country to save money on healthcare? How are such savings possible? Can it really be safe for patients to do such a thing?

The book had obviously hit a huge nerve, and the need for information was varied and vast: Fully insured patients who had been in chronic pain for a decade had been turned down for a hip replacement. Employers who could no longer afford their health plans were seeking alternatives. Uninsured Americans were aging into expensive and financially ruinous medical procedures.

Canadians and Britons were tired of the months-long waits for "covered" surgeries. Sons and daughters of patients were trying to figure out how to pay for their loved ones' otherwise unaffordable care. The list goes on.

In the nearly two years that have passed since the release of the First Edition of *Patients Beyond Borders,* I have traveled to a dozen countries and visited more than 100 hospitals, meeting with surgeons, healthcare administrators, and their patients. Nearly every encounter reinforced the facts that our medical world is indeed becoming smaller and that healthcare consumers from all countries now have choices in quality medical care that did not exist even five years ago. That's why I wrote *Patients Beyond Borders* and why we are incorporating new information into the revised and expanded Second Edition you now hold in your hands.

In less than two years since the publication of the First Edition, much has changed in the medical travel arena. There were fewer than 50 JCI-accredited hospitals when our initial research began; now there are more than 160. That number is expected to double by 2010, offering patients seeking high-quality care abroad an even wider array of choice and comfort. Information has become more available — and trustworthy — as the medical travel road becomes four-laned. More countries are joining the ranks, offering excellent facilities and infrastructure to the international patient. Indeed, as employers, insurers, hospitals, and large third-party players become more involved in global healthcare, the idea of heading abroad for medical care is becoming as ordinary as owning a German or Japanese automobile.

What's New in the Second Edition?

For those who read the First Edition and are wondering what's new in this edition, here are the highlights:

- Fourteen new destinations in eight new countries: Israel, Jordan, New Zealand, Panama, the Philippines, South Korea, Taiwan, and Turkey

- Dozens of new hospitals, health travel agents, hotels, and recovery accommodations

- The latest, up-to-date, checked, and verified contact information for top hospitals worldwide

- Information on the English-language-friendly hospitals most recently accredited by JCI

- New information on getting low-cost medical care in the United States

- All new cost comparisons and price information (gathered from direct surveys of a large sample of hospitals in 22 countries)

- All new glossary and index

- Expanded answers to health travelers' frequently asked questions:

  - Can I sue?

  - Can I carry prescription medications through customs?

  - How can I prevent medical complications such as deep vein thrombosis (DVT) when traveling long distances by air?

  - How I can safely transfer my medical records out of the country?

  - Will my insurance cover my treatment abroad?

  - What immunizations do I need?

  - How can I best protect myself against complications post-procedure?

Beginnings

Despite all that has changed since the First Edition of *Patients Beyond Borders* hit the bookstore shelves, I still think back to what started it all: when my father, age 72 at the time, announced he was heading off to Mexico for extensive dental work. I well remember my first reaction upon hearing his plans: a mixture of bewilderment and fear, then resignation, knowing that despite my protestations, he was going anyway. In spite of my concerns — some of them quite real — I'm pleased to report a happy ending. Dad and his wife, Alinda, selected a US-trained dentist in Puerto Vallarta and spent around $11,000 — which included two weeks noodling around the Pacific Coast. They returned tanned and smiling, Dad with new pearly whites and Alinda with an impromptu skin resurfacing. The same procedures would have cost them $24,000 in the US.

After his treatment, when I told the story of my father's trip, most friends responded with the same shock and disbelief that I had felt initially. Then, when I explained the quality of care and the savings, more often than not those same folks followed me out the door, asking for Dad's email address. I even had an airport customs agent abandon his post and follow me to the boarding gate, seeking additional information for his son, who he had just learned required heart surgery.

Not long afterward, I developed an infected root canal and found myself following my father's example. My research led me abroad for extraction and implant work. While pleasantly surprised at the quality of care, the prices, and the all-around good experience of the trip, I nonetheless made a number of mistakes and created unnecessary difficulties and discomforts for myself. Had I done some simple things differently, my trip would have been more successful and more economical.

In seeking additional data on medical travel, I found no reliable source of information. Everybody had something to sell or a political axe to grind. Books, magazine articles, and newspaper reports seemed more like tourists' brochures than health-travel references. Thus the idea for *Patients Beyond Borders* was born: a well-researched guide, written in plain English, which would offer an impartial look at contemporary medical travel, while helping prospective patients ask the right questions and make informed choices.

As we contemplate our options in an overpriced, overburdened US healthcare environment, nearly all of us will eventually find ourselves seeking alternatives to costly treatments — either for ourselves or for our loved ones. Americans are in the midst of a global shift in healthcare service: in a few short years, big government investment, corporate partnerships, and increased media attention have spawned a new industry — medical tourism — bringing with it a host of encouraging new choices, ranging from dental care and cosmetic surgery to some of the more costly procedures, such as hip replacement and heart surgery. Those patients who take the time to become informed about our changing healthcare world will be pleasantly surprised by a smorgasbord of affordable, high-quality, American-accredited medical options abroad. Those who do not may find themselves grappling with an ungainly, prohibitively expensive healthcare system and a rising absence of choice.

There is no single type of health traveler. In researching and writing *Patients Beyond Borders,* I talked with wealthy women from Beverly Hills who, despite their affluence, prefer the quality of treatment and attention they receive in Brazil or South Africa to medical care California-style. I met a hardworking couple from Wisconsin who, facing the prospect of refinancing their home for a $65,000 hip operation here in the US, headed to India instead. I interviewed a Vietnam vet who wearied of long waits and red tape. He said "bon voyage" to this country's ever-deteriorating healthcare system and headed overseas for treatment.

From these patients' experiences, and many more like them, you'll learn when and how health travel abroad might meet your medical and financial needs. And you'll become a more informed healthcare consumer — both here and abroad.

You Deserve an Impartial Perspective

This new phenomenon of medical tourism — or international health travel — has received a good deal of wide-eyed attention of late. While one newspaper or blog giddily touts the fun 'n sun side of treatment abroad, another issues dire Code Blue warnings about filthy hospitals, shady treatment practices, and procedures gone bad. As with most things in life, the truth lies somewhere in between.

In short, I've found the term "medical tourism" is something of a misnomer, often leading patients to emphasize the recreational more than the procedural in their quest for medical care abroad. Unlike much of the hype that surrounds contemporary health travel, *Patients Beyond Borders* focuses more on your health than on your travel preferences. Thus, throughout this book, you won't see many references to the terms "medical tourism" or "health tourism." In the same way business travelers don't normally consider themselves tourists, you'll begin to think more in terms of medical travel and health travel.

My research, including countless interviews, has convinced me: with diligence, perseverance, and good information, patients considering traveling abroad for treatment do indeed have legitimate, safe choices, not to mention an opportunity to save thousands of dollars over the same treatment in the US. Hundreds of patients who have returned from successful treatment overseas provide overwhelmingly positive feedback. They persuaded me to write this impartial, scrutinizing guide to becoming an informed international patient. I designed this book to help readers reach their own conclusions about whether and when to seek treatment abroad.

What Exactly *Is* Medical Tourism?

Last year, more than 180,000 Americans packed their bags and headed overseas for nearly every imaginable type of medical treatment: tummy tucks in Brazil, heart valve replacements in Thailand, hip resurfacing surgeries in India, addiction recovery in Antigua, fertility diagnosis and treatments in South Africa, thalassotherapy in Hungary, or restorative dentistry in Mexico.

Currently, at least 28 countries on four continents cater to the

> Currently, at least 28 countries on four continents cater to the international health traveler, with more than 2 million patients visiting hospitals and clinics each year in countries other than their own.

> If the notion of complex medical procedures in far-flung lands seems intimidating, don't feel alone.

international health traveler, with more than 2 million patients visiting hospitals and clinics each year in countries other than their own. The roster of treatments is as varied as the travelers.

If the notion of complex medical procedures in far-flung lands seems intimidating, don't feel alone. That's why I wrote this book, drawing from the varied experiences of hundreds of patients who, for dozens of reasons, have beaten a well-worn path to successful treatments abroad.

Why Go Abroad for Medical Care?

Cost savings. Most people like to get the most for their dollar. The single biggest reason Americans travel to other countries for medical treatment is the opportunity to save money. Depending upon the country and type of treatment, uninsured and underinsured patients, as well as those seeking elective care, can realize 15–85 percent savings over the cost of treatment in the US.

> "I took out my credit card instead of a second mortgage on my home."

Or, as one successful health traveler put it, "I took out my credit card instead of a second mortgage on my home."

As baby boomers become senior boomers, costs of healthcare and prescriptions are devouring nearly 30 percent of retirement and pre-retirement incomes. With the word getting out about top-quality treatments at deep discounts overseas, informed patients are finding creative alternatives abroad.

Case Studies: Margaret S. and Doug S.

Margaret S., a patient from Santa Ana, California, was quoted $6,600 for a tooth extraction, two implants, and two crowns. One of the 120 million Americans without dental insurance, Margaret had heard of less expensive dental care abroad. Through a friend, she learned about Escazú, Costa Rica, known for its excellent dental and cosmetic surgery clinics. Margaret got the same treatment in Costa Rica for $2,600. Her dentist was a US-trained oral surgeon who used state-of-the-art instrumentation and top-quality materials. Add in airfare, lodging, meals, and other travel costs, and this savvy global patient still came out way ahead.

Doug S., a small-business owner from Wisconsin, journeyed with his wife, Anne, to Chennai, India for a double hip resurfacing procedure that would have cost more than $55,000 in the US. The total bill, including travel for him and his wife, lodging, meals, and two-week recuperation in a five-star beach hotel, was $14,000. "We were treated like royalty," said Doug, "and I'm riding a bicycle for the first time in six years. We could not have afforded this operation in the US."

Big Surgeries: Comparative Costs

Procedure	US Cost	India	Thailand	Singapore	Malaysia	Panama*	South Korea	Taiwan
Heart Bypass	$70,000– 133,000	$7,000	$22,000	$16,300	$12,000	$10,500	$31,750	$27,500
Heart Valve Replacement with Bypass	$75,000– 140,000	$9,500	$25,000	$22,000	$13,400	$13,500	$42,000	$30,000
Hip Replacement	$33,000– 57,000	$10,200	$12,700	$12,000	$7,500	$5,500	$10,600	$8,800
Knee Replacement	$30,000– 53,000	$9,200	$11,500	$9,600	$12,000	$7,000	$11,800	$10,000
Facelift	$10,500– 16,000	$4,800	$5,000	$7,500	$6,400	$2,500	$6,650	$8,500
Gastric Bypass	$35,000– 52,000	$9,300	$13,000	$16,500	$12,700	$8,500	$9,300	$10,200
Prostate Surgery (TURP)	$10,000– 16,000	$3,600	$4,400	$5,300	$4,600	$3,200	$3,150	$2,750

*Doctor's fees not included.

The above costs are for surgery (except as noted), including the hospital stay in a private, single-bed room. Airfare and lodging costs are governed by individual preferences. To compute a ballpark estimate of total costs, add $5,000 for you and a companion, figuring coach airfare and hotel rooms averaging $150 per night. For example, a hip replacement in Bangkok, Thailand, would cost about $18,000, for an estimated savings of at least $15,000 compared to the US price.

Dentistry: Comparative Costs in Popular Destinations

Procedure	US Cost	Mexico	Costa Rica	Hungary	Thailand
Implant	$2,200	$1,500	$725	$1,400	$2,150
Crown	$1,750	$495	$400	$590	$540
Porcelain Veneer	$900	$390	$350	$620	$285
Dentures (Upper & Lower)	$5,000	$2,700	$1,600	$1,500	$1,000
Inlays & Onlays	$1,500	$360	$350	$500	$235
Surgical Extraction	$365	$235	$195	$265	$60
Root Canal	$600	$265	$190	$120	$165

The estimates above are for treatments alone. Airfare, hospital stay (if any), and lodging vary considerably. Savings on dentistry become more dramatic when "big mouth-work" is required, involving several teeth or full restorations. Savings of $15,000 or more are common.

Better quality care. Veteran health travelers know that facilities, instrumentation, and customer service in treatment centers abroad often equal or exceed those found in the US. Governments of countries such as India and Thailand have poured billions of dollars into improving

> Governments of countries such as India and Thailand have poured billions of dollars into improving their healthcare systems, which are now aggressively catering to the international health traveler.

their healthcare systems, which are now aggressively catering to the international health traveler. VIP waiting lounges, deluxe hospital suites, and staffed recuperation resorts are common amenities, along with free transportation to and from airports, low-cost meal plans for companions, and discounted hotels affiliated with the hospital.

Moreover, physicians and staff in treatment centers abroad are often far more accessible than their US counterparts. "My surgeon gave me his cell phone number, and I spoke directly with him at least a dozen times during my stay," said David P., who traveled to Bangkok for a heart valve replacement.

> "My surgeon gave me his cell phone number, and I spoke directly with him at least a dozen times during my stay."

Excluded treatments. Even the most robust health insurance plans exclude a variety of conditions and treatments. You, the policyholder, must pay these expenses out-of-pocket. Although health insurance policies vary according to the underwriter and individual, your plan probably excludes a variety of treatments, such as cosmetic surgeries, dental care, vision treatments, reproductive/infertility procedures, certain nonemergency cardiovascular and orthopedic surgeries, weight-loss programs, substance abuse rehabilitation, and prosthetics — to name only a few. In addition, many policies place restrictions on prescriptions (some quite expensive), post-operative care, congenital disorders, and pre-existing conditions.

Rich or cash-challenged, young or not-so-young, heavily or only lightly insured — folks who get sick or desire a treatment (even one recommended by their physician) often find their insurance won't cover it. Confronting increasingly expensive choices at home, nearly 40 percent of American health travelers hit the road for elective treatments. In countries such as Costa Rica, Singapore, Dubai, and Thailand, this trend has spawned entire industries, offering excellent treatment and ancillary facilities at costs far lower than US prices.

Specialty treatments. Some procedures and prescriptions are simply not allowed in this country. Either Congress or the FDA has specifically disallowed a certain treatment, or perhaps it's still in the testing and clinical trials stage or was only recently approved. Such treatments are often offered abroad. One example is an orthopedic procedure known as hip resurfacing, for most patients a far superior, longer lasting, and less expensive alternative to the traditional hip replacement still practiced in the US. While this procedure has been performed for more than a decade throughout Europe and Asia, it was only recently approved in the US, and its availability here remains spotty and unproven. Hundreds of forward-thinking Americans, many having suffered years of chronic pain, have found relief in India, where hip resurfacing techniques, materials, and instrumentation have been perfected, and the procedure is routine.

Shorter waiting periods. For decades, thousands of Canadian and British subscribers to universal, "free" healthcare plans have endured waits as long as two years for established procedures. "Some of us die before we get to the operating table," commented one exasperated patient, who journeyed to India for an open-heart procedure.

Here in the US, long waits are a growing problem, particularly among war veterans covered under the Veterans Administration

Act, for whom long queues are becoming far too common. Some patients figure it's better to pay out-of-pocket to get out of pain or to halt a deteriorating condition than to suffer the anxiety and frustration of waiting for a far-future appointment and other medical uncertainties.

More "inpatient-friendly." As US health insurance companies apply increasing pressure on hospitals to process patients as quickly as possible, outpatient procedures are becoming the norm. Similarly, US hospitals are under huge pressure to move inpatients out of those costly beds as soon as possible. Medical travelers will welcome the flexibility at the best hospitals abroad, where they are often aggressively encouraged to spend extra time in the hospital post-procedure. Staff-to-patient ratios are usually lower abroad, as are hospital-borne infection rates.

The lure of the new and different. Although traveling abroad for medical care can be challenging, many patients welcome the chance to blaze a trail, and they find the creature comforts often offered abroad a welcome relief from the sterile, impersonal hospital environments so often encountered in US treatment centers. For others, simply being in a new and interesting culture lends distraction to an otherwise worrisome, tedious process. And getting away from the myriad obligations of home and professional life can yield healthful effects at a stressful time.

What's more, travel — and particularly international travel — can be a life-changing experience. You might be humbled by the limousine ride from Indira Gandhi International Airport to a hotel in central New Delhi or struck by the simple, elegant graciousness of professionals and ordinary people in Thailand, or wowed by the sheer beauty of the mountain range outside a dental office window in Mexico. As one veteran medical traveler put it, "I brought back far more from this trip than a new set of teeth."

Who Should Read *Patients Beyond Borders*?

You'll benefit from reading this book if

✦ You're one of 85 million uninsured or underinsured individuals who wish to explore less expensive options for a treatment often covered by health insurance.

✦ You're one of 120 million Americans without a dental plan and wish to take advantage of the full range of affordable dental procedures in other countries.

✦ You wish to pursue an elective treatment (such as cosmetic surgery, in vitro fertilization, or homeopathy) not normally covered by health insurance policies.

✦ You're exploring one of many treatments either not offered or not approved in the US.

✦ You feel a friend or family member might benefit from learning more about health travel, yet that person might lack the confidence or focus to launch an inquiry.

✦ You plan to join a family member or friend for treatment abroad (see Chapter Seven, "For Companions").

What *Patients Beyond Borders* Will (and Won't) Do for You

Patients Beyond Borders isn't a guide to medical diagnosis and treatment, nor does it provide medical advice on specific treatments or caregiver referrals. Your condition, diagnosis, treatment options, and travel preferences are unique, and only you — in consultation with your physician and loved ones — can determine the best course of action.

> Your condition, diagnosis, treatment options, and travel preferences are unique, and only you — in consultation with your physician and loved ones — can determine the best course of action.

Should you decide to investigate traveling abroad for treatment, we *do* provide you with all the resources and tools necessary to become an informed medical traveler, so that you'll have the best possible travel experience and treatment your money can buy.

Our job is to

✦ help you become a knowledgeable, confident health traveler;

✦ assist you in planning and budgeting your trip and treatment;

✦ provide you with up-to-date information about the most popular, widely used treatment centers;

✦ make your in-country visit as comfortable and hassle-free as possible;

✦ recommend good lodging and recovery accommodations; and

✦ provide tips, tricks, and advice for a successful medical travel experience — before, during, and after treatment.

Your job is to

✦ consult with your local doctor(s) to ensure you've reached a satisfactory diagnosis and recommended course of treatment;

✦ decide, based on your research and the material featured in this book, whether you wish to travel abroad for treatment; and if so,

✦ select a travel destination, treatment center, and physician based on the information you find in this book and elsewhere.

It's a truism: every journey begins with the first step. Health travel is no exception. Once you've taken that first step toward learning more, you'll find that your friends, family, this book, and a trusty Internet connection will speed you on your way.

How to Use This Book

Before you dive into Part Two, "The Most-Traveled Health Destinations," you'll want to carefully read Part One, "How to Become a Savvy, Informed Medical Traveler." It provides you the basic resources and tools you'll need to do your research and make an informed decision.

Chapter One, "What Am I Getting Into? Some Quick Answers for Health Travelers," addresses the questions and concerns most often voiced by patients (and their loved ones) considering a medical journey abroad.

Chapter Two, "Planning Your Health Travel Journey," helps you design your trip step by step. The chapter provides data and advice culled from interviews with hundreds of patients and treatment centers. You'll learn how to cut through the chaff quickly to find the right clinics, determine physician accreditation, narrow your destination choices, choose the right companion, and more.

Chapter Three, "Budgeting Your Treatment and Trip," walks you through the financial basics of a medical trip and gives you the tools you need to prepare an estimated budget. Our "*Patients Beyond Borders* Budget Planner" helps you determine specific cost-savings and avoid financial surprises.

Chapter Four, "Choosing and Working with a Health Travel Planner," shows you how to avoid hassles and save money by finding and engaging the right health travel agent.

Chapter Five, "While You're There," provides valuable information on what to expect from your treatment center and physician, plus general tips for dealing with local cultures, language barriers, and more. A section on communicating while on the road includes pointers on using cell phones and computers to communicate with physicians in-country, as well as loved ones back home.

Chapter Six, "Home Again, Home Again," helps you get settled in post-treatment, offering practical advice on working with your hometown doctor, shaking off the "post-treatment blues," coping with discomforts and complications, and getting back on your feet.

Chapter Seven, "For Companions," is written especially for those caring family members or friends who accompany patients on health journeys.

Chapter Eight, "Dos and Don'ts for the Smart Health Traveler," helps you avoid common speed bumps and potholes on the health travel road.

Part Two, "The Most-Traveled Health Destinations," features 37 destinations in 21 countries, with up-to-date information on hospitals and clinics, specialties, accreditation, recovery centers and recuperation resorts, transportation, communication, and more. You'll use the information in this section to get a good idea about where to travel for your particular procedure and what to expect for the costs of common treatments.

Part Three, "Resources and References," provides additional sources of medical travel information and helpful links, plus a glossary of commonly used medical terms.

As you work your way through decision-making and subsequent planning, remember that you're following in the footsteps of tens of thousands of health travelers who have made the journey before you. The overwhelming majority have returned home successfully treated, with money to spare in their savings accounts.

Still, the process—particularly in the early planning—can be daunting, frustrating, even a little scary. That's normal, and every health traveler we interviewed experienced "the Big Fear" at one time or another. Healthcare abroad is not for everyone, and part of being a smart consumer is evaluating all the impartial data available before making an informed decision. If you accomplish that in reading *Patients Beyond Borders*, we've achieved our mission.

Let's get started.

PART ONE

How to Become a Savvy, Informed Medical Traveler

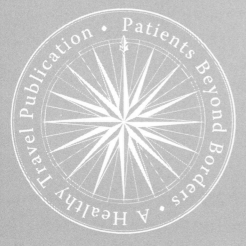

What Am I Getting Into? Some Quick Answers for Health Travelers

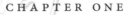

Is Healthcare Overseas Safe?

Interestingly, the friends and family members of patients considering healthcare abroad ask this question more often than do the patients themselves. In fact, at least one friend or family member is virtually guaranteed to balk at the thought of your heading overseas for treatment. Most of these concerns are unfounded. They usually arise either from a lack of knowledge or from cultural myopia.

Although no medical procedure is 100 percent risk free anywhere in the world, the best hospitals and clinics abroad maintain health and procedural standards equal to, or higher than, those you encounter in the US. Many hospitals abroad are accredited by the same US agency (the Joint Commission) that certifies hospitals here. (For more information on hospital ac-

> Many hospitals abroad are accredited by the same US agency (the Joint Commission) that certifies hospitals here.

creditation and safety standards, see Chapter Two, "Planning Your Health Travel Journey.")

It's not hard to find overseas physicians, dentists, and surgeons who received their medical training and degrees at first-rate medical schools in the US, Great Britain, Canada, Switzerland, or Germany. All the countries listed in *Patients Beyond Borders* enforce strict governmental and private standards for healthcare, hospital, and clinic certification.

Finally, many hospitals — particularly the larger institutions in Asia and Southeast Asia — boast lower morbidity rates than in the US, particularly when it comes to complex cardiac and orthopedic surgeries, for which success rates higher than 98.5 percent are the norm.

If Healthcare in Other Countries Is So Good, How Can It Be So Cheap?

This question is best answered by another question: why is US healthcare so expensive? High facilities costs, unpaid hospital bills totaling billions of dollars, high-priced medical education, costly research, and excessive malpractice litigation all add up to exorbitant prices for healthcare in the US.

In addition, US physicians who perform elective and specialty procedures — such as cosmetic surgeries, in vitro fertilization, and certain hip, spine, and cardiac procedures — command astronomical fees from patients willing and able to pay, leaving those of more modest means in the lurch and seeking alternatives.

Healthcare in other countries is also less costly because standards of living are more modest, doctors and staff command lower wages, government-subsidized healthcare keeps private healthcare costs down, and malpractice attorneys are, if not docile, at least considerably more restrained.

Some Facts about Medical Costs and Medical Travel

Every 38 seconds in the US someone files for bankruptcy in the aftermath of a serious health problem," reports Elizabeth Warren of Harvard Law School in the *International Medical Travel Journal*.

"We spend so much more money on healthcare in the United States than other industrialized countries primarily because our prices are so much higher," says Gerard Anderson, a professor in the Department of Health Policy and Management at the Johns Hopkins Bloomberg School of Public Health.

- US healthcare spending per capita is 2.5 times greater than the median of countries in the Organization for Economic Cooperation and Development (OECD).

- The US is now ranked fourth highest among OECD countries for hospital spending per capita.

- The US spends 3.6 times what the median OECD country spends for outpatient care. Most of the difference is attributable to higher spending on physician services.

- Last year, more than 180,000 Americans packed their bags and headed overseas for medical treatment.

- Currently, at least 28 countries on four continents cater to the international health traveler.

- More than a million patients worldwide visit hospitals and clinics each year in countries other than their own.

- By 2010 medical travel is expected to be a $40-billion business, with some 2–3 million patients annually seeking care outside their principal country of residence.

How Much Can I Save?

Your savings will depend on your treatment, your selected destination, and your travel and lifestyle preferences. Patients who travel to India for complex heart bypass surgeries will probably save more than $50,000 or more over the price in the US. People traveling to Costa Rica for reconstructive dentistry or extensive breast and abdominal cosmetic surgery can save $10,000 or more.

A good rule of thumb is "the $6,000 Rule": If your US specialist quotes you a price of $6,000 or more for a treatment, chances are good that one or more foreign countries can offer you the same procedure and quality for less, even including your travel and lodging expenses. If your US quote is less than $6,000, you're probably better off having your treatment at home.

Is It Safe to Travel Overseas?

For many, a medical trip is their first journey abroad. That can be a scary prospect. Post-9/11 news is fear inducing enough to make any novice international traveler think twice about packing a suitcase. Yet it's easy to forget that most other countries enjoy far lower crime rates than ours. In fact, many citizens outside the US are afraid to travel to this country because of the well-publicized rates of violent crime here.

Your own behavior will determine much of your experience abroad. If you follow the common sense rules of courtesy and observe cultural norms, you should be safe in any country featured in this book. Outcomes have proven that's true. Hundreds of thousands of international health travelers return home safe and sound each year.

Health travelers can be further reassured because, from the moment of arrival in another country until departure on a homebound plane, most are under the near-constant supervision of a hospital, health travel broker, tour agency, or other third-party agent. Most health travelers are met at their airport arrival gate and whisked to an American-style hospital or hotel.

> If your US specialist quotes you a price of $6,000 or more for a treatment, chances are good that one or more foreign countries can offer you the same procedure and quality for less, even including your travel and lodging expenses.

From that point, they're usually under someone's care in a treatment center, getting a bite in a restaurant, or resting in a cozy hotel room.

What Medical Treatments Are Available Abroad?

Although nearly every kind of treatment is possible abroad, most Westerners head overseas for orthopedics (hip replacement, knee replacement, spinal work); cardiovascular surgery (bypass, valve replacement, heart transplant); cancer diagnosis and treatment; dental care (usually more extensive cosmetic or restorative surgery); or cosmetic surgery. In addition, US patients seek specialty treatments (such as fertility and in vitro fertilization procedures), weight loss procedures (such as bariatric surgeries), and therapies not yet allowed in this country (such as certain stem cell treatments). In Part Two of this book, you'll discover a range of treatment specialties and superspecialties that run the full medical gamut.

What all those treatments have in common is great expense. The huge savings to be garnered abroad can outweigh the challenges of traveling overseas for treatment.

How Do I Know Where to Travel for Treatment?

Most countries are known for a particular category of treatment, and your diagnosis will distill your list of choices down to a handful of destinations. If you're seeking cosmetic surgery, Brazil, Costa Rica, and South Africa rank among the most popular destinations. Dentistry will have you exploring Mexico, Costa Rica, or Hungary. The more expensive, invasive surgeries, such as open-heart surgery or a knee replacement, make a longer trip to India, Thailand, Singapore, or Malaysia well worth the cost, time, and distance of travel.

To get a preliminary idea of where you're likely to be heading, refer to the *"Patients Beyond Borders* Treatment and Country Finder" at the beginning of Part Two. Use Chapters Two and Three (on planning and budgeting your trip), along with your own travel and lifestyle preferences, to pinpoint your country of choice.

 Action Item: **Consult the "Treatment and Country Finder" in Part Two to find out where you can save the most on the treatment you want.**

Can Someone Go with Me? I Don't Like Traveling Alone.

That's good, because we don't recommend you travel alone. We've found that most health travelers fare better with a companion in tow — a spouse, family member, or friend. Companions don't greatly increase the overall costs of a trip, and they can actually save you time and money in the end, because they are looking out for your interests every step of the way. For more information on traveling with family or friends, see Chapter Seven, "For Companions."

Even if you cannot travel with a companion, or prefer not to, you won't be going it alone in-country. If you're staying in a hospital, the quality of care and attention you'll receive in the better centers is truly remarkable, with low nurse-to-patient ratios and a host of staffers, orderlies, physician's assistants, and dieticians in and out of your room with great frequency. You'll make fast friends during your stay.

If you're not planning to travel with a companion, we strongly recommend you engage the services of a health travel agency that offers concierge services. A good agent is with you almost daily, particularly at the more stressful junctures, such as arrival in-country, medical consultations, and immediately before and after a surgical procedure. For more information on agents, see Chapter Four, "Choosing and Working with a Health Travel Planner."

What If They Don't Speak English?

Every country catering to international health travelers offers a host of English-speaking physicians, staff, and third-party agencies. If English is your native tongue and you're uncomfortable speaking another language, then insist on English. If a hospital or clinic you've contacted can't furnish English-speaking doctors, don't be embarrassed. Politely thank them and move on. Your continued research will lead you to professionals who can converse in your native tongue.

How Realistic Is the "Vacation" Part of the Trip?

That depends on the type of treatment you're seeking, how much time you have, and how comfortable you feel combining leisure travel with the medical side of your trip. Most patients who take a vacation as part of a healthcare journey are either planning to travel anyway or have allocated a good deal of additional time for recreation as well as recovery. (There's a big difference, which we cover in Chapter Five, "While You're There.")

Throughout this book, we encourage patients to focus more on their treatment and recovery than on tourism, even for the less invasive procedures. Web sites and health travel brochures peppered with zealous promotion ("Enjoy Fabulous Rainforest Vacation While Recovering from Your Tummy Tuck!") ignore the realities of health travel. Long flights, post-treatment recovery, and just plain being alone in a faraway place can be overwhelming, even for the most optimistic health traveler.

> We encourage patients to focus more on their treatment and recovery than on tourism, even for the less invasive procedures.

Think of your medical journey more as a business trip than a leisure junket. Consider socking away some of your savings for a separate vacation you and a loved one can take after the primary challenge of managing your immediate health need is behind you. Then, by all means, break out the champagne at a far-flung exotic hideaway and celebrate your health and good fortune.

What If Complications Arise after I Return Home?

Depending on your treatment, your physician or surgeon will usually strongly advise you to stay in-country for at least a few days post-treatment. Your doctor will want to make sure that your treatment went well, your medications are working as they should, you're settling into any recommended physical therapies, and required follow-ups are going according to plan. Thus, by the time you board the plane home, your risk of complications will be greatly reduced.

In the unlikely event that you develop complications after returning home, you'll need to decide whether to make a return trip or continue your treatment at home. Some procedures, such as dental work, are guaranteed; so it may well be financially worthwhile, albeit inconvenient, to return. If you choose not to, most overseas dentists and surgeons are happy to talk with your hometown physician to discuss complications and recommend further action. For more information on complications and other post-treatment considerations, see Chapter Six, "Home Again, Home Again."

Prior to traveling abroad for treatment, be sure to let your local doctor(s) know your plans. It's better to alert them beforehand than to surprise them after the fact.

Will My Health Insurance Cover My Overseas Medical Expenses?

As of this writing, probably not. While the largest US employers and healthcare insurers — not to mention our ever-vocal politicians — struggle with new models of coverage, most plans do not yet cover the costs of obtaining treatment abroad. Yet, with healthcare costs threatening to literally bust the economy, pressures for change are mounting. Recognizing that globalization of healthcare is now a reality—and that the US is falling behind—insurers, employers, and hospitals are now aggressively beginning to form partnerships with payers and providers abroad. By the time you read this book, large insurers may already be offering coverage (albeit limited) across borders. You may want to check with your insurer for the latest on your coverage abroad.

> *Action Item:* **Check with your health insurance company (if you have one) to see if all or part of your overseas treatment is covered.**

Can I Sue?

The US is well known as Earth's most litigious nation. For better or worse, most countries outside the US do not share our attitude toward personal and institutional liability. While all countries listed in *Patients Beyond Borders* have established channels of legal recourse, the intricacies of working with foreign statutes, legal systems, and counsel make such action impractical except in the most egregious cases.

The best defense is a good offense. International patients should focus on success rates, accreditation, and other quality assurance measures that help to mitigate the chances of complications that would trigger legal claims. Here's another good rule of thumb: if legal recourse is a primary concern in making your health travel decision, you probably shouldn't head abroad for medical treatment.

There are, however, some legal options you might consider if your care goes wrong. For a full discussion, see "Medical Travel and Medical Malpractice" in Chapter Six.

Can I Finance My Treatment?

Increasingly, established hospitals abroad and some health travel agents offer financing plans in the form of loans or delayed payment. Ask your agent or clinic for details.

Most hospitals, clinics, and health travel brokers accept credit cards, but many charge an additional fee to cover their processing costs. Ask beforehand.

Nearly all hotels, restaurants, retailers, and businesses abroad happily accept major credit cards. Automatic teller machines (ATMs) are common in most cities and towns, and it's fun to watch your cash come out in an unfamiliar currency.

Planning Your Health Travel Journey

First Things First: Seek Guidance

As you've probably learned from previous trips, an expert guide can teach you things and take you places you would not have otherwise discovered. Consider Part One of *Patients Beyond Borders* your "health travel planning companion," a trusty side-kick to help ease the burdens of your journey. You'll progress more safely and easily if you draw upon the collective wisdom of those who have traveled successfully before you.

Although each journey varies according to the traveler's preferences and pocketbook, good planning is essential to the success of any trip. That goes double for the medical traveler. In this chapter, you'll learn how to become an informed global patient. If you decide that a medical trip is right for you, we'll help you gain confidence about finding the right destination, selecting the best clinic and physician, and working with others to help ensure your success.

 Action Item: **Research several physicians, clinics, or hospitals that offer the treatment you need. Don't snap up the first option you find.**

Trust Yourself

Most likely, you're considering health travel because you want an elective treatment, such as a cosmetic, dental, or reproductive procedure, or because you've been diagnosed with a condition that requires surgical intervention, such as orthopedic or cardiovascular surgery. Whatever the reason, a condition you want or need treated — usually coupled with a desire or need for substantial cost savings (and for some, a sense of adventure or a wish to try something new) — is what brought you to this point.

Other factors may be influencing your decision as well. It's no secret that contemporary economic and medical trends in the US have spawned overworked practitioners, crowded hospitals, and vast variations in the quality of care available to all but the wealthiest citizens. Your dad's or grandmother's friendly, chatty, all-knowing family doctor has become a medical oddity, supplanted by a bevy of busy assistants, hurried consultations, arms-length testing, hasty diagnoses, and increasingly faulty treatment. As a result, the traditional trusting patients of yesteryear, who unquestioningly put their lives in the hands of the medical system, are a rapidly disappearing breed.

Today, patients are urged to educate themselves, take a proactive stance, and ask questions. Our medical system is based on market principles. This makes you a consumer of healthcare. As a consumer, you should remember "buyer beware" in all your choices.

If you're holding this book in your hand right now, chances are you've left the old world of blind faith and have appropriately adapted to modern medical times, evolving into a curious, assertive, informed patient. Congratulations! Your prognosis for becoming a successful health traveler is vastly improved.

Knowledge is power, and the more thought you put into weighing your options, the more confidence you'll gain in reaching the decision that's best for you and your loved ones. Even if you only skim the rest of *Patients Beyond Borders*, read this chapter carefully and thoroughly. At the end of it, you'll have answered enough questions to know whether, when, and where to travel for your medical care.

Plan Ahead

Okay. You're beginning to recover from the heart-stopping quote your medical specialist laid on you two weeks ago. You've talked with friends and family about heading abroad for treatment. They're skeptical but reluctantly willing to trust your judgment. Truth be told, you're still a tad skeptical yourself, but you're willing to consider medical travel as an option.

Long before you pack your bags, you have a lot to do and a logical progression of decisions and events to work through. The first item of business is to plan ahead, as far in advance as you can. Three months prior to treatment is good. Six months ahead of time is great. One month is not so good. Here's why:

✦ **The best overseas physicians are also the busiest.** That's a fact everywhere. Just as here in the US, doctors, surgeons, and specialists abroad work 24/7, and their schedules are often established a month or more in advance. If you want the most qualified doctors and the best care your global patient money can buy, give the doctors and treatment centers you select plenty of time to work you into their calendars.

✦ **The lowest international airfares go to those who book early.** As veteran international travelers know, ticket prices rise savagely as the departure date draws closer. Most punishing of all are last-minute fares, reserved for family tragedies, rich jetsetters, and busy corporate executives. Booking at least 60 days prior to treatment allows you to avoid the unhappy upward spiral of air travel costs.

If you're planning to redeem frequent-flyer miles, try to book at least 90 days in advance, even if you're not 100 percent certain of your treatment date. At this writing, most airlines don't charge for schedule changes on frequent-flyer fares, and you're better off reserving a date — then changing it later — than being stuck without any reservation at all.

> Plan ahead, as far in advance as you can. Three months prior to treatment is good. Six months ahead of time is great. One month is not so good.

Similarly, for paid fares, it's usually better to reserve your trip as far in advance as you can, giving your best guess at a schedule. Then, budget in the $100 penalty in case you need to change your flight itinerary.

✦ *Peak seasons can snarl the best-laid plans.* International tourism is again on the rise. If you want or need to travel during the busy tourist season for your chosen region, start planning your global health trip four to six months in advance.

✦ *Preparation is a big part of planning.* When you paint your living room wall, you know that preparation is half the effort; by the time you pick up the paintbrush, you're halfway done. The same is true with health travel. Before you can book your flight or reserve your hotel room, you must first confirm your treatment appointment. Before you do that, you'll need to decide which country you want to visit, which physician(s) will suit your needs, and much more.

While such planning is not rocket science, an organized approach in the preparation stages will save you time and money in the end. In the following pages, we provide a guide to that organized approach.

Set Your Mind to It

As you plan, your mindset is as important as any set of skills. So cultivate and practice the following:

An open mind. Our twenty-first-century world is increasingly becoming a global village, with American cultural influences leading the charge. Still, contrasts abound: different time zones (they're sleeping while we're working); different accents (English can take on many forms, some of them barely comprehensible to Americans); different clothes (burkas, turbans, exotic neckwear); different table manners (never eat with your left hand).

Those with a strictly US-centric cultural bias may have trouble absorbing and accommodating such diversity. You need an open mind to accept that other points of view and ways of life are not only valid, but in some respects perhaps more refined than ours. After all, our culture is adolescent compared to thousands of years of Indian or European civilization.

Patience. As you embark on your health journey, you'll find that patience is indeed a virtue, particularly in the planning stages.

For one thing, the pace abroad is generally slower — and more cordial — than in the US. While here you might expect your inquiry returned within three hours, you may not hear back from a hospital in Bangkok for three days. Be patient. Call or email a second time. If you don't get an answer in a week, move on. There are plenty of hospitals and clinics in the world willing and able to work with you. Finding the right one is a systematic process, sometimes involving false starts.

And what about that receptionist in Mumbai who always wants to know how your family is doing? Well, it's customary in many cultures to talk for a few moments about your personal life, beginning with inquiries about family and loved ones. Take a deep breath and chat it up. You'll be glad you did when you're working with an in-country doctor who's willing to spend an hour with you as part of the clinic's normal routine.

Persistence. When planning any international trip, you'll encounter a host of tasks, contingencies, and sometimes setbacks. Health travel is no exception. When your phone calls and emails are not returned as quickly

> As you embark on your health journey, you'll find that patience is indeed a virtue, particularly in the planning stages.

as you would like, remember that delays don't necessarily arise from a lack of professionalism. The pace of business in a foreign country can often be slower than Americans anticipate.

So, be flexible and persistent in your planning. If Plan A isn't working, move to Plan B. You'll sometimes find yourself at Plan D, only to discover that Plan B worked out after all, although not on your expected timetable.

Generally, the early planning stages require the most perseverance. Once you're in-country, you'll be pleased to see other people sweating the details.

Email and Internet Searching

Although you needn't be a computer whiz, you'll gain a huge advantage from an Internet connection for two important purposes:

Communication. As annoying and inefficient as telephones are in daily life, they are exponentially more so when you're trying to conduct business from afar. Email, on the other hand, knows no time zones, lowers the language barrier, and provides an efficient information trail for contacts, recommendations, and myriad other details you'd otherwise be obliged to somehow remember.

Email is vital for making initial inquiries, following up on research, confirming and reconfirming appointments, booking airline and hotel reservations, and keeping records of your transactions with physicians and staff. You needn't be a great journalist or business correspondent; if you can email successfully with your kids in Duluth or your Aunt May in Oklahoma, you'll do fine.

Research. What a world we live in, where all earthly knowledge is now truly at our fingertips! The rise of the Web and the refinement of search engines such as Google, MSN, and Yahoo have enabled anyone with an Internet connection to obtain reliable research results quickly and easily.

Primary to successful health travel planning is a basic ability to gather and sort information. The Internet offers some big keys to the research kingdom. Indeed, ten years ago, medical travel as we know it would have been possible only for those with professional knowledge or inside information. Today, the power of that knowledge is available to us all.

For some of us, however, these new Internet tools are as bewildering as they are powerful. If you don't like doing the required digging, or if you aren't confident in your research skills, perhaps a family member or friend is willing to help. Make your fact-finding a shared project — perhaps working with a younger member of your circle who can show off his or her computer prowess. Although *Patients Beyond Borders* provides sufficient guidelines to get anyone started in finding the right fit for particular treatment needs, the specifics of where to go and which doctor to engage are up to the individual. Making such decisions requires doing your homework, and the Internet is a great homework tool.

Action Item: **Get help with Internet research if your skills are less than stellar.**

Chutzpah!

During the planning stages, make sure you maintain the will to keep moving forward, the courage to do things a little differently, and the confidence that you're making the right choices. Along your health journey you're likely to encounter US physicians who aren't happy that you're heading overseas for treatment, friends and relatives who think you're nuts (even if they didn't previously), and days of genuine self-doubt. But stick with it. Don't let other people talk you out of your quest because of their ignorance, anxiety, or competitive zeal. If you do your homework and follow the guidelines in this book, you'll make the right decisions.

Nixing the Nonresponders

Sad but true: not everyone in the medical travel business keeps up with their contacts and correspondence. Telephone calls are not always returned; emails are not always answered. Some otherwise excellent hospitals and health travel agencies may be guilty of responding in an untimely or haphazard manner — or in some cases, not at all.

What should you do if you don't receive a reply to your initial inquiry? Three things:

1. Ask yourself whether the failure to communicate is indicative of the quality of service and care you can expect. For major hospitals and well-established agencies, the nonresponse may be a one-time lapse. In that case . . .

2. Try again. If you don't get a response the second time, move on to a provider who wants your business. With so many hospitals in so many countries to choose from, think of the inquiry phase as part of the screening process in your search for the best fit.

3. Report nonresponders to us by email at info@patientsbeyond borders.com, and we'll do our best to warn other medical travelers and to encourage those less-than-conscientious service providers to clean up their act.

THE TWELVE-FOLD PATH TO ENLIGHTENED HEALTH TRAVEL PLANNING

The following is culled from hundreds of interviews with patients and treatment center staff members around the world. Follow the steps and advice outlined here and you'll streamline your planning, organize your trip well, select the best physician(s), communicate effectively with staff and agents, save money, and prepare to pack your bags with confidence.

Step 1: Confirm Your Treatment Options

1 Doctors generally recommend a range of choices for a given condition, then leave it up to you and your family to settle upon a course of action, based on their recommendations. After all, the buck stops with your body, especially these days, and no one other than you can or should make those important health-related judgment calls. Most physicians respect that, and that's why they usually stop short of advising you what specific course of treatment to take. That's wise, because your body is your own, and so are such vital decisions. Most physicians respect their patients' autonomy.

If you have doubts about your diagnosis or feel dissatisfied in your relationship with your physician or specialist, don't be timid about seeking a second — or even third — opinion. At the very least, a second opinion expands your knowledge base about your condition. The more you and your hometown health team learn about — and discuss — your condition, diagnosis, and treatment options, the more precisely and confidently you'll communicate with your overseas practitioners.

 Action Item: **Request copies of all local consultations and recommendations in writing, along with cost estimates for treatment. Then begin a file for all paperwork related to your treatment and travel.**

As you sort through your treatment options and consider courses of action, you'll want to learn as much as you can about your condition. You'll get better care from your overseas practitioners if you are a knowledgeable and responsive patient.

It works both ways: your experiences and challenges as an informed medical traveler will sharpen your skills on the home front, better equipping you and your loved ones to survive and flourish in the increasingly complex morass of our contemporary healthcare system.

Becoming Informed Here and Abroad

Toward becoming the best possible patient both at home and abroad, we highly recommend you buy, beg, or borrow and read—cover to cover—*You: The Smart Patient: An Insider's Guide for Getting the Best Treatment* by Michael F. Roizen and Mehmet C. Oz. These two physicians have written a witty, often irreverent, and highly useful guide to becoming an informed patient, whether in your doctor's office or dentist's chair, on the surgeon's table, or in an emergency room. This 400-page consumer bible is packed with information on patients' rights, surgical precautions, second and third opinions, health insurance plans, medical records, and precautionary advice that falls outside the scope of *Patients Beyond Borders*.

Step 2: Narrow Your Destinations

2 Once you've resolved what treatment you're looking for, refer to the *"Patients Beyond Borders* Treatment and Country Finder" at the beginning of Part Two. This handy reference will help you locate the destinations cited throughout the book that offer the care you're seeking. In addition, you may also want to consult the Web or other trusted sources you may know.

Your searches will likely produce a dozen or so places that offer, for example, excellent dental care. Great! Choice is good. You can then narrow your search based on your circumstance and personal preferences. For example, if you have a choice in travel times, you may prefer a cooler climate in Eastern Europe over the coastal humid heat of Cape Town, South Africa. Or perhaps you speak a little Spanish and are more comfortable conversing with Costa Ricans than Croatians. For sheer travel convenience, a patient living in California or Oregon may prefer Mexico as a destination for dental treatment, while Costa Rica makes more sense to a Florida or Georgia resident.

The point is to narrow your options based on your travel preferences, geography, budget, time requirements, and other variables. Part Two, "The Most-Traveled Health Destinations," provides a wealth of information on the most widely visited regions and treatment centers.

To help narrow your options, ask yourself these questions:

✦ When do I want — or need — to travel?

✦ If I'm taking a companion, when can he or she travel?

✦ How much do I mind a ten-hour flight? An 18-hour flight?

✦ Do I have a preference for a hotter or cooler climate?

✦ If I'm planning on leisure activities while abroad, what types most interest me? Hiking? Museum-hopping? Shopping? Beaches? Night life?

✦ How much cultural diversity can I tolerate?

For Big Surgeries, Think Big

If you're heading abroad for a liposuction or tooth whitening, you can skip this. However, if you're going under the knife for major surgery, including

- open-heart surgery of any kind
- any type of transplant
- invasive cancer treatment
- orthopedic surgery
- spinal surgery of any kind

you want to be certain you're getting the best. Your life is at stake. For big surgeries, you should head to the big hospitals that have performed large numbers of *exactly* your kind of procedure, with the accreditation and success ratios to prove it. A JCI-accredited hospital — such as Apollo in Delhi or Bumrungrad in Bangkok — carries the necessary staff, medical talent, administrative infrastructure, expensive instrumentation, and institutional follow-up to pull off a complex larger surgery. They make it look easy. They've done thousands of jobs like yours. It's almost routine. You want that. (**Note:** For more information on the Joint Commission International, see "The What and Why of JCI." See also "Alternatives to JCI.")

Be sure to ask about success and morbidity rates *for your particular procedure;* find out how they compare with those in the US. Also ask your surgeon how many surgeries *of exactly your procedure* he or she has performed in the past two years. While there are no set standards, fewer than ten is not so good. More than 50 is much better.

Step 3:   Engage a Great Health Travel Agent

3 Good news: if you don't want to do all the planning, research, and booking work yourself, you don't have to. The medical travel industry has recently given rise to the specialty services of the health travel planner. A qualified agent is usually a specialist in a given region or treatment, with the best doctors, accommodations, and in-country contacts at his or her fingertips.

Once you've settled on your health travel destination, it pays to seek out the services of that locale's best health travel agent. Agents usually pay for themselves in convenience and cost savings. They are usually well worth the relatively modest fees they typically charge.

The better health travel agents do all the work of a traditional travel agent and more, including some or all of the following:

✦ *Match you with the appropriate clinic and physician(s).* By far the most important service a health travel agent provides is that of matchmaker. The best agents have years of experience with treatment centers, physicians, and healthcare staffs, and they are in a position to toss out the bad apples and find the best fit for you among many choices. Because the agency's success depends on references from satisfied customers, top agents work hard to make the physician-patient relationship a good match from the start.

✦ *Arrange and confirm appointments.* Once you've selected or approved a physician, the agent can handle the details of making appointments for consultations, tests, and treatment.

Agents know all the assistants and aides; they can push the right buttons to fast-track your arrangements.

✦ *Expedite the transfer of your medical information.* Your agent can work with you and your physicians at home and abroad to relay medical data, including history, x-rays, test results, recommendations, and other documentation. Agents can help you get data into the right format for emailing or help you determine the best way to ship documents.

✦ *Book air travel.* Agents sometimes have arrangements with airlines for good deals on airfares, and booking international flights is usually a standard part of an agent's service offering.

✦ *Obtain visas.* For a relatively modest fee, a health travel agent can help you avoid the hassles of purchasing a visa (if required), updating your passport, procuring tourist cards, and hounding the appropriate embassy for service.

✦ *Reserve lodging and other accommodations.* These folks can work with your budget and lifestyle preferences to put you in touch with hotels closest to your treatment center; they'll often book reservations and arrange amenities such as private nursing care. Many agents have forged partnerships with hotels for discounted rates.

✦ *Arrange in-country transportation.* Most agencies either provide transportation from the airport to your hotel or treatment center, or they work directly with the hotel or hospital to arrange your transport. If transport is required between your hotel and treatment center, they'll also help with those arrangements.

✤ *Help manage post-treatment procedures.* Agents can be hugely helpful at the point of discharge from your treatment center, ensuring that your exit paperwork and other documentation are in order.

✤ *Help with recovery and recuperation.* Little publicized and often overlooked are the recovery resorts, surgical retreats, and recuperation hotels that can make a week or two of post-treatment more bearable — sometimes even enjoyable. Agents know all about facilities in their area and work in close partnership with the better ones. The international travel services coordinator at your hospital can also help on this front.

✤ *Help with leisure activity planning.* If you and your companion are up for a pre- or post-treatment trip, most agents offer assistance with side trips, car rentals, hotels, restaurants, and other travel amenities.

For more information on health travel agents in your preferred destinations, see Chapter Four, "Choosing and Working with a Health Travel Planner." For information on specific agents, see the "Health Travel Agents" sections in Part Two.

Low-Cost Surgery in the US: An Option for You?

While thousands of patients are traveling abroad for health-care — and dozens of agencies are helping them do it — another new trend is peeking over the horizon, and it may prove as attractive to cash-strapped patients as international health travel. At least one agency that we know of has started negotiating price breaks with hospitals—often physician-owned—right here at home. North American Surgery, Inc. is a health travel agent, although of a decidedly different sort. Its mission is to expedite low-cost surgeries at fully accredited hospitals and surgical centers in the US.

Richard Baker, the founder of North American Surgery (www .northamericansurgery.com; 1 866 496.2764), got the inspiration for his agency when a woman who needed a hip replacement called his office in Vancouver from her home in Wisconsin. She asked if she might get cheaper surgery in Canada. Her only other option, it seemed, was India. Canadians themselves face long waiting lists, so there are few opportunities for US citizens to cut into the queue, but Baker thought outside the box. He started contacting US hospitals to identify sources of high-quality, deeply discounted surgery. In the end, the woman had her surgery at Northern Michigan Regional Hospital. While the price, $19,000, was slightly higher than the total cost of the medical journey to India, Baker's client was happy. She found crossing a single time zone far preferable to a trip to the other side of the world.

That experience was the genesis of North American Surgery. Since then, Baker reports that hundreds of his clients have received high-quality, low-cost surgeries at hospitals and clinics listed on North American Surgery's roster. Baker has continued to negotiate even lower prices since he first opened shop. The surgery that cost his Wisconsin client $19,000 is now available for as little as $14,000.

Whether other agencies will spring up to follow Baker's lead remains to be seen. Will US hospitals respond with lower prices as they face increasingly stiff competition overseas? Until that question is answered, health travelers should check out all their options both at home and abroad.

Step 4: Choose a Reliable, Fun Companion

 This is such an important component of successful health travel that we've dedicated an entire chapter to it, Chapter Seven, "For Companions."

Folks who journey to far-flung places for medical treatment generally fare much better with a companion than if they go solo. Whether a mate or friend or family member, the right companion can provide great help and support before, during, and after treatment. Together, you and your companion may also add in some fun and adventure when your health permits.

Most health travelers choose either a good friend or spouse as companion. If you have the luxury of choice, make sure the two of you won't be packing a lot of emotional baggage for the trip. The successful medical journey requires large and prolonged doses of support. In an ideal world, you should get on fabulously with your capable, reliable, organized, and fun companion.

If you've already found a willing and able companion, you are blessed. Be sure to involve him or her in the early planning stages. That's the best way to cement the relationship and to learn at the outset if you'll be compatible. Ask your companion to accompany you to your hometown doctor's appointments, help with second opinions, and make initial international inquiries. You'll begin to work as a team. If you don't feel comfortable at the early stages, find a cordial, diplomatic way to part company.

And always remember to be as supportive and complimentary of your companion as you can possibly be. Your companion is a treasure. Cherish the relationship.

How can you choose the right companion? Three words: Capable. Organized. Fun.

Above all, travel with an individual you can count on in any number of circumstances. From taking notes in your doctor's office to talking your way past a snarly customs agent to fetching a post-surgery prescription, you'll be immeasurably aided and comforted by having someone beside you who will take the job seriously and stay with the program.

> The successful medical journey requires large and prolonged doses of support. In an ideal world, you should get on fabulously with your capable, reliable, organized, and fun companion.

Good organizational skills are essential. No job description is complete without that requirement, and the same holds true for your companion. He or she will remind you to bug the travel agency for your passport renewal application, help you organize and email your medical documentation, keep track of your in-country appointments, monitor your post-treatment prescription regimen, encourage you to follow your doctor's orders, and assist with myriad other tasks that call for sustained bouts of left-brain activity.

Step 5: Find Dr. Right

5 For most folks considering a medical trip abroad, this step is the most challenging—and perhaps the most emotionally charged. If you follow a few basic suggestions and caveats, however, you'll find the process far less mysterious and daunting. Remember, the final choice in selecting a physician—like the decision of whether to travel at all—remains always in your hands.

Here are some tips to aid you in your search:

+ **Insist on English.** While this advice may sound provincial and harshly xenophobic, if English is your only tongue, then insist that the parties you're working with speak English. Your health is too important to risk important information getting lost in translation.

Don't settle for poor English. Do your best to listen and understand, but if you find yourself constantly asking people to repeat themselves, don't blame yourself. Hospitals, clinics, and agents who cater to an international clientele will have English-speaking staff. If not, then apologize graciously for your lack of language skills, and move on.

+ **Seek Dr. Right, not Dr. Personality.** Okay, if a practitioner candidate is downright rude to you, then move on, but otherwise, give your physician some "personality latitude," at least initially. Focus on skill sets, credentials, and accreditations, not charm.

Even here in the US, many of the finest medical practitioners are technicians. While they may love what they do and be quite good at their chosen specialty, their personal presentation skills may be lacking. This is doubly true where language and cultural differences create additional social awkwardness.

Use your judgment and give the charm factor — or lack of it — the benefit of the doubt. If credentials and other criteria check out, and if you're otherwise comfortable with your choice, then charm and personality can probably take a back seat.

✦ **Expect good service.** Although patience is often required when corresponding with international healthcare providers, rudeness should never be excused, and no culture condones it. If anything, you're likely to encounter greater courtesy and graciousness abroad than here. If parties on the other end appear rude or indifferent, move on.

In corresponding with hospitals and clinics overseas, you will often find yourself directly in contact with your physician or surgeon. The good news is that you're engaged in a real dialogue with the professional who will be treating you. The downside is that he or she is probably very busy. Expect delays — sometimes two or three days — for return email or phone calls. If it's been longer, then politely, but firmly, request a response.

Ten "Must-Ask" Questions
for Your Physician Candidate

Be sure to make the following initial inquiries, either of your health travel agent or the physician(s) you're interviewing. Note that for some of these questions, there's no right or wrong answer. Your initial round of inquiry will help establish a dialogue. If the doctor is evasive, hurried, or frequently interrupted, or if you can't understand his or her English, then either dig deeper or move on.

1. *What are your credentials? Where did you receive your medical degree? Where was your internship? What types of continuing education workshops have you attended recently?* The right international physician either has credentials posted on the Web or will be happy to email you a complete résumé.

2. *How many patients do you see each month?* Hopefully, more than 50 and less than 500. The physician who says "I don't know" should make you suspicious. Doctors should be in touch with their customer base and have such information readily available.

3. *To what associations do you belong?* Any worthwhile physician or surgeon is a member of at least one medical association. Particularly in regions where formal accreditation is weak, your practitioner should be keeping good company with others in the field. For example, if you're seeking cosmetic surgery in Mexico, your surgeon should be a member of the Mexican Association of Plastic, Reconstructive, and Aesthetic Surgery. It's also a plus to see physicians who are members of, or affiliated with, American medical or dental associations.

4. *How many patients have you treated who have had my condition?* There's safety in numbers, and you'll want to know them. Find out how many general procedures your hospital has performed. Ask how many of your specific treatments for your specific condition your doctor has personally conducted. While numbers vary according to procedure, five cases are not good. Fifty or 200 are much better.

5. *What are the fees for your initial consultation?* Answers will vary, and you should compare prices with other physicians you interview. Some consultations are free; some are deducted from the bill, should you choose to be treated by that physician; some are a straight nonrefundable fee. In any event, it pays to have this information in advance.

6. *May I call you on your cell phone before, during, and after treatment?* Direct and personal access to your doctor is foreign to the American experience. Yet most international physicians stay in close, direct contact with their patients, and cell phones are their tools of choice. When physicians aren't treating patients, you'll find cells or headsets glued to their ears.

7. *What medical and personal health records do you need to assess my condition and treatment needs?* Most physicians require at least the basics: recent notes and recommendations from consultations with your local physician or specialist, x-rays directly related to your condition, perhaps a patient history, and other health records. Be wary of the physician who requires no personal paperwork.

8. *Do you practice alone, or with others in a clinic or hospital?* "Safety in numbers" is a good bet on this front. Look for a physician who practices among a group of certified professionals who have a broad range of related skills. For example, your initial consultation might reveal that you need a dental implant instead of bridgework, and it just so happens that Dr. Guerrero down the hall is one of the country's leading implantologists. Or, on a return visit, your regular doctor might be on vacation, but Dr. Cho who's available in the clinic can access your history and records, check your progress, and help you determine your next steps.

For surgery:

9. *Who's holding the knife during my procedure? Do you do the surgery yourself, or do your assistants do the surgery?* This is one area where delegation isn't desirable. You want specific assurances that all the trouble you went through to find the right surgeon isn't wasted because the procedure will actually be performed by your practitioner's protégé.

10. *Are you the physician who oversees my entire treatment, including pre-surgery, surgery, prescriptions, physical therapy recommendations, and post-surgery checkups?* For more extensive surgical procedures, you want the designated team captain. While that's usually the surgeon, check to make sure.

Step 6: Get to Know Your Hospital or Clinic

6 At this point, you've probably chosen a date and destination for your treatment, settled on one or two physicians you like, and perhaps you or your health travel planner have even scheduled a consultation. Excellent! You've made great headway, and most of the heavy lifting is behind you.

Before you start booking air travel and accommodations or planning the more relaxing parts of the trip, you'll be wise to do some additional sleuthing, beginning with your treatment center. Although detail-driven, this investigation is not as daunting as it sounds, and most of your research involves simple fact-checking. Here's what to do and how:

✦ **Check hospital accreditation.** If you're looking into a treatment that requires hospital care, check to see whether the center is JCI-accredited. (See "The What and Why of JCI," below.) While JCI accreditation is not essential, it's an important new benchmark and the only official American seal of approval for international hospitals and clinics. Learning that your treatment center is JCI-approved lends a comfort to your research process, and the remainder of your searching and checking need not be as rigorous. That said, many excellent hospitals abroad, although not JCI-approved, have received local accreditation at the same standards as American-approved treatment centers. (See "Alternatives to JCI," below.)

✦ **Check for affiliations and partnerships.** Did you know that many of the best overseas hospitals enjoy close partnerships with US universities and medical centers? For example, Harvard Medical School has a center in Dubai in the United Arab Emirates, where its Institute for Postgraduate Education and Research promotes cross-national collaboration on key education and research projects. The Dubai Harvard Foundation for Medical Research seeks to support a regional community of leaders in medicine and the life sciences.

✦ **Learn about success rates.** Although smaller clinics don't offer such information, the larger and more established hospitals freely publish their "success rates" or "morbidity rates." These are usually calculated as a ratio of successful operations to overall number of operations performed. For larger surgeries (such as cardiovascular and orthopedic), success rates of 98+ percent are on par with those found in the US. For the more common surgeries, you should further investigate any rates under 98 percent.

✦ **Learn about number of surgeries.** Most large hospitals will happily furnish information on numbers of surgeries performed. Generally, the more the better, as there's safety in numbers on this front. For example, India's Wockhardt hospitals have amassed a record of more than 40,000 cardiac surgeries and 75,000 interventional cardiology procedures. You will rest easier on your outbound flight knowing that your destination hospital has performed large numbers of procedures with high success rates.

> For larger surgeries (such as cardiovascular and orthopedic), success rates of 98+ percent are on par with those found in the US.

The What and Why of JCI

When you walk into a hospital or clinic in the US, chances are good it's accredited, meaning that it's in compliance with standards and "good practices" set by an independent accreditation agency. In the US, by far the largest and most respected accreditation agency is the Joint Commission. The commission casts a wide net of evaluation for hospitals, clinics, home healthcare, ambulatory services, and a host of other healthcare facilities and services throughout this country.

Responding to a global demand for accreditation standards, the Joint Commission launched its international affiliate agency in 1999, the Joint Commission International (JCI). In order to be accredited by the JCI, an international healthcare provider must meet the same set of rigorous standards set forth in the US by the Joint Commission.

At this writing, more than 160 hospitals outside the US have been JCI-approved, with more coming on board each month. This is good news for the medical traveler, who can walk with greater confidence into a JCI-accredited facility, knowing that standards are high and that staff, procedures, instrumentation, and administrative infrastructure are monitored regularly.

Please note that many very fine hospitals and clinics throughout the world are not yet JCI-accredited, and it's sometimes more difficult for some of these organizations to receive approval for highly specialized or experimental treatments. However, if you're considering one of these hospitals, you'll want to ask some tough questions about accreditation and standards.

A general rule of thumb for a global patient, particularly if you're planning on major surgery, is to first seek out JCI-approved sites. Then, when you've settled on a JCI-approved hospital, don't stop there. Rigorously scrutinize your physician's or surgeon's educational background, certification, and affiliations.

JCI's Web site carries far more information than you'll ever want to explore on accreditation standards and procedures. To view a current roster of JCI-accredited hospitals abroad, go to www.joint commissioninternational.org; in the left column, click "JCI Accredited Organizations."

Alternatives to JCI

When researching hospitals and clinics abroad, you'll often come across the phrase "ISO-accredited." Based in Geneva, Switzerland, the International Organization for Standardization (ISO) is a 157-country network of national standards institutes that approves and accredits a wide range of product and service sectors worldwide, including hospitals and clinics. ISO mostly oversees facilities and administration, *not healthcare procedures, practices, and methods.* That's of limited value in terms of your treatment.

Other organizations around the world set standards and accredit hospitals, and some may be as careful in their procedures and protocols as JCI — or not. JCI is the only organization that demands the equivalent of US health standards in hospitals accredited abroad. Other organizations that accredit in non-JCI countries include the International Society for Quality in Health Care (ISQua), the Australian Council of Healthcare Standards, the Canadian Council on Health Services Accreditation, the Irish Health Services Accreditation Board, the Council for Health Services Accreditation of Southern Africa, the Japan Council for Quality in Health Care, and the Egyptian Health Care Accreditation Organization. If you are considering a hospital accredited by one of these organizations, it pays to investigate the criteria the organization applies and determine to your own satisfaction that the standards are sufficient and appropriate to your needs.

Step 7: Follow Up with Credentials

7 Once you've located one or two suitable physicians, be sure to obtain their résumés. Many physicians post such data on the Web. If your candidates don't, then request that they or your health travel agent send you full background information, including education, degrees, areas of specialty, number of years in practice, number of patients served, and association memberships.

✦ *Get references, recommendations, and referrals.* If possible, speak with some of the doctor's former patients to get their feedback. Understandably, many former patients wish their privacy respected, and international law protects us all in that regard. Thus, it's often difficult for a physician to put you in direct contact with a former patient.

If you're unable to talk with former patients, ask the physician to provide you with testimonials, newspaper or magazine articles, and letters of recommendation — in short, anything credible that will help you assess this individual's expertise. If you're using the services of a health travel agency, ask your representative to check credentials and backgrounds of physicians to help you narrow your search.

Specifically, here's what you're looking for:

✦ *Education.* Universities, medical schools attended, degrees held and when awarded. Any special achievement awards or honors.

✦ **Certification.** Exactly what is this physician licensed to practice? If you're having implants done, then you want a certified implantologist's fingers in your mouth.

✦ **Professional history.** How long has he or she been practicing, and where? If a surgeon, how many surgeries have been performed and what types of procedures? Information on presentations, publications, honors, and awards gained along the career path will help you evaluate a doctor's talent, performance, and commitment to his or her trade.

✦ **Affiliations.** With what medical and related associations is the physician affiliated? Information about community involvement is useful as well.

✦ **Continuing education.** Mandatory in many countries, continuing education helps a physician stay abreast of new trends in his or her field. Most good physicians travel at least once a year to accredited conferences and workshops. Find out where your doctor goes and how often.

✦ **Patient references and letters of recommendation.** Nearly as useful as professional histories are reference letters or letters of recommendation from patients, colleagues, or other credible sources.

If you haven't engaged the services of a health travel agent, ask your candidate physician or medical staff to email you a copy of the doctor's résumé or CV. If you want to take your search a step further, contact the universities, associations, and references listed in the résumé to verify its authenticity.

For more information, see "Ten 'Must-Ask' Questions for Your Physician Candidate" earlier in this chapter.

Step 8: Gather Your Medical Records

8 Once you've established a relationship or scheduled a consultation with one or more overseas physicians, they'll probably ask to see supporting information about your medical needs. Such data usually include the following:

✦ reports or written recommendations from your local specialist related to your condition

✦ x-rays or imaging reports from your specialist's office or your radiology lab

✦ test results from your specialist's office or third-party laboratories

Depending upon your treatment, some physicians may ask for additional data, including your general medical history, health record, or pathology reports from previous treatments.

Some patients are timid about requesting health information from their doctors. If you're one of those people, it's important for you to know that as of April 2003, any physician, surgeon, specialist, hospital, or laboratory you visit is *required by law* to provide you with copies of any and all medical information they've compiled about you. These data include consent forms, consultation records, lab reports, test results, x-rays, immunization history, and any other information compiled as a result of your

> Any physician, surgeon, specialist, hospital, or laboratory you visit is *required by law* to provide you with copies of any and all medical information they've compiled about you.

visits. Although most won't require payment for making copies, your doctor or laboratory has the right to charge you a nominal fee for this service.

These days more and more medical information is going digital, particularly all-important x-rays and other imaging data. When you request your medical records, ask the staff to email you the data in digital form and to provide you with a hard copy as well. If you can obtain only hard-copy documents, then have them scanned.

If you're uncomfortable with technology and computers, perhaps your companion or friend or family member can tweak the paperwork into the form of an electronic file (scanning is not time-consuming for those who know how). A full-service copy shop or office supply center can convert hard-copy paperwork to digital files for a nominal fee, and you'll save real money on international courier rates if you transmit via email instead. Overseas physicians generally prefer digital records, particularly x-rays, which are easier to study and manipulate in this form.

Continuity of Care—Critical to Success

Continuity of care can be a challenge for patients who travel for medical procedures, say Steven Gerst, MD, and John Linss of MedicaView International (www.medicaview.com). Typically, the patient's primary physician diagnoses the condition and then suggests treatment. When the patient chooses to travel to another location or country to receive the treatment, the primary physician is too often left out of the process.

Similarly—and amazingly enough—many traveling patients engage a facility to perform a procedure without speaking directly to the surgeon before arriving. The patient and the hospital's international patient services coordinator may use email for preliminary communications. There may also be a telephone call or two with the coordinator. But the surgeon may not become actively involved until the patient arrives at the facility.

Too many patients make the assumption that a diagnosis is the "end of the story" and that contact with the coordinator is all that is required. *They could not be more wrong!*

Establish Communication!

If you're the patient, insist that you must speak to the surgeon who will perform the procedure *before* you schedule your travel. You may communicate via teleconference, videoconference, or voice over Internet protocol (VOIP).

It is equally important that you establish communication between your primary (hometown) doctor and your in-country surgeon so that follow-up care is prearranged. Because of time and language differences, this advance planning may be difficult, but it is essential. Complications and misunderstandings can arise if your doctors are not communicating properly. For example, after a knee replacement or a kidney transplant, many concerns and complications can arise during the long period of recuperation. Lack of communication can result in unnecessary hardships and potential returns to surgery.

Once you choose to go outside your physician's primary network, few mechanisms currently exist to encourage and facilitate ongoing consultations. *You must establish your own.* Critical information about your case can be lost if you don't. *Be proactive!* Here and abroad, it is usually up to you, the patient, to keep the dialogue going between your physicians.

Persistence is important, and the time-delayed effectiveness of email comes in handy—once you get the doctors in the habit of emailing each other and you. A secure online collaboration tool is even better because it can keep all communications in one place where it is available to all participants at any time.

Have Your Most Current Medical Records

Once you have established contact with an overseas doctor (or surgeon) and facility, provide them with your most current medical records. If you have a chronic condition and you've finally said "enough," your medical records may be a year or more old. If they are, visit your physician to obtain new laboratory tests, x-rays, MRI images, CT scans—whatever your overseas provider needs.

Medical records can be transmitted in two ways: you can send paper copies or disks by postal service, or you can send electronic documents via a secure online service. An online service is preferable for several reasons. First, it gets the records in the hands of the surgeon more quickly. Second, it creates a secure repository that can be accessed by both your physician and your surgeon. Third and most important, digital records create a foundation for after-care collaboration.

Collaboration Between Your Local Doctor and Your Overseas Surgeon

Transferring your medical records may get your local doctor communicating with your overseas doctor for the first time. This communication can be achieved though email, telephone, or a private group set-up in an online environment specifically designed for that purpose. Often such an environment is part of an online repository system that provides a secure place for collaboration between the doctors via protected blog, chat, email, and VOIP.

The next collaboration between doctors should occur after surgery. The surgeon should notify your hometown physician, preferably through an online system, of the details of the surgery and the aftercare protocol.

Once you return home and are again under the care of your physician, collaboration and consultation should continue. This collaboration should carry on until you are released from care with a clean bill of health.

Complete Documentation

Frequently, when such a repository system is not utilized, patients return home lacking the complete documentation their local physician needs to oversee ongoing care. The absence of information compromises a physician's effectiveness and threatens a patient's health.

Be sure to ask the surgical facility if access is available to an electronic system of medical record-sharing and physician collaboration. If not, request that your overseas healthcare providers subscribe to one to ensure that you can keep your at-home physician informed.

At a minimum, make sure your in-country facility provides you with complete records when you return home. Also make sure you keep your hometown physician involved from the first day. Good continuity of care is essential for a successful outcome.

Remember, as a patient, you need to take responsibility for the quality and consistency of the care you receive. If you don't, no one else will!

Step 9: Plan Your Recuperation and Recovery

9 For patients abroad, the days or weeks spent post-treatment can be particularly difficult. Perhaps you were on the road vacationing prior to treatment, and now you're eager to head home. Or seemingly urgent work challenges are piling up back at the office. Or you're just feeling far away and becoming homesick.

Any surgeon, dentist, or other medical specialist can tell you that if complications are going to develop, they're most likely to occur in the first few days following treatment. That's the time when your body is doing everything it can to compensate for the stress and trauma of your treatment. Rest and a healthful lifestyle are essential during recovery, but in these busy, overworked times, many people don't take recuperation as seriously as they should. At the first glimmer of normalcy, everyone wants to be off and running again.

Do yourself and your loved ones a big favor: follow your doctor's post-treatment orders, allowing your body and spirit time to return to health. It's not that much more time out of your life. For extensive dental work, recovery is usually a matter of a few days. Even the more invasive surgeries have you back to something approaching normalcy within a couple of weeks.

You might be surprised — and encouraged — to learn that many international health travelers enjoy recovery and recuperation accommodations not available in the US. Recovery resorts, surgical retreats, hospital residences, and a host of other options are available at many of the destinations featured in this book. Services offered include

+ **on-site medical staff** to assist with bathing, getting in and out of bed, physical therapy, medication, and more
+ **gyms** and other accommodations for physical therapy and daily exercise
+ **room service** for meals and laundry
+ **Internet access**
+ **liaison with hospitals**

Another big plus for recovery accommodations is the company you keep. The guests are people like you who have recently undergone treatment. There's comfort in sharing experiences, and dinner-table conversations with fellow patients can yield a wealth of medical tips and travel advice. If recovery retreats are not offered in your region of choice, ask your health travel planner or hospital for recommendations on hotels or apartments near your treatment facility.

Step 10: Create Your Health Travel Vacation

10 For most health travelers, a vacation takes a back seat to treatment and recovery. Many simply don't have the time or the motivation to tack a vacation onto an already time-consuming health travel trip. Some patients require more invasive procedures with longer recovery, and the planning alone (not to mention the usual discomforts of recuperation) knocks a beached-whale Riviera jaunt clean out of the picture.

Medical travelers planning for less demanding treatments, such as light cosmetic surgery or nonsurgical dentistry, should take a brief inventory of their treatment schedule and time requirements. Ask the following questions:

+ How many appointments does my treatment require?

+ How long should I remain near my treatment center during my stay?

+ How long is my expected recuperation period?

Unexpected tests, appointment reshuffles, and travel delays can eat up leisure time. As a rule, the treatment part of your trip will probably be three or four days longer than your appointment schedule indicates.

Whether you can squeeze in a vacation or not, the most important consideration is your health. Focus on your treatment and try not to bite off too much. Remember that you can always take a vacation later, happily spending the money you saved by being treated abroad. And if you find yourself feeling up to a little sightseeing post-procedure, you can usually schedule tours while in-country, with 24-hours notice. This approach allows you to avoid cancellation fees should you have to back out of an excursion you booked in advance.

Step 11: Book Air Travel and Accommodations

11 Why isn't this the first step? Although it may seem counterintuitive to book your travel and accommodations last, remember that you must first determine where you want to go, select a treatment center and physician, and schedule your consultations or procedure. Only at that point does it make sense to begin contacting airlines and hotels; otherwise you're likely to spend needless effort and expense changing itineraries.

You can see now why planning ahead is so important to successful medical travel. Some airlines and most hotels levy stiff penalties for changes and cancellations. That's another reason why it pays to begin your initial planning 60–90 days prior to your expected departure date and to book your flight *after* you've scheduled your treatment.

When it's time to book air travel and hotels, your health travel agent can provide information on good hotels and recovery accommodations near your treatment center. Some agents have standing arrangements with airlines for special discounts, so ask about favored rates before you book.

Be sure also to give your health travel representative a good idea of your budget. You might be surprised to learn that hotel rooms in developing countries can cost as much as the best accommodations in New York. Confirm rates and amenities before pulling out your credit card.

The same holds true for airfares. First-class and business-class fares are usually quite punishing; they're best paid by jetsetters, corporate executives, and frequent flyers. If you don't mind traveling coach or economy class, you'll save a bundle.

If you're making your travel plans on your own, ask your in-country physician to recommend some hotels nearby. Some of the larger hospitals have partnerships with hotels at discounted rates. Such information is often posted on their Web sites.

Just Ask

When it comes to asking for special assistance from the airlines, many travelers believe they must be severely handicapped to request a wheelchair or some other service. And some folks are just shy about asking for help or embarrassed to be wheeled around airport corridors and jetways.

Get over it! If you're heading to India for hip surgery and you've been in chronic pain for three years, there's no shame in requesting a wheelchair, and every airline we contacted ministers happily to medical travelers. In the same vein, if you're still feeling the effects of surgery on your homebound trip, it's perfectly reasonable to request wheelchair assistance.

Airlines ask that you or your companion request a wheelchair 48 hours prior to your flight. Then, when you arrive at the airport, check in with the skycap at curbside, where a wheelchair is usually nearby. Remember to tip folks a few dollars for assisting you; they'll appreciate the gesture and remember you the next time your paths cross.

Step 12: Triple-Check Details and Documents

12 In addition to ensuring that the kids, dog, and other loved ones are looked after in your absence, it's crucial on a medical trip to remember to take everything that you and your companion will need. Unlike forgetting your favorite tie or blouse, leaving important documents behind can create unnecessary hassles on the other side of the world.

Make sure you have all your paperwork in order, including travel itinerary, airline tickets or etickets, passports, visas, immunization records, and plenty of cash for airport taxes and other unexpected expenses. Be sure to pack all medical records, consultation notes, agreements, and hard copies of email correspondence. Also remember to take the telephone numbers, fax numbers, and email addresses of all your contacts, at home as well as in-country.

Pack Smart

You've likely heard the cardinal rule of international travel: pack light. Less to carry means less to lose. Don't worry if you leave behind some basic item like toothpaste or deodorant. Once abroad you can always buy essential items you may have forgotten, and picking up socks or toothpaste is a great excuse for you or your companion to hit the local market.

That said, below are several items you absolutely, positively shouldn't forget:

- passport
- visa (if required)
- travel itinerary
- airline tickets or eticket confirmations
- driver's license or valid picture ID (in addition to passport)
- health insurance card and policy
- enough cash for airport fees and local transportation upon arrival
- credit card(s)
- ATM card or traveler's checks
- immunization record
- hard copies of all appointment schedules and financial agreements
- prescription medications you're taking and copies of written prescriptions
- hard-to-find over-the-counter drugs you're taking
- alcohol-based hand-sanitizing gel (for cleaning hands while traveling)
- your medical records, current x-rays, consultations, and notes
- phone numbers, postal addresses, and email addresses of people you need or want to contact at home or in-country
- travel journal for notes, expense records, and receipts

CHAPTER THREE

Budgeting Your Treatment and Trip

First Things First: Consider Your Treatment and Travel Preferences

As with any other trip, your health travel costs will depend largely upon your tastes, lifestyle preferences, length of stay, side trips, and pocketbook. A patient flying first-class and staying at a deluxe hotel can naturally expect less of a savings than one who spends frequent-flyer miles and lodges in a nearby — and perfectly satisfactory — guesthouse.

To set reasonable expectations and avoid surprises, you should calculate an estimate of your trip's cost. This chapter offers advice, tips, and milestones that will help you plan.

To derive an estimate of your health travel costs and savings, we suggest you use the "*Patients Beyond Borders* Budget Planner" at the end of this chapter. As you get an idea of each separate cost, a realistic estimate will emerge.

Don't feel pressured to fill in every line item in your Budget Planner. Focus on the big expenses first, such as treatment and airfare, and then fill in the remainder as your planning progresses. You probably won't use all the categories. For example, some countries don't require a visa; or, you may stay only at a hospital and never visit a hotel. The Budget Planner simply lists all the common health travel expenses. As you plan, you can fill in the blanks that apply to you and arrive at a rough estimate of your total costs — and your savings!

As you complete the items in your Budget Planner, consider the following:

Passport and Visa

If you don't have a passport and are purchasing one for the first time, budget around $200 for fees, photographs, and shipping. If you're renewing your passport, budget around $150.

Depending on where your travels take you, visa expenses can run from $0 (for those countries that do not require visas) to around $120.

> Air transportation will likely be your biggest nontreatment cost. It pays to shop hard for bargains.

To avoid punishing rush charges and needless pre-treatment anxiety, take care of your passport and visa purchases early — passports at least two months in advance of your trip, and visas at least 30 days prior.

Airfare

Unless you're driving to Mexico (automobile travel can sometimes have undesirable post-treatment drawbacks!), air transportation will likely be your biggest nontreatment cost. It pays to shop hard for bargains. If you're okay flying coach, by all means do so; business- and first-class international travel are wildly expensive.

If you have a *trusted* travel agency, use it, although with caution. Most have side deals with airlines, and their commissions and fees can cut into your savings.

If you're comfortable using the Internet, take advantage of one of the many discount online travel agencies, such as Orbitz (www.orbitz.com), Expedia (www.expedia.com), Travelocity (www.travelocity.com), or CheapTickets (www.cheaptickets .com). Or, go to individual airlines' Web sites, where you can sometimes snag special Internet fares.

Auction and deep-discount services, such as Priceline (www .priceline.com), take a little more knowledge and patience. Exercise buyer caution with the lesser-known "cheap-trip" agencies.

Action Item: **Keep your budget current. As your plans change, so will your cost estimate.**

International Entry and Exit Fees

They're usually around $30 US per person, and they may be due at your in-country airport upon arrival, departure, or both. Most countries will not accept credit cards or checks for these fees, only cash. In some countries the fees must be paid in dollars, pounds, or marks. Local currency is not accepted. Some countries do not levy these fees.

Rental Car

When traveling, some people feel they can't manage without a car. It's the American way! Yet international car rentals are expensive, big-city parking is a hassle, and driving in a foreign country can land you in the hospital well ahead of your scheduled stay.

Even the most adventurous health traveler should think twice about driving a car while full of sutures and post-operative medications, especially on the left side of the road.

It's better to use taxis or limousines. They're comparatively inexpensive and, despite the overworked horror stories, cab drivers are generally cooperative when you follow the basics found in any travel guide.

As a medical traveler, your transportation needs — at least immediately pre- and post-treatment — are likely to be limited to hotels and restaurants. The hospital, hotel, or your health travel agent usually provides local transportation free or at modest cost.

If you're planning to head out of town on a post-treatment

vacation, then renting a car is fine. Just be sure that you, your companion, or your agent books the car in advance, as sometimes a conference, festival, or other special event can deplete rental inventories fast.

Other Transportation

Transportation to and from the destination airport will probably be handled by the hospital, your health travel agent, or the hotel where you or your companion will reside. You should budget for the cost of transportation to and from your US airport, as well as in-country transportation costs. Taxis and buses are usually not expensive; $150 should cover nearly any two-week trip.

Companions

Most health travelers we interviewed were glad that a friend or family member accompanied them. In addition to providing love, support, and a shoulder to cry on during difficult moments, companions can attend to myriad details. Many of those who traveled alone wished they'd had a companion or assistant during those inevitable trying times even the healthiest of tourists experience.

You should budget for the additional airfare and meals for your companion and—depending on whether you'll be doubling up—lodging. Items you can usually share include local taxi rides, mobile phone, and computer and Internet services. Items you can't share include passport and visa costs, airfare, airport fees and taxes, rail fares, meals, and entertainment.

Treatment

Treatment costs vary widely, depending upon the procedure, pre-ferred country, room choice, service options, and post-treatment care. In Part Two of this book, each destination features a com-parative cost-of-treatment chart, which provides cost estimates for the typical and specialty treatments available there. While these figures are not hard and fast, they'll give you a good idea of what to expect.

When you are considering a treatment center or physician, request the cost details in writing (email is okay), including the prices for basic treatment plus ancillaries, such as anesthesia, room fees, prescribed medications, nursing services, and more. Other useful questions include these: Are meals included in my hospital stay? Do you supply a bed for my companion? Is there an Internet connection in the room or lobby?

If you're using a health travel agency, make sure your agent gets specific answers in writing to these important questions, along with a firm cost estimate for treatment and ancillary fees. Then, once you've decided to head abroad, check, double-check, confirm, and reconfirm your hospital's and physician's quotes.

Lodging During Treatment

These costs are straightforward and are largely a function of your tastes and pocketbook. If you're not staying in a hospital or treatment center, search for a hotel or treatment retreat near the hospital. Long cross-town treks can be time-consuming, hot, frenzied, and costly. Your doctor or your treatment center's staff can provide you with a list of preferred hotels nearby.

You may wish to take advantage of the specialty lodging the region offers. Be sure to ask your agent or treatment center about surgical retreats or recovery lodging facilities recommended by, or affiliated with, the hospital.

Post-Treatment Lodging

Unless you're undergoing nothing more than tests or light dental work, it's a good idea to stick around for at least a week post-treatment, instead of jumping on the first plane out. Your physician will want to keep an eye on how your recovery is progressing. We highly recommend you take advantage of this important period to gain strength, guard against complications, and adjust to new medications, physical therapies, and lifestyle changes.

Many hospitals offer nearby recuperation resorts or other facilities, which include resident nurses and other staff who can assist you with your post-treatment needs.

> Many hospitals offer nearby recuperation resorts or other facilities, which include resident nurses and other staff who can assist you with your post-treatment needs.

Many of these facilities are four- or five-star hotels in excellent — sometimes exotic — settings, and your stay there can be the most memorable and relaxing part of your trip. Ask your treatment center or agent about such facilities in your region.

Whether you're recuperating in a recovery resort or hotel, budget $150–$350 per day to cover lodging, meals, post-treatment services, and tips.

Meals

If you're staying in a hospital, most of your meals will probably be provided, and the food is often surprisingly good. Many overseas hospitals also offer reasonable meal plans for companions. Ask the facility or your agent about costs. Otherwise, budget your dining out according to taste, both for you and for your companion. Any reputable travel guide can give you a good idea of costs in a given country. And, of course, avoid street food and restaurants of questionable repute. You don't want to complicate your medical travels with a rising bout of "Delhi Belly" just prior to treatment.

Tips

Tipping protocols vary according to country; check your travel guide on recommended tipping for taxi drivers, baggage handlers, waiters, and maids. A two-week trip shouldn't set you back more than $100 in tips.

We spoke with many patients who were so happy with the quality of service they received that, upon departure, they left an envelope on the bed with $20–$100 in local currency for nurses, aides, and service personnel. While a tip is entirely up to you, the gesture is generally much appreciated when handled discreetly.

Leisure Travel

Many health travelers plan a vacation for either before or after treatment. While this expense isn't strictly a part of your health travel, you may want to add the costs of vacation-related lodging, transportation, meals, and other expenses into your estimated budget.

The $6,000 Rule Revisited

We've mentioned it elsewhere in this book, but it's worth stating again: A good monetary barometer of whether your medical trip is financially worthwhile is the *Patients Beyond Borders* "$6,000 Rule." If your total quote for US treatment (including consultations, procedure, and hospital stay) is $6,000 or more, you'll probably save money traveling abroad for your care. If it's less than $6,000, you're likely better off having your treatment at home.

The application of this rule varies, of course, depending on your financial position and lifestyle preferences. For some, a $500 savings might offset the hassles of travel. Others might be traveling anyway, so savings considerations are fuzzier.

Patients Beyond Borders Budget Planner

Item	Cost	Comment
IN-COUNTRY		
Passport/Visa	$200.00	For passport and visa, non-expedited
Rush charges, if any:		
Treatment Estimate		
Procedure:		
Hospital room, if extra:		Often included in treatment package
Lab work, x-rays, etc:		
Additional consultations:		
Tips/gifts for staff:	$100.00	
Other:		
Other:		
Post-Treatment		
Recuperation lodging:		Hospital room or hotel
Physical therapy:		
Prescriptions:		
Concierge services:		Optional
Other:		
Other:		
Airfare		
You:		
Your companion:		
Other travelers:		
Airport exit fee:	$25.00	
Other:		
Other:		
In-Country Transportation		
Taxis, buses, limos:	$100.00	
Rental car:		
Other:		
Other:		

Patients Beyond Borders Budget Planner (*continued*)

Item	Cost	Comment
Room and Board		
Hotel:		
Food:		
Entertainment/sightseeing:		
Transportation:		
Other:		
Other:		
"While You're Away" Costs		
Petsitter/housesitter:		
Other:		
Other:		
IN-COUNTRY TREATMENT SUBTOTAL		
HOMETOWN		
Procedure:		
Lab work, x-rays, etc:		
Hospital room, if extra:		
Additional consultations:		
Physical therapy:		
Prescriptions:		
Other:		
Other:		
HOMETOWN SUBTOTAL		
TOTAL SAVINGS:		Subtract "In-Country" Subtotal
		from "Hometown" Subtotal

Patients Beyond Borders Sample Budget Planner

Item	Cost	Comment
IN-COUNTRY		
Passport/Visa	$200.00	For passport and visa, non-expedited
Rush charges, if any:		
Treatment Estimate		
Procedure:	$9,000.00	
Hospital room, if extra:		Often included in treatment package
Lab work, x-rays, etc:	$45.00	
Additional consultations:	$200.00	
Tips/gifts for staff:	$100.00	
Other:		
Other:		
Post-Treatment		
Recuperation lodging:	$1,100.00	Hospital room or hotel
Physical therapy:		
Prescriptions:	$65.00	
Concierge services:	$300.00	Optional
Other:		
Other:		
Airfare		
You:	$880.00	
Your companion:	$880.00	
Other travelers:		
Airport exit fee:	$25.00	
Other:		
Other:		
In-Country Transportation		
Taxis, buses, limos:	$100.00	
Rental car:		
Other:		
Other:		

Patients Beyond Borders Sample Budget Planner (*continued*)

Item	Cost	Comment
Room and Board		
Hotel:	$1,500.00	
Food:	$650.00	
Entertainment/sightseeing:	$500.00	
Transportation:		
Other:		
Other:		
"While You're Away" Costs		
Petsitter/housesitter:	$300.00	
Other:		
Other:		
IN-COUNTRY SUBTOTAL	$15,845.00	
HOMETOWN		
Procedure:	$55,000.00	
Lab work, x-rays, etc:	$375.00	
Hospital room, if extra:	$4,400.00	
Additional consultations:		
Physical therapy:	$400.00	
Prescriptions:	$500.00	
Other:		
Other:		
HOMETOWN SUBTOTAL	$60,675.00	
TOTAL SAVINGS:	$44,830.00	Subtract "In-Country" Subtotal from "Hometown" Subtotal

Is Your Medical Trip Tax Deductible?

What do tortillas, taxi rides, and treatments have in common? All these expenses may be tax deductible as part of your health travel. Depending upon your income level and cost of treatment, some or most of your health journey can be itemized as a straight deduction from your adjusted gross income.

In brief, if you're itemizing your deductions, and if IRS-authorized medical treatment and related expenses amount to more than 7.5 percent of your adjusted gross income, you're allowed to deduct the remainder of those expenses, whether they were incurred in Toledo, Ohio, or Toledo, Spain.

For example, if your adjusted gross income is $90,000, then any allowed medical expense over $6,750 ($90,000 x 7.5%) becomes a straight deduction. Suppose, for example, that your medical trip cost you a total of $14,000 including treatment, travel, lodging, and, of course, a two-week surgeon-recommended stay in a five-star beachfront recuperation resort. For that trip, you could deduct $7,250 ($14,000 – $6,750) from your adjusted gross income.

Examples of typical tax-deductible items include

- any treatment normally covered by a health insurance plan
- transportation expenses, including air, plane, train, boat or car travel
- lodging and in-treatment meals
- recovery hotels, surgical retreats, and recuperation resorts

Of course, your expenses must be directly related to your treatment, and many specific items are disallowed. (See below to learn more about allowed expenses.)

Be sure to save all your receipts. That's often easier said than done in foreign lands. Hotel and treatment bills are sometimes not computer-generated overseas, and just try getting a receipt from a three-wheel taxi operator in New Delhi. Receipts or not, keep a detailed expense log, noting time, date, purpose, and amount paid. Ask for letters and other documentation from your in-country healthcare provider, particularly any recommendations made for outside lodging, special diets, and other services.

For more information, you can go straight to the source. Go to www.irs.gov, click on "individual," then search for "medical deductions." You can also call the IRS directly at 1 800 829-1040. Believe it or not, most IRS customer service representatives are friendly and competent, and if you are sufficiently persistent, you'll eventually be put in touch with a medical tax specialist. As always with such matters, you should consult your tax advisor with questions or concerns.

Action Item: **Research IRS rules on allowable deductions for healthcare and health travel.**

A Typical Medical Expense and Tax Spreadsheet

When it comes to taxes, we're no experts, nor are we professionally or legally qualified to advise you. That said, readers often ask us how exactly the medical deduction works. Here's our best shot, a theoretical scenario of Robert Thrifty, a patient who traveled to Delhi, India, for hip resurfacing surgery. His allowable expenses went something like this:

- 90-day Visa to India: $140

- Immunization: Yellow fever $72

- Birmingham Hip Resurfacing Treatment: $9,000

- Hospital Room (four days): $350

- In-Hospital Meals: $110

- Recovery Retreat (physician recommended): $1,750

- Physical Therapy (physician mandated): $200

- Prescriptions (physician mandated): $65

- Transportation (airfare): $1,450

- Transportation (other): $200

- Total: **$13,357**

When Robert sat down to complete his tax return, his initial Adjusted Gross Income (AGI) totaled $83,000.

Adjusted Gross Income: $83,000

In order to calculate his medical deduction, Robert first calculated 7.5 percent of his AGI. (Don't ask us how the IRS came to this figure. It's just the one they use.)

$$7.5\% \times \$83,000.00 = \$6,225$$

Then, Robert subtracted his $6,225 medical expense baseline from his actual trip costs.

$$\$13,357 - \$6,225 = \$7,126$$

Finally, Robert calculated his new, improved Adjusted Gross Income of $75,874:

$$\$83,000 - \$7,126 = \$75,874$$

Naturally, if your income were lower or if your allowable health travel expenses were higher, you'd gain even more. But the calculation process is the same in all cases.

If the above is clear as mud, then a good rule of thumb is this: if your Adjusted Gross Income is less than $100,000 and your allowable medical expenses are more than $10,000, then you probably have a tax benefit worth pursuing.

Before you submit your return, consult your tax advisor or the friendly folks at the IRS on this important tax provision.

CHAPTER FOUR

Choosing and Working with a Health Travel Planner

The New Good Old Days of Hitting the Road

You may remember the pre-Internet days of the friendly local travel agent, when you or your parents picked up the phone and called — or actually visited — the small office of an agency that took care of all your vacation planning needs. If you didn't know where you wanted to travel, your agent helped you find a destination. If you knew where you wanted to go, then your trusty agent helped you book flights, hotels, and tours, matching accommodations and amenities to your budget and lifestyle preferences. And best of all, the agent's services were usually free — the costs borne by airlines, hotels, and tour companies.

Those days are long gone, the travel agent having, for the most part, lost trade to the Web, which appears to be slowly strangling us with the joys of ubiquitous, dehumanized self-service.

So, you ask, why bother to work with an agent who specializes in medical travel, when Expedia, Travelocity, CheapTickets, and dozens of other reliable Web sites now serve all our travel needs?

As you'll see below, the answer lies in getting the best available healthcare. Health travel planners can usually ensure a superior, personalized medical travel experience, and no general travel agent or Internet service will be able to offer that service anytime soon.

What Is a Health Travel Planner?

They answer to many names: brokers, facilitators, planners, expediters. Throughout this book, we use the phrase "health travel planner" or "health travel agent" to mean any agency or representative who specializes in helping patients find medical treatment abroad. Agents, representatives, and agencies come in all shapes and sizes. Some are departments of larger agencies; others are family-run businesses. Some are located in the country of treatment and specialize only in cosmetic surgery or orthopedics; others provide general services for multiple destinations.

As larger numbers of travelers head abroad for medical care, the health travel industry will mature, offering new infrastructure and amenities that only larger corporations can bring. At the moment, however, most health travel agencies are small, dedicated businesses with lean budgets and small staffs. All have their unique characteristics, along with distinct pros and cons. This chapter will help you match your needs and interests to those agents who can best meet them.

Why Use a Health Travel Planner?

Convenience. Some health travelers like to take it all on themselves, searching the Web and other sources to check destination opportunities, hospitals' accreditation, physicians' credentials, and patients' references; and to research and arrange air travel, hotel accommodations, airport pickups and dropoffs, sightseeing, and more. But if you're like many working people today, you're too busy to make such arrangements solo, particularly if you're not accustomed to sorting through all the complexities of international travel. Planners help with all that and more, leaving you additional time to make the important decisions and to care for yourself pre-treatment.

Experience. While health travel agents are not generally licensed physicians, most have long-standing affiliations with in-country treatment centers and practitioners. They cannot provide you advice on your particular treatment, and many will not recommend one particular physician or surgeon over another. However, all of the agents mentioned in Part Two of *Patients Beyond Borders* maintain a dossier of their preferred hospitals, clinics, physicians, and surgeons, and they can readily provide you with a list of healthcare providers to match your requirements.

From the hundreds of hospitals and thousands of physicians in a given country, reputable agents have selected practitioners who are tops in their respective specialties, often working within the walls of the most prestigious hospitals. After all, the reputation of any agency depends on delivering consistent treatment success and a high level of patient satisfaction. Any agent who doesn't is soon out of business.

Savings. Most health travel planners have worked hard to negotiate better-than-retail rates with hospitals, clinics, physicians, hotels, and sometimes airlines. They'll save you additional money on local transportation by providing airport pickup and dropoff, as well as transport to and from your clinic. Some agents are also hooked into tour companies, so they can provide discounts on in-country vacations and sightseeing as well.

Collaboration. Whether in the planning stages or in-country, the health traveler is more often than not a "stranger in a strange land." Unless you're unusually adventurous or have a MD degree yourself, it's good to have a planner to help you work through the complexities of your treatment options and to act as an intermediary between you and your local doctor,

> The reputation of any agency depends on delivering consistent treatment success and a high level of patient satisfaction. Any agent who doesn't is soon out of business.

your in-country practitioner(s), and all the third parties involved in your trip. Sometimes it's just good to have a shoulder to cry on, or a caring but dispassionate third party who's "been there and done that" and can reassure you that all will turn out well.

A good health travel agent works in collaboration with you, your companion, and your family, incorporating your treatment needs, budget, and lifestyle preferences into one package designed to result in the most healthy, comfortable experience possible.

What a Health Travel Planner Does

Although not all agents offer the same services, here's what you can generally expect:

> A good health travel agent works in collaboration with you, your companion, and your family, incorporating your treatment needs, budget, and lifestyle preferences into one package.

Planning and Budgeting

+ *Information exchange.* Once you've established a working relationship, your planner will begin sending you information on hospitals and physicians who can meet your treatment needs. Agents can supply data on hospital accreditation as well as physician's credentials, board affiliations, number of surgeries performed, association memberships, and ongoing training.

+ *Match you with the appropriate physician(s).* By far the most important service a health travel agent provides is that of matchmaker. The best planners have years of experience with treatment centers, physicians, and staffs. They long ago sorted out the bad apples and are now in a position to find the best options for you among a variety of choices. Because the agency's success depends on references from satisfied customers, top agents work very hard to make the physician-patient relationship a good match from the start.

✦ *Arrange and confirm appointments.* Once you've selected or approved a physician, your planner can easily handle the details of making appointments for consultations, tests, and treatment. Agents also know the assistants and aides who can pull the strings and push the buttons you need.

✦ *Teleconsultation.* Once you've narrowed your search to a few candidates or settled on a physician, surgeon, or dentist, most agents will arrange a telephone consultation with your selected practitioner during which you can share information about your condition, review your medical history and needs, and discuss your procedure. You'll be able to get a feel for your practitioner's working style and assess the "chemistry" between you.

✦ *Travel arrangements.* Most planners help arrange the best flight schedules and fares, and some have pre-negotiated discounts with airlines or affiliated tour agencies.

✦ *Obtain visas.* For a relatively modest fee, a health travel agent can handle the hassles of purchasing a visa (if required), updating your passport, procuring tourist cards, and hounding the appropriate embassy for service.

✦ *Reserve lodging and make living arrangements.* Agents will work with your budget and lifestyle preferences to put you in touch with several hotels close to your treatment center. They'll often book hotel reservations and make arrangements for local travel. For an additional fee, they can organize "concierge services," such as take-out food from restaurants, tickets for events, dry-cleaning and laundry services, and more.

✦ *Expedite the transfer of your medical information.* Your planner can work with you and your physicians at home and abroad to relay medical data, including history, x-rays, test results, recommendations, and other documentation. Agents can help you get data into the right format for emailing or help you determine the best way to ship documents.

In-Country

✦ *Arrange in-country transportation.* Most agencies either provide transportation from the airport to your hotel or treatment center, or they work directly with the hotel or hospital to arrange transport. If transport is required between your hotel and treatment center, they'll also help with those arrangements.

✦ *Communication.* An agent can usually arrange for the use of a cell phone for in-country calls. For more information on telephone and Internet options, see "Operator, Information: Staying in Touch While on the Road" in Chapter Five.

✦ *Consultation.* Most agents will arrange for you to be accompanied on your first face-to-face consultation, where you'll be guided through your health assessment, including tests, blood work, scans, and other pre-treatment procedures. The agent's representative will help answer any questions about your treatment before confirming the date for your procedure.

✦ *Pre-treatment.* An agent's representative will accompany you on appointments up to the day of surgery.

+ *Hospital admission.* Upon your arrival, an agent's representative will usually meet you to help with check-in and registration.

+ *Post-treatment.* Your agent or representative will check on you from time to time and arrange for you to be transported to any medical appointments you might have scheduled.

+ *Hospital discharge.* Prior to your heading home, your agent will usually be available to help assess your fitness for travel, as well as to ensure that all your exit paperwork — including post-treatment instructions, records, notes, scans, prescriptions, and receipts — is in order.

+ *Help with leisure activity planning.* If you and yours are up for a pre- or post-treatment excursion, planners can often help you with side trips, car rentals, hotels, restaurants, and other travel amenities.

Back Home

+ *Aftercare and follow-up.* Once you've returned home, most agents are happy to help with any difficulties you might experience, particularly if complications arise. It's helpful to have someone on the other end when your hometown doctor requests an x-ray from your trip or you have misplaced your prescription and notes for physical therapy.

Many physicians guarantee their work, particularly in the specialties of dentistry and cosmetic surgery. In the unlikely event that post-treatment complications make a return trip necessary, your planner acts as a liaison to arranging travel, appointments, and follow-up treatment.

Fees, Packages, and Payment

There are probably as many different fee and "package" arrangements as there are health travel agents. Most agents offer packages, which include various bundles of services priced according to what is included. Package prices depend most on your specific medical treatment. For example, one agent serving medical travelers to India offers the following complete knee replacement packages:

Basic Package

✦ surgery

✦ all directly related medical expenses

✦ two-day hospital stay

✦ consultations before and after surgery

✦ prescription medications and post-operative services

✦ support team during your stay

Deluxe Package

✦ surgery

✦ all directly related medical expenses

✦ seven-day hospital stay

✦ consultations before and after surgery

✦ pre-operative exams and tests

✦ prescription medications and post-operative services

✦ lodging in a five-star hotel for one person for seven days, with breakfast

✦ transport between airport, hotel, and hospital

✦ cell phone for local and international calls (500 minutes)

✦ support team during your stay

Action Item: Some planners offer "all-in-one" package deals, which are fine. However, at tax time, you may need to show your itemized cost breakdown, including treatment, lodging, meals, transportation, and health travel agent fees. Spreadsheets are universal these days. Ask your planner to give you a detailed expense log.

Costs and payments are usually handled in one of three ways:

✦ **Membership, up-front fee required.** This arrangement requires a patient to pay a nonrefundable membership fee (usually $50–$300) before any services are rendered. The membership fee is usually folded into the package price should you engage that agent.

✦ **Package, advance deposit required.** In this arrangement, an agent provides enough information to get you well along your path: data on specific treatment centers and physicians, advice on medical records and in-country procedures, and perhaps even a telephone consultation with your physician or surgeon. At that point, if you decide to engage the agent, you'll be asked to submit a deposit, perhaps 25–50 percent of the price of the entire package. Another payment is due prior to surgery, and the remainder is payable when you leave the hospital.

✦ **_Pay as you go, direct to third parties._** A handful of planners act more as referral services than full-blown brokers, providing you information about hospitals and physicians, airfares, and vacation opportunities, without doing much of the real legwork. They usually charge you a commission or a set fee on any service you engage.

If you're dealing with a reputable agent, all these fee structures ultimately get you to the same place. Beware, however, of agents asking 100 percent up front. You want to see evidence of performance, meet all the parties personally, and know that your hard-earned dollars are going where they should before you make full payment. Always, always request — and check — at least two references or some other hard evidence of an agent's ability to produce results.

Bill Me Later

While a deposit of up to 50 percent of the total package cost is usually required, you should try to reserve at least 25 percent of the total bill for final payment. In other words, as with most other services, don't pay the entire bill until you're satisfied and all the services you've been promised have been provided.

Most planners accept credit cards, but before you use yours, ask your agent about any surcharges associated with credit card payments. If paying with a credit card, be sure to alert your bank or credit card company to any overseas transactions, so their fraud department doesn't mistakenly shut you down just when you most need your card.

What to Look for in a Health Travel Planner

The health travel agency industry is growing, and more and more planners are springing up monthly, with varied experience and credentials. As of this writing, the health travel industry is unregulated, and any individual can hang a health travel shingle, "open for business." Thus, if you decide to work with an agent, particularly one who's not been directly recommended by a trusted source, you should do some checking:

✦ **Is there a language barrier?** As with physicians and other in-country contacts, if you're having trouble with translation or feel awkward communicating, look for help from a different source.

✦ **Request client references.** Any qualified agent should be able to furnish detailed letters of reference from at least two former clients. Agents may require you to keep such information confidential.

Check, Please

An agent's self-promotion on a Web site is not sufficient evidence of competence. Ask for at least two references from treatment centers or former patients. You'll also see the names of the better agencies popping up on hospital Web sites and in travel blogs. They'll be mentioned in newspaper and magazine articles and by in-country travel booster associations.

- **Obtain professional references.** As you work with a potential planner but before you write your first check, you should contact one or two potential treatment centers and ask if they've worked with the agency in the past and would recommend its services.

- **Request direct contact with your overseas physician.** Just as a general travel agent isn't an airline pilot, a health travel agent is not a physician. Agents are facilitators, not doctors. Most agents are more than happy to put you in touch with one or more treatment centers and physicians. They'll work collaboratively to help you make the best choice among available options.

- **What services are provided?** Of all the services a health travel planner offers, the most important are related to your treatment. Start your dialogue by asking the fundamental questions: Do you know the best doctors? Have you met personally with your preferred physicians and visited their clinics? Can you give me their credentials and background information?

What about accommodations? Do you provide transportation to and from the airport? To and from the treatment center? If an agent is knowledgeable and capable with these details, the rest of the planning usually goes easily from there.

- *What's all this going to cost?* Don't wait until you get your final bill to discover the agent's fee structure. Ask the important money questions up front: What are your fees? How and when are payments made? Which credit cards do you accept? Are there any extra or hidden costs?
- *How's the chemistry?* Usually after the first couple of conversations and email exchanges and after you've done some checking around about a planner, either you'll reach a comfort level or you won't. If you're beginning to sense a good working rhythm and feel the planner genuinely has your interests at heart, you can feel confident about moving forward with the relationship.

Domestic or Abroad?

Some agents serve several destinations, while others specialize in a single country, with in-country offices or point people. Either scenario is fine, as long as the good service that's promised on the Web site is actually being delivered.

Advantages of an agency based in your home country include local time zones and cultural familiarity. On the other hand, in-country agents give you the benefits of being on-the-scene, in close touch with treatment centers, physicians, lodging, and other third-party services.

If you choose to work with an agency headquartered in your home country, make sure you'll have a contact available in-country to work out the details and smooth your trip.

When *Not* to Use a Health Travel Planner

Don't use an agent if your initial requests for information are not promptly answered, if the agent doesn't reasonably follow through on commitments, or if you aren't treated well. Difficulty deciphering your agent's communications is a red flag, too.

If a trusted friend or other source has referred you to a specific clinic and physician, then half the work is done, and you may want to consider forgoing an agent's services, particularly if the hospital or clinic provides similar services through an international patient center or coordinator.

> If you choose to work with an agency headquartered in your home country, make sure you'll have a contact available in-country to work out the details and smooth your trip.

However, even if you have a great direct reference, you might still experience difficulty communicating with a busy physician and staff. If so, it might be prudent to find an agent willing to work with your recommended physician and capable of providing a variety of services to help ease your planning burdens.

For Best Results . . .

Seek quality and service over price. While cost is a big reason most health travelers head abroad for treatment, avoid the "penny wise, pound foolish" trap. A few hundred dollars in additional fees can buy a wealth of experience, information, comfort, and quality service. If you're saving thousands on your

> A few hundred dollars in additional fees can buy a wealth of experience, information, comfort, and quality service.

treatment, the extra expenditure won't be noticed; in fact, in hindsight it will likely be appreciated.

As the medical tourism industry grows, new health travel agencies are popping up monthly, with all the usual promises of unmatched service and untold savings. When you find a planner whose references check out and with whom you appear to be striking up a good working relationship, that's a good time to quit shopping around and hunker down to serious trip planning.

Get it in writing. Prior to engaging an agent formally, get a good understanding of the services offered and the compensation expected. If your agent doesn't furnish a written agreement or letter of engagement, then a simple email from you, confirming roles, responsibilities, costs, and timelines, will prevent disagreements down the road.

The Write Stuff

Some planners use contracts or simple letters of engagement; others are less formal, and it's all word of mouth. Don't settle for a handshake; it may come back to haunt you! That said, agents are usually individuals or family businesses, and a 20-page contract backed by a bevy of lawyers won't be forthcoming. If you can't wangle a formal agreement, then take the time to send a confirming email that spells out work expectations, timelines, and financial arrangements. If you've already reached a comfort level with your agent's abilities and credentials, that email confirmation is usually good enough.

Respect boundaries. Health travel planners are facilitators and information providers, not servants. Agents frequently complain about customers overstepping the bounds of courtesy, expecting concierge services for free, or demanding medical advice and extra amenities not covered in their agreement. The best planners are also the busiest — and the most sensitive to your needs. Respecting the relationship will usually get you the best service.

Remember: the ultimate responsibility always rests with you to settle upon a physician and treatment center and to make key decisions about your trip.

Stay vigilant. Once you've decided to engage the services of an agent, you'll be doing yourself a disservice to let him or her do all the work. It's your health at stake. Whether at home or abroad, the buck stops with you.

Thus, continue to check and double-check everything. When your agent recommends two or three physicians, research their credentials, double-check their board affiliations, and ask for patient references. Confirm a recommended hospital's standing and stature (e.g., accreditation, number of surgeries performed) and follow up any references supplied.

If you engage the services of a health travel planner, frequently consult Chapter Two, "Planning Your Health Travel Journey," and Chapter Five, "While You're There," to ensure that you and your agent share the same understandings about all aspects of your travel and treatment.

Follow up periodically. While a good planner can work wonders, relieving you of huge travel and planning burdens, even the best planner can fall behind or miss a beat. So check in with your agent from time to time and always end your conversation with an understanding of the next steps. Be sure to find out when you can expect to hear from your agent again.

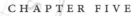

While You're There

First Things First: Arm Yourself with Information

Now that you have settled on a destination, made appointments with one or more physicians, booked your airfare and hotel, and arranged transportation, the hard part is behind you — except, of course, for your treatment itself. You'll find that once you arrive in-country, you will be greeted graciously, with help and support from hotel and hospital staff, your health travel agent, and sometimes even a friendly bystander.

But before you embark on an airplane journey overseas, you should read, ask questions, and learn as much as you can about your destination. *Patients Beyond Borders* can't begin to provide all the important information you need about international travel — much less the specifics of your chosen destination. Yet we do want to point you to a few important basics to get you started. Everything else you need is readily available through a number of sources. (See "Getting the Information," below.)

If you've not done much international travel prior to booking your health journey, keep in mind that you need not be a seasoned travel veteran to have a successful trip. In fact, most American international tourists board their outbound flight in blissful ignorance of their destination's culture, customs, and language — and they do just fine. Armed with multiple credit cards, they rent a car or hire a limousine at the airport and head for a US-owned beach resort, without giving a thought to the country they're visiting. Many scarcely speak to a local resident, except perhaps to mumble a few words during shopping sprees or dining out.

> Knowing a little something about the culture, history, geography, and language of your host country will buy you boatloads of goodwill and appreciation.

Health travel is different. Unlike that dimly recollected junket to Las Vegas last summer, you're now far more concerned about practical matters. Getting things done cooperatively and efficiently will help you and your companion preserve your physical *and* mental health. And most health travelers are interested in saving money when it's prudent to do so.

By pre-arrangement, you'll be interacting closely with local physicians, staff, health planners, and others who live and work in-country. Thus, knowing a little something about the culture, history, geography, and language of your host country will buy you boatloads of goodwill and appreciation. A small investment of time and effort in learning something about your destination will help you make the right choices and become more confident and proficient when you arrive in-country.

Getting the Information

Travel guides. You've probably seen at least one edition of *Lonely Planet, Insiders' Guide, Frommer's, Fodor's,* or some of the other popular travel series. A host of travel guides has been published for every city and country featured in *Patients Beyond Borders.* Most of the general information (e.g., history, currency, banking, and transportation) is essentially the same in all the books. *Lonely Planet* books are generally written for a younger crowd, with information for backpackers as well as five-star travelers. *Frommer's* guides are aimed at an older audience, but like *Lonely Planet, Frommer's* is budget conscious, although somewhat stodgier then its hip counterpart.

It's a good idea to thumb through the pages of various guides in your local bookstore or library and choose the format and presentation that best fits your tastes. Avoid titles like *Rough Guide* . . . and *Off the Beaten Path.* . . . Save them for your dream adventure vacation.

Since books are not cheap, you might want to head to your local library to borrow three or four titles on your destination of choice. Or search the Amazon customer reviews, which offer individual readers' surprisingly erudite, accurate assessments of a book's strengths and shortcomings; then purchase the one or two that sound best.

Be sure to take at least one travel book with you on the trip — it will become your travel bible — filled with notes, dog-eared pages, business cards, phone numbers, email addresses, and random scribblings. It's a good idea to purchase both a country guide and a city guide. The latter will contain a wealth of detailed information not found in a general reference. Of course, if you're planning a side trip or vacation, you might want a travel guide for those destinations as well. However, if you are a real lover of books, you may be wise to curb your enthusiasm. Books are heavy to carry, and they seem to grow more so the farther you travel.

Maps. While most travel guides contain country and city maps, they are often difficult to read. The print is small and the maps lack detail. If you want or need to know your precise location or if you are planning side trips, a small investment in an oversized street map or road map will yield a large return.

When in-country, bookstores are usually your best bets for high-quality maps and road atlases, but they can be difficult to find, and sellers are frequently out of stock. For that reason, it's often a good idea to buy a map before you travel. Some passport and visa services sell maps at a reasonable price (check online for various services). Amazon has a good supply; just go to www.amazon.com and search for **<city> map** or **<country> map.**

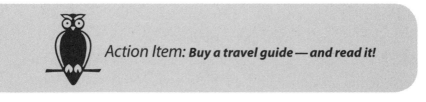

*Action Item: **Buy a travel guide — and read it!***

General Guidelines and Cautions

Here are a few general travel tips and guidelines that will help get you started.

Safety and security. The overriding concern of most patients new to global health travel is safety. That's understandable. In the past five years, this old world has seen several terrorist plots at UK airports (a frequent medical tourist stopover), a military coup in Bangkok (one of the most-traveled medical tourist destinations), peoples' rebellions in Oaxaca and Mexico City (popular with dental travelers), rioting in Budapest (a popular dental and cosmetic surgery destination), and never-ending strife in Israel (an important destination for reproductive and infertility procedures) — to mention only a few.

> As a medical traveler, you'll be too busy achieving your health goals to be booking risky nights out on the town, hazardous wilderness tours, or adventurous side trips of uncertain outcome.

Obviously, we live in a troubled world. Yet, this fact remains: of the 500,000 Americans who traveled overseas for medical treatment in the last five years, not one has died as a result of violence or hostility. As you read this chapter, you'll learn that most health travelers are quite sheltered. They're chauffeured from the airport to the hospital or hotel, personally driven to consultations, given their meals in their rooms, and chauffeured back to the airport when it's time to go home — all with good reason, as the primary purpose of health travel is to undergo medical treatment. As a medical traveler, you'll be too busy achieving your health goals to be booking risky nights out on the town, hazardous wilderness tours, or adventurous side trips of uncertain outcome.

Currency, credit cards, and banking. Much has changed in our new era of electronic banking, and currency is no exception. Check your local travel guide for specifics. Check with your health travel broker and hospital beforehand to determine accepted forms of payment.

✦ **Cash.** Despite the dollar's slide, good old American greenbacks — albeit devalued — are usually the best way to get the most for your money, without all the surcharges and hassles that come with traveler's checks and credit cards. If you want to bring cold hard cash to cover your entire trip and treatment, be sure that you are confident about carrying that much money. Check with your hotel staff or hospital administration beforehand to determine whether they offer room or lobby safes.

Remember that most countries have restrictions on the amount of cash you are allowed to bring, or at least require that you declare it. Check beforehand.

✦ **Traveler's checks.** These outdated instruments are still accepted by most hotels, hospitals, and restaurants — but usually only for a fee. Be sure to check first with your treatment center on the types of traveler's checks accepted.

✦ **Credit cards.** As convenient as they are, credit cards may not always be your best method of payment, particularly for large transactions (such as settling your hospital bills). Some establishments tack on service charges as high as 10 percent — negating the value of any frequent-flyer miles you might want to earn. Then, adding insult to injury, upon your return, your bank statement may reflect an additional 2–5 percent fee on each transaction. If possible, avoid using your credit card for cash advances, as banks charge big commissions on those. Check with your bank or credit card company before you leave home about its policies concerning international transactions.

✦ **ATMs.** Popping up on nearly every overseas street corner are the ubiquitous ATMs now so indispensable to Americans. ATMs usually offer exchange rates equal or close to the day's official rate. Prior to departing, check with your bank on its ATM surcharges, if any.

✦ **International wire transfers.** Avoid them. They are prone to frustrating, bungled attempts at one end or the other. Also avoid black markets and moneychangers.

✦ **Hotel safes.** Most of the hotels and hospitals recommended in this book offer personal safes where you can stash your cash, passport, airline tickets, and other important belongings. Just remember to clean out your safe as you pack for departure! One dental patient reported getting to the airport still woozy on painkillers, fumbling for tickets and money, and becoming hysterical before realizing he had forgotten to empty his safe. He made the plane, a little poorer and a little more gray-haired, after a hectic taxi ride back to the hotel.

✦ **Change.** When traveling on your own — as you might when shopping for gifts — be sure to take lots of small bills or coins. You don't want to be seen on the street sorting through a pile of large bills, and most vendors can't or won't break them, leaving you standing there while they trot next door for change. Yet large bills are what you usually get from ATMs, banks, and money exchange offices. Ask for smaller denominations. Your hotel desk or hospital cashier can break big bills. Keep a change purse, and keep it full!

✦ **Water.** The last thing you need as a patient — pre- or post-treatment — is a case of "green apple quickstep." Even in most parts of Europe, it's a good idea to request bottled water. Check to ensure that the cap's seal is unbroken, as plastic bottles are sometimes "recycled" by enterprising vendors, then filled with local tap water.

✦ **Food.** One of the most oft-heard comments from "on the road" patients is about the food. Surprisingly, the complaint isn't about the quality of the hospital meals. Indeed, the heart of the problem is that institutional meals abroad tend to be *too* robust, particularly post-treatment. Patients just out of surgery, who are taking antibiotics, painkillers, and other pharmaceuticals, should not be sampling exotic new taste delights. Until you are well on your way to recovery, ask your hospital dietician for the blandest food possible, and pass the tray of spicy tandoori chicken to your companion!

Outside the hospital, avoid "greasy spoons" and street vendors. While veteran travelers and locals have no trouble with street food, American digestive systems are not primed to withstand the flora that often thrives in native dishes. The better restaurants and best hotels are safer places to eat, but even there, it's best to choose only cooked foods. Fresh fruits and salads, as appetizing as they appear, may be washed in tap water. Say no to ice in drinks, too. It's often made with local water, and the last thing the health traveler needs is a case of vomiting or diarrhea to impede recovery.

Dress. If you're staying in a hospital, comfort is your first priority, and your gown will be about as elegant a fashion statement as you'll make. Once on the outside, you should respect local customs for dress. As a nearly universal rule, shorts are frowned upon except at the beach. And shirtless men are almost never seen in town, even in the hottest climates. When walking the city, check out what the folks on the streets are wearing; if you're comparably dressed, you'll be fine.

Note for women: Make sure you take a scarf to Middle Eastern countries, India, and Southeast Asia, as well as some Mediterranean countries like Greece and Turkey. There may be times when you are expected to cover your head. Also, sleeveless garments, tank tops, and camisoles are frowned on; unless you're heading to the beach, leave them home. Cover your arms in-country.

Getting around town. Ground transportation varies depending upon your destination — from rickshaws and bicy-

> Note for women: Make sure you take a scarf to Middle Eastern countries, India, and Southeast Asia, as well as some Mediterranean countries like Greece and Turkey. There may be times when you are expected to cover your head.

cles to motorcycles, buses, and stretch limousines. Generally, your best bet is a good old-fashioned motorized sedan taxi. They come in different shapes and sizes and are usually reliable. Be sure you use only authorized, licensed, or certified taxis. Your local travel guide or hotel concierge can give you specific information on finding the right services at the right price. Taxi drivers and honesty don't always coincide. Agree on the price — or insist on using the meter — *before* getting into the car. Also, make sure your driver understands your destination; if not, find a driver who does. Carry the address and phone number of your hotel, hospital, or recovery resort with you at all times so you can show your driver where you need to go or phone your hotel if necessary.

Remember to tip, although in many countries the 15 percent that's customary in the US is not always expected.

Operator, Information: Staying in Touch While on the Road

When in-country, most folks want to communicate with friends, family, and coworkers back home, and good communications with your caregivers and medical staff are also essential during your stay.

Gone are the days of postcards and telefax, now largely replaced by email, cell phones, instant messaging, and other helpful tools. If you're already using email and cell phones at home, you'll no doubt be comfortable with them in-country once you learn a few new ways of doing things.

Email. The most hassle-free and least expensive way to keep current with loved ones and coworkers is via email. Most countries featured in this book offer excellent Internet access, either free or very cheap. If you take your laptop, avoid traditional dial-up and modem connections. Dialing out from far-flung places can often be more trouble than it's worth, and high-speed access is available nearly everywhere you're likely to visit.

Before leaving on your trip, ask your email or Internet service provider how to log onto your email account using the Web. Follow their instructions to access your email account on the Web and note your username and password, which may be different from those you ordinarily use. If you can't access your email using a Web browser (such as Internet Explorer or Mozilla), consider setting up a temporary email account with one of the many free Web-based services. The three most popular are Hotmail (www.hotmail.com), Yahoo (www.yahoo.com), and Google (www.gmail.com). You can easily cancel the account after you return home.

You'll have no trouble finding Internet access abroad. Most hotels now of-

> If you take your laptop, avoid traditional dial-up and modem connections. Dialing out from far-flung places can often be more trouble than it's worth, and high-speed access is available nearly everywhere you're likely to visit.

fer high-speed wireless or Ethernet connections, either in your room or in the lobby. If you choose not to take a laptop, many hotels have terminals in their lobbies with Internet connectivity, but the price is often high and the wait may be long. It's usually cheaper and easier to find an Internet café on the street, if you're healthy enough to venture out.

Internet cafés. They abound abroad. They're usually inexpensive, with reliable, fast connections. Internet cafés can be a welcome change of scene from your hotel or treatment center, and they'll sometimes afford you an opportunity to meet and chat with a fellow traveler. Your hotel or treatment center staff can tell you where the nearest Internet café is located. Or, you can do a Google search by entering the search terms **<internet café> <city> <country>**. Expect to pay $2–$6 an hour in an Internet café, with modest extra charges for printing.

> Internet cafés can be a welcome change of scene from your hotel or treatment center, and they'll sometimes afford you an opportunity to meet and chat with a fellow traveler.

The more advanced or adventurous computer user can also deploy a wide range of telecommunications services including VOIP (voice over Internet protocol), instant messenger, Web video chat, and more.

Mobile phones. If you want to hear your loved ones' voices from afar, do a little research into the country you'll be visiting before you leave home. International telecommunications standards vary, as do costs and quality of service.

Your best bets are purchasing or renting a "GSM-enabled" phone, buying an international calling card, or both.

The right mobile phone can be a great travel companion and medical assistant. Not only does a mobile phone allow you to circumvent the hassles of international telephone calling cards, it's usually the way overseas physicians and other caregivers prefer to communicate with their patients. Thus, your in-country calls are likely to be as important as calls back home, making a cell phone nearly essential during your stay.

But before you invest in an international mobile phone, check with your health travel agent or hospital. These folks often offer mobile phones as part of their service package, and it's much easier to use a phone that's provided for you than to go through the hassle of do-it-yourself.

If a phone is not provided for you, you may want to purchase or rent a GSM-enabled phone, along with a prepaid SIM card for the country you'll be traveling in. Before you do, however, check the cell phone you already own; if it's less than a year old, chances are it is GSM-enabled. Contact your mobile phone service provider to find out if your phone is GSM-enabled. If it is, ask to have it "unlocked." Insist if necessary. Unlocking your phone will allow you to use it much less expensively in any other country.

If you do not have a GSM-enabled phone and your stay abroad is a month or less, we suggest you buy an inexpensive, unlocked GSM phone. They are now available for under $100, along with a prepaid SIM card. That way, you can give your cell phone number to friends and loved ones *before* you leave. Although buying a phone is more expensive than other options, you can circumvent numerous hassles and the dauntingly steep learning curve that goes along with mastering the public pay phone system in many countries overseas. Also, purchasing a GSM-enabled phone is still cheaper than dialing from your hotel room, calling collect, or using a credit card.

Here are a few additional tips for using mobile phones internationally:

✦ Don't let your local mobile phone service talk you into using their GSM plan, which may well be expensive, without allowing you to make in-country, local calls to your physician and other caregivers easily.

✦ If you purchase a GSM phone abroad, be careful about signing up for a plan that might commit you to a year or more of service. Before you pull out your credit card, read the fine print.

✦ If you decide to rent a GSM phone, either in the US or abroad, you'll probably be tied into the rental company's calling plan, which can sometimes prove significantly more expensive — even for local, in-country calling. As a rule, if you plan to use your international phone *only* for emergencies, renting may be prudent. Otherwise, purchase a phone; it will come in handy on your next trip abroad!

✦ Even if you can't use your normal cell phone abroad, pack it anyway. Many folks find that upon returning, a cell phone is useful in communicating from the airport or on the way home. Make sure to switch it off before packing, so the battery doesn't lose its charge.

International calling cards. If you've ever used international calling cards, you know there's a large and often bewildering array of options, with pros and cons for each.

If you choose to purchase a calling card in-country, chances are you'll be buying a card that you "swipe" through a pay phone, much as you swipe a credit card at your local grocery store. You'll be asked for your authorization code, and after giving it, you can input the phone number. Other calling cards ask you to input a local toll-free phone number and then enter your access code. While these cards are more versatile, you're faced with a whole lot of numbers.

A newer alternative to purchasing calling cards in-country is to sign up on the Internet for an international calling card service, prior to departing. After you register, calling card access information and a PIN code are emailed to you. You can also check your billing status online, add credit to your account, and utilize a host of other services. A simple Web search of **<telephone calling cards>** will bring up dozens of such companies.

If you're having no success with calling cards, remember that you can always head to a pay phone, access the international operator, and call collect. While that's a much more expensive option, you'll at least get through. Or, as a last resort, you can call from your hotel room. It's extremely expensive, but it gets the job done. Just remember to keep calls from your room brief.

Additional tips for using telephones abroad:

✦ If you want to place international calls directly from your hotel room or use the phone line to dial out on your computer, inquire about the rates before you connect. As with US hotels, you'll pay a high premium for such services.

✦ Never call from a pay phone or other calling center that takes Visa or MasterCard without first checking the rates. They're usually rip-offs (including Verizon and other big names), and charges of $3–$5 a minute are common.

✦ When using an international calling card from a pay phone, try to find a quiet place and avoid calling from the streets, particularly if you are hard of hearing or use a hearing aid. Hotel lobbies are usually quieter.

✦ Many Internet cafés offer reasonably priced international telephone service, a great alternative to calling cards.

Communicating with Your In-Country Caregivers

Voice. Most folks who travel abroad for treatment are stunned to find that physicians and surgeons are generally far more easily accessible than are their doctors in the US. When you're in-country, your doctor's preferred method of communication may be the cell phone, which can be used for voice, voice messaging, and text messaging.

As part of your early planning and screening for the right doctor, be sure to ask for his or her cell phone number and ask if it's okay to call with questions or concerns. If it's not okay, then ask how the doctor prefers to stay in touch; ask also for the names and contact information of key staff members. While email is great during the early planning stages, once in-country you'll want to be assured of immediate direct contact and prompt responses to your queries.

Remember that while caregivers abroad are generally friendlier and more accessible than their US counterparts, they are nonetheless quite busy. Keep your phone conversations concise and have a good idea what you want to say before you call.

Text messaging. Knowing how to use text messaging on your mobile phone is a real plus when communicating with your caregivers. In brief, text messaging is email for mobile phones. It's more widely used abroad than traditional email. Keep your text messages concise, e.g., "Doctor Alvarez, please call me back soon. I have a problem."

> While email is great during the early planning stages, once in-country you'll want to be assured of immediate direct contact and prompt responses to your queries.

Going under the Knife? Pre- and Post-Surgery Tips and Cautions

Be informed about general and specific pre-treatment precautions. If your physician has not already briefed you (usually in writing), be sure to ask about food, alcohol, pharmaceuticals, and physical activities that may not be allowed prior to surgery. Ask also about the aftercare regimen you will need to follow. Although all surgeries come with similar general precautions, take the time to learn the instructions *specific to your treatment.*

Get There Good to Go

Did you know that patients planning to undergo LASIK eye treatment must not wear contact lenses for two weeks prior to the operation? Imagine disembarking from a 23-hour trip to Bangkok, walking into your doctor's office for your initial consultation wearing contacts, and hearing that for the first time!

The point is this: take the time to learn about the dos and don'ts for your specific procedure. Don't assume that your physician has already told you everything you need to know—or that you heard, understood, and remembered all of the instructions your healthcare provider gave you. Ask about pre-treatment precautions specific to your procedure. And ask well in advance. As with passports and visas, the earlier the better.

The healthier you are before your treatment, the better your chance of a positive outcome. Prior to your procedure, follow these steps:

- **Stop smoking,** as it impedes the healing process. Smoking also damages your air passages, which makes lung infections more likely. If you're planning major surgery, and particularly cosmetic surgery, your physician will insist that you stop smoking prior to the procedure.
- **Maintain a healthy weight.** Overweight patients are more prone to infection.
- **Inform your doctor of any current or recent illness.** A cold or the flu can lead to a chest infection and other complications. Let your physician or health travel agent know if you don't feel well.
- **If you're diabetic,** make sure that your blood sugar levels are under control.

Ask questions; voice concerns. Too often, patients are timid about asking questions or raising concerns. Or, smitten by a nostalgic notion of yesterday's paternal, omniscient physician, patients trust their doctors to provide them with all necessary information. Remember, times have changed, doctors are busy, and being chronically overbooked is now a routine part of their work.

Thus, especially as medical travelers, you and your companion have a right — and an obligation! — to ask questions. If things don't feel right, voice concerns politely and firmly. Don't allow a procedure to move ahead until you feel good about the answers you receive.

If your surgeon doesn't provide much information, ask questions like these:

✦ How long is my recovery period?

✦ How much pain will I experience?

✦ What kinds of physical therapy will I require?

✦ How will I know when it's safe to take a long flight home?

✦ When I return home, how will I know when it's safe to return to my normal routine?

Your doctor should welcome such questions. If you don't understand the answers, or if you don't clearly understand your doctor's English, ask that the explanation be repeated. It's okay to be something of an annoyance. It's your health at stake, and getting this information right is essential to your well-being.

Be germ-obsessed. Whether on the streets or in a de-luxe hospital suite, cleanliness is a common worry among health travelers. And no wonder: overworked horror stories abound of children drinking sewer water; cows, camels, and monkeys fouling the streets; and kitchen personnel preparing food with unwashed hands and untreated water.

Food- and water-borne pathogens are a significant concern, both here and abroad. In the US, the Centers for Disease Control and Prevention estimate that nearly 100,000 patients die each year from "hospital-acquired infection" (HAI) alone. That doesn't count the millions of cases of food poisoning acquired at home and while eating out. At least one-third of such cases are preventable by simple measures and precautions. The good news is that of all the patients, staff, and visitors who walk a given clinic's floors each year, fewer than 5 percent become infected, and far fewer die.

Although standards of cleanliness vary among countries (some, like Thailand, consider our hygienic standards inferior), infection rates in nearly all accredited hospitals abroad generally rank on par with, or a little lower than, rates in the US.

Thus, whether here or there, risk does exist, however slight, and it pays to be vigilant, following a few simple precautions when in the hospital and before and after treatment:

✦ Make sure you wash your hands thoroughly, particularly after using the toilet. If necessary, remind your companion, physician, nurse, and other hospital staff to do likewise before and after attending to you. They should wear gloves. If they don't, insist that they do.

✦ Inform your nurse if the site around the needle of an IV drip is not clean and dry.

✦ Ask that hair around the site of a surgical incision be clipped, not shaven. Razors cause tiny lacerations where infections can invade.

✦ Tell your nurse if bandages or other dressings aren't clean and dry or if they are sticking to incisions. Ask that discolored, wet, or smelly dressings be changed.

✦ Ask staff members to check on tubes or catheters that feel displaced or may be malfunctioning.

✦ Do deep-breathing exercises to prevent chest infections.

> Although standards of cleanliness vary among countries, infection rates in nearly all accredited hospitals abroad generally rank on par with, or a little lower than, rates in the US.

✦ Ask relatives or friends who have colds or are unwell not to visit. If your companion contracts a cold or flu, postpone visits or keep them as brief as possible. Watch out for unclean clothing, floors, or instruments, and bring such breaches of hygiene to the attention of physicians or staff.

✦ Eat only cooked foods, even in the hospital. Drink only bottled water and say no to ice.

Manage post-treatment discomfort and complications. You've been out of surgery for two days, you hurt all over, your digestive system is acting up, and you're running a fever. Was the dinner you just ate simmered in sewer water? Have you somehow contracted an antibiotic-resistant staph infection? Will you die here, alone and unloved, a stranger in a strange land?

Coping with post-surgery discomfort is difficult enough when you're close to Mom's chicken soup. Lying for long hours in a hospital bed, far away from home, family, and Monday night football — that's often the darkest time for a health traveler.

Knowledge is the best antidote to needless worry. As with pre-surgery preparation, ask lots of questions about post-surgery discomforts *before* heading into the operating room. Be sure to ask doctors and nurses about what kinds of discomforts to expect following your specific procedure.

If your discomfort or pain becomes acute, bleeding is persistent, or you suspect a growing infection, you may be experiencing a complication that is more serious than mere discomfort and that requires immediate attention. Contact your physician without delay.

Follow doctor's orders. That advice holds for post-treatment as well as pre-treatment. Physicians here and abroad complain long and loud about patient noncompliance. A large number of patients — 40 percent or more according to some reports — simply will not follow the programs prescribed for them. Patients don't take their pharmaceuticals, despite clear instructions on the bottle. They don't attend physical therapy sessions, despite inarguable research that shows dramatically improved recovery rates when physical therapy is deployed. Patients don't follow instructions for bed rest, choosing instead to head back to the office prematurely or hop onto a riding lawn mower before they should. If that sounds like you, rethink your strategies — and comply! Your body, mind, and loved ones will thank you. So will your doctor.

Before Leaving the Hospital: Get All the Paperwork

Wonderful! Your treatment was a success! You've rested a little, and you're now more than eager to leave the hospital for the comforts of home or of that five-star recovery retreat you booked on the Bay of Bengal. Not so fast! Impatient to be gone, and often suffering the woozy side effects of surgery and post-operative pharmaceuticals, patients too often find themselves back at home later, missing important documents that could have more easily been obtained on site. So before you hightail it out of your hospital or clinic, be sure that you have all of your important documents.

Generally, larger hospitals provide complete medical documentation as part of the standard exit procedure. However, some smaller clinics may rely more on verbal instructions, and they are less likely to build and maintain a dossier on your case.

Regardless, be sure that you have the following in your possession before you walk out of the hospital (ideally, prior to making final payment):

> Before you hightail it out of your hospital or clinic, be sure that you have all of your important documents.

✦ *Any x-rays your surgeon and staff may have taken.* Try to get all x-rays and images in digital form (.jpg or .tif files), as well as hard copy.

✦ *Any pre- or post-operative photographs.* If your doctor doesn't take them, you might ask your companion to snap a few close-ups. While not entirely complimentary, photographs provide additional visual information for your specialists back home, as well as backup should complications arise.

✦ *Any test results* from exams, blood work, or scans.

✦ *Post-operative instructions* (e.g., diet and physical activity precautions, bed rest, bandaging, bathing). If your doctor doesn't furnish you with such instructions, ask for them. If you can't obtain written instructions, arrange a time to talk with your doctor and take careful notes.

✦ *Prescribed medication(s) and the written prescription(s), including instructions on dosage and duration.* If the pharmaceutical is a brand name manufactured in a country outside the US, be sure to ask your doctor what the comparable prescription is in the US. Your doctors at home may not know, and they'll feel more confident prescribing for you if you can provide them with documentation from your overseas practitioners.

✦ *Physical therapy recommendations or prescriptions,* including full schedules and instructions.

✦ *Exit papers* that indicate your discharge with a clean bill of health.

✦ *Insurance claim forms,* if you've determined that your treatment is covered by a particular plan or for a particular hospital.

✦ *Receipts for payment,* particularly if you paid in cash.

Action Item: Alert your doctor prior to treatment that you'll be requesting copies of all images, instructions, and notes. Then a medical staffer can arrange to have duplicates made for you. Alerting your doctor serves notice that you're serious about wanting documentation, and the staff will be more likely to assemble and duplicate all materials as treatment proceeds.

Speaking of paperwork, be sure to keep a journal near your bed, so that you or your companion can easily jot notes and keep them in a central place. Keep lists of questions so you don't forget to ask them. Record all verbal instructions and important observations for future reference.

Leisure Time: Before or after Treatment?

Since the recent dawn of contemporary medical travel, the media have had a field day promoting the image of sophisticated, devil-may-care patients jetting overseas for treatment, then heading to exotic resorts for two-week romps. Truth is, few health travelers match that description. The overwhelming majority of health travelers we interviewed had focused on researching, locating, and receiving quality healthcare at significant cost savings. Vacation and leisure time played second fiddle.

The decision of when or whether to include a vacation as a part of a medical journey depends upon a number of important variables. Thus, before booking a week at that yummy-looking mountain rainforest spa retreat, consider the following:

Intensity of treatment and length of recovery period. While promoters of health travel may imply otherwise, there's a big difference between tooth whitening and a hip replacement. Or, in the words of one physician, "Minor surgery is what other people experience." When it's you, it's major, and even a simple tooth extraction or brow lift involves pain, swelling, post-treatment care, pharmaceuticals, and possible complications.

If you're undergoing surgery, focus on your recuperation. If your surgeon or health travel agent recommends a specialized recovery accommodation nearby, take that advice seriously. Recovery lodges often offer 24-hour nursing services and rapid, on-call physician care should you develop complications. Even if you're planning only minor surgery (such as simple oral treatment or light cosmetic surgery), build in at least three days of recovery immediately following your treatment before heading out on a vacation.

> In the words of one physician, "Minor surgery is what other people experience."

Also remember that for many surgeries — and for *all* cosmetic treatment — you are required to avoid exposure to the sun for at least two weeks.

Remember also that air travel too soon after surgery increases the risk of deep vein thrombosis (DVT), which is the formation of a clot, or thrombus, in one of the deep veins, usually in the lower leg. The immobility of long flights increases DVT risk, as does recent surgery. You can take preventive measures, including wearing compression stockings and moving about while on planes and trains. Ask your doctor about how soon after surgery you can undertake a long, sedentary trip. (For more on DVT, see Chapter Six.)

Your availability. Most health travel journeys take at least ten days: three or so for consultation and treatment and at least seven for recovery. Thus, if you or your companion works for a living, an extended stay may be out of the question. On the other hand, if you are retired or you have vacation days accrued, building leisure activities into the trip could be good medicine.

> If money is tight, perhaps you're wiser to plan shorter, simpler, cheaper vacations at some other time, when you are feeling your best.

If you don't have at least three weeks to travel, reconsider combining treatment with pleasure and focus on what's most important — your health!

Your pocketbook. The idea of saving a lot on airfare because "you're already there" is attractive. An added vacation may feel like a free bonus. But vacation expenses add up, and you're still spending real cash for every vacation day you take. Are you sure you want to spend the money you saved by getting healthcare overseas on a vacation you would never have taken otherwise? If money is tight, perhaps you're wiser to plan shorter, simpler, cheaper vacations at some other time, when you are feeling your best. Maybe the money you saved on treatment can be put to better use if saved for later. Patients who opt out of long, potentially stressful vacation trips tacked on to their health travel tend to return home in a better frame of mind — and with fewer complications.

Your personal preferences. Some health travelers we interviewed had no problem taking a week's vacation in-country before heading into the hospital for treatment. Others worried the entire time. "All I did was fret about the procedure and all the unknowns before me," said one patient, who underwent a successful knee replacement in Malaysia. "I would have been better off postponing the fun part for another time."

> Most successful health travelers focus their efforts on taking care of their bodies, recovering successfully, and returning home happy and well.

Your companion. When planning your medical journey, consider your companion's interests as well as your own. One patient found that her companion — although a great friend and ally and a huge contributor to her successful heart surgery — was not the ideal fun-mate. While in Austria, they had different notions about how to spend their leisure time. Carol liked playing the blackjack tables at Casino Wien; Jennifer preferred chamber music at the Conservatory.

Your first priority. We found the most successful health travel vacationers were either veteran medical travelers who knew the ropes or patients who had lots of time on their hands — at least a month — to tack a vacation onto their treatment and full recovery period.

If you fall into neither of those categories, consider earmarking some of your medical savings for some delayed gratification — in the form of an unfettered, fully relaxing vacation once you've successfully recovered. Why rush it, when in truth a successful medical treatment and a fun vacation usually make for strange bedfellows? For the moment, know that most successful health travelers focus their efforts on taking care of their bodies, recovering successfully, and returning home happy and well.

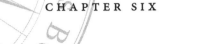

CHAPTER SIX

Home Again, Home Again

Beating Those Home-Again Blues

It's something of a paradox: arriving home from a long trip is at once joyful — and challenging.

After all, you've just been to a new and exciting place. Perhaps the richness of the culture, the cordiality of the people, or the quality of the healthcare you received surprised you. You may have delighted in learning a thing or two about a new land. Maybe you even picked up a bit of wanderlust on the road.

On the downside, you're probably experiencing the expected discomforts of surgery, the side effects of pharmaceuticals, and the annoyances of jet lag.

You'll likely return home exhausted, only to face backlogged bills, clogged email, endless voice-mail messages, demanding kids, and a dirty house. Take a deep breath and try to relax. It's important to pace yourself, particularly your first few days back home, allowing yourself time to settle back into a routine. It's even more important if you're not completely healed and you need additional recovery time.

Communicate Your Needs to Family Members

Yay! Dad's home! He went all the way to India for a knee replacement and came back alive to tell about it. In all the hub-bub, family members also need to know that the returned health traveler might still need prescriptions filled, physical therapy, follow-up consultations with physicians, additional tests, x-rays, and lab work. You may be unable to get back to your full, pre-treatment load of tasks and responsibilities — at least not right away. Let family members know how they can help. Accommodations — as simple as a son who does his own laundry for a while or a mother-in-law who brings over a casserole — can make a world of difference.

Action Item: **Within a day or two after returning from your trip, review your exit documentation carefully with your family and loved ones and clearly communicate the help you need to complete a successful recovery. If possible, form a plan of who will do what, whether it's tracking down a medication, giving you a lift to the local occupational therapy center, or simply loading the dishwasher after dinner.**

Touch Base with Your Local Doctor

If you followed our advice in previous chapters, you informed your local doctor or specialist about your health trip *prior* to departure. When you sent your medical records abroad, you established the basis for a continuing communication between your local healthcare provider and your overseas physician (see "Continuity of Care" in Chapter Two).

Shortly after your return, pay a brief visit (or send an email) to your healthcare provider's office and let everyone there know that you're back. Chances are you'll have specific needs, based on your overseas physician's instructions or recommendations. You might need an antibiotic prescription refilled or six weeks of physical therapy approved. Thus, it's best to touch base as soon as you reasonably can, both as a courtesy and for practical reasons.

Most physicians will be understanding and cooperative, particularly if you've brought home complete, accurate paperwork. If for some reason you find your physician uncooperative or uncommunicative, then consider seeking an alternative healthcare provider sooner rather than later. So make that call to your hometown doc soon after returning home.

Anticipate Longer Recovery Periods

Whether treated here or abroad, most patients can expect recovery periods of three months — sometimes even more — for large, invasive surgeries. For less intensive treatments, recovery periods range from a few days to several weeks. Regardless of the intensity of your treatment, don't be surprised if you find that you need what seems like a long time to feel fully yourself again, particularly after a long trip.

It's easy, for example, to underestimate the effects of jet lag. In fact, seasoned travelers know that, for every one hour of time zone difference, travelers should allow one day to fully recover from jet lag. For a trip to Asia, that's nearly two weeks! Typical jet lag discomforts include feelings of disorientation, fatigue, and general tiredness, inability to sleep, loss of concentration, loss of drive, headaches, upset stomach, and a general feeling of unwellness.

> Seasoned travelers know that, for every one hour of time zone difference, travelers should allow one day to fully recover from jet lag.

Add symptoms of jet lag to the list of unavoidable post-treatment discomforts, and your body's inner voices will be pleading with you to take things easy, at least during the first week after your return.

At home, some patients feel timid about asking for help, particularly if they managed to work a vacation or extended recovery period into the medical trip. Yet the fact remains that the healing body needs a great deal of rest and attention. Don't be afraid to voice a gentle reminder that you're still recuperating.

Hold on to Your Paperwork

Remember all that paperwork and assorted gobbledygook the hospital gave you prior to your departure? Forms, instructions, prescriptions, notes, and recommendations *ad nauseum* — keep it all! Take it with you when you visit your local doctor, who's likely to find those documents more informative and reliable than your personal account of the trip. If your physician wants to keep any of the documents, ask for a copy for your files.

> *Action Item:* **Comply with your doctors' instructions before, during, and after any procedure. Every single one of them.**

Stay with the Program

We've said it elsewhere in the book: pre- and post-procedure, it's all about compliance, compliance, compliance.

If you've just had dental surgery, you might be instructed to use a special antiseptic rinse twice a day. Do so. Or after an orthopedic procedure, patients are usually required to undergo a rigorous physical therapy program. Do that, too. Nearly all procedures come with a regimen of antibiotics and other prescriptions, sometimes lasting weeks. That means you!

Granted, it's no fun to take those big horse capsules or drag yourself to that physical therapy appointment when you really need to clear those 400 emails sitting in your inbox. But consider the alternative: after all that work and investment and travel, do you really want to develop complications that could cost you extra time and money — if not your life?

Fully inform your family members and close friends about your post-treatment procedures and regimens.

Fully inform your family members and close friends about your post-treatment procedures and regimens. Loved ones should encourage you to do everything you can to get better, and they should help you follow your program in every way possible. Pepper your calendar and to-do list with reminders — of your medications, appointments, therapy sessions, and other health-promoting activities.

Get Help or Farm Out the Work

If you've come this far in your health travel experience, chances are you're one of those people who "do it all." You're good at planning and problem-solving, juggling many balls at once, keeping myriad tasks and projects in the air, and managing to walk the tightrope of a complex contemporary life. That's why an otherwise challenging, difficult journey turned out so well. You managed it!

> For the first month or so after your trip, demand less of yourself and work back gradually into your normal routine.

Now that you're home, cut yourself some slack. Don't try to return immediately to your pre-treatment pace. If housecleaning was one of your daily chores, use some of your treatment savings to hire a temporary maid service. If you need to repair a lawn mower so you can cut the grass, send it into the shop. You get the idea. For the first month or so after your trip, demand less of yourself and work back gradually into your normal routine.

Stay Mentally and Socially Active

During long recovery periods, it's easy to become bored, isolated, and listless, falling into a rut of watching endless TV or surfing the Internet for hours on end. If your recovery doesn't allow you to be as physically active as you'd like or to return to work immediately, try to stay as emotionally fit as possible. Get a friend to bring you a stack of your favorite reading materials from the local library. Invite friends and family members to watch a good movie with you. Take up chess again, or Dungeons and Dragons, or whatever activity keeps you stimulated. Studies show that patients who stay mentally and socially active post-treatment recover better and faster than those who become couch potatoes.

> Studies show that patients who stay mentally and socially active post-treatment recover better and faster than those who become couch potatoes.

If Complications Develop . . .

If your overseas doctors played your treatment by the rules, they probably insisted that you remain in-country for at least a few days following your procedure. The main reason was to observe your progress and monitor your condition for any signs of complications, which are more serious than the usual discomforts experienced post-surgery. Most complications arise within a week after surgery. While 95 percent of all surgical patients experience no post-treatment complications, every patient should be able to recognize the warning signs and promptly seek medical help.

Post-Treatment: Normal Discomfort or Something More Complicated?

Prior to your surgery, your doctor should thoroughly explain the procedure and tell you about any discomforts you can expect after being wheeled out of the operating unit. Discomforts differ from complications. Discomforts are predictable and unthreatening. Complications, while rarely life-threatening, are more serious and may require medical attention.

These are some common discomforts you can expect following your surgery:

+ minor local pain and general achiness

+ swelling (after dentistry)

+ puffiness (after cosmetic surgery)

+ bruising, swelling, or minor bleeding around an incision

+ headaches (side effect of anesthesia)

+ urinary retention, or difficulty urinating (side effect of anesthesia and catheters)

+ nausea and vomiting, headache, dry mouth, temporary loss of memory, lingering tiredness (all common side effects of anesthesia)

+ hunger and under-nutrition

Most surgically induced discomforts recede or disappear altogether during the first few days after treatment, as the body and spirit return to normal. Be sure to report discomforts that persist or become more pronounced, as they might be early warning signs of more serious complications.

Complications vary according to each type of surgery, and you should be aware of the more common ones. Complications are scary, and many doctors would rather not go into morbid detail about them unless pressed. Complications are rare; most arise in less than 5 percent of total cases — and generally among patients who are aged or infirm in the first place. So while it's wise to be informed and vigilant, there's no need to worry yourself sick anticipating the worst.

Common symptoms of complications include:

✦ infection, increased pain, or swelling around an incision

✦ abnormal bleeding around an incision

✦ sudden or unexplained high fever

✦ extreme chest pain or shortness of breath

✦ extreme headache

✦ extreme difficulty urinating

If you experience any of the symptoms listed above, call your hometown physician immediately.

The Straight Dope on Pharmaceuticals

True or false: When traveling, it's okay to bring small amounts of prescription drugs back into the US.

True or false: It's legal to order prescriptions from reputable online pharmacies in Canada and Mexico.

Believe it or not, false on both counts, though with some favorable caveats.

Many international travelers like to purchase their favorite prescription medications less expensively while abroad. While it's *technically* illegal (and clearly stated as such on both the FDA and US Customs Web sites), consumer activists have turned the issue into a political hot potato. Consequently, at this writing, customs inspectors and FDA personnel are loathe to bust Granny with her two vials of benazepril, and in most instances they turn a blind eye to folks entering the US with prescription drugs purchased abroad. Thus it's become a gray area, with FDA inspectors empowered to use "general discretion" when prescription drugs are apprehended by customs agents. Most often, the offending pharmaceuticals are simply confiscated, and the traveler must decide whether it's worth all the red tape required to petition for their return.

The overwhelming number of tourists who carry pharmaceuticals purchased abroad cross the border with no trouble, their medications usually unnoticed. The best advice is to use common sense. You're far less likely to be hassled for carrying $100 worth of amoxicillin than if your suitcase is seen bursting with enough tramadol to supply the streets of Los Angeles for a year. And as always, if you're carrying drugs that are illegal in the US—prescription or otherwise—you may be subject to arrest, as well as seizure of the prohibited items.

Similarly, it's *technically* illegal in the US to purchase any pharmaceutical of any kind from any mail-order pharmacy outside the US, even from Canada or Mexico. Again, highly vocal activists have prevailed politically, and only a small fraction of prescriptions purchased from foreign countries are seized. In those cases, the pharmacies often double-ship the order, so the buyer usually doesn't even know the purchase was interrupted.

Until the laws change, you're advised to use good judgment on this issue as well. Purchase only from reputable pharmacies, using legitimate prescriptions from your physician. And anticipate the outside chance you'll be among the few every year who are inconvenienced by FDA border seizures.

It's perfectly legal to purchase prescriptions online from authorized mail-order pharmacies anywhere in the US.

For specifics about importing controlled substances, call 1 202 307.2414. For additional information about traveling with medication, contact your nearest FDA office or write to the US Food and Drug Administration, Division of Import Operations and Policy, Room 12-8 (HFC-170), 5600 Fishers Lane, Rockville, MD 20857. For further information on prescription drug rules and regulations, contact the FDA's Center for Drugs, 1 888 INFO.FDA or www.fda.gov/cder.

Medical Travel and Medical Malpractice

If you experience severe complications and do not receive the follow-up care you think you need or deserve, then you may want to consider legal action.

"Unlike the American legal system, legal recourse and remedies are generally limited abroad for patients who experience bad outcomes in foreign facilities," report attorneys Amanda L. Hayes and Natasha A. Bellroth of Global MD (www.yourglobalmd.com). "Moreover, a patient's ability to sue a foreign physician or facility for medical malpractice is limited by the availability of an appropriate forum in which to bring a lawsuit."

For example, say Hayes and Bellroth, assume that American patient John Smith travels to India for hip replacement surgery at ABC Hospital and suffers a bad outcome that was caused by his surgeon's negligence. Let's review Mr. Smith's options for pursuing a judicial remedy:

- In order to sue ABC Hospital in the US, a US court must be able to exercise jurisdiction over ABC Hospital, an Indian corporation with no offices or employees in the US. US courts may only assert general or specific personal jurisdiction over a foreign entity when the foreign entity's presence or dealings where the suit is brought justify requiring the company to defend suit there.

- Assuming that the case proceeds to judgment against ABC Hospital in the US, Mr. Smith will face an uphill battle to enforce an American judgment in India. If Mr. Smith wins a large punitive damage award from an American court, he will be disappointed to learn that punitive damages are rarely awarded outside of the US (another reason for the high cost of US healthcare) and are unlikely to be enforced (in any of the countries currently attracting American medical tourists).

- Alternatively, Mr. Smith may try to sue ABC Hospital in India, which will require that Mr. Smith hire a lawyer in India and perhaps travel back to India to attend the proceedings. Even if Mr. Smith prevails against ABC Hospital in India, he will probably only be able to recover his actual damages (the provable out-of-pocket cost of harm caused by negligence, e.g., medical bills incurred for corrective surgery and time away from work), as few countries award punitive damages to successful plaintiffs.

- Mr. Smith may seek to arbitrate his claim against ABC Hospital before an international tribunal. For example, the International Court of Arbitration of the International Chamber of Commerce may provide Mr. Smith with a viable and likely more cost-effective way to hold ABC Hospital accountable for its negligence. Generally, an agreement to arbitrate claims must be in place before the relationship commences. Mr. Smith should have confirmed prior to surgery that ABC Hospital had agreed to arbitration of potential future claims and to where those proceedings would occur.

Each alternative forum presents its own unique set of challenges. There is no ideal solution that would put judicial recourse against a foreign entity on par with the remedies available against a US hospital or physician. There are, however, practical measures that Mr. Smith might have taken before he traveled to India that would have helped him to manage the risk in the unlikely event of a bad outcome:

- For example, Mr. Smith might have purchased insurance (a health travel agency should be able to point the patient to available policies) designed specifically to protect him from the financial consequences of foreseeable complications and unforeseeable medical malpractice. Such insurance could have helped Mr. Smith eliminate the cost of legal action while compensating him up to the amount of his purchased policy's limit.

- In addition, had Mr. Smith paid for his procedure with a major credit card, his card company may have allowed him to recover the cost of a disappointing treatment by disputing the charges.

- Finally, Mr. Smith could have made sure that the health travel agency that planned his procedure had a clear and reasonable protocol in place with the treating facility on how to deal with bad outcomes and complications. Ideally, the hospital would have agreed to absorb costs associated with making Mr. Smith whole again (return flight, accommodations, and corrective procedure) and compensate him if he could not be satisfied.

Ultimately, there is no perfect way to compensate a patient—either domestically or abroad—who has suffered an imperfect outcome after a medical procedure. The good news is that informed patients can take preventive measures to protect themselves before they travel abroad for care so that they do not end up in the hands of imperfect healthcare insurance and judicial systems. Foreign hospitals are eager to prove that they have surgeons and technical facilities of high quality that rivals and even exceeds that in the US. Your independent research will reveal that sophisticated foreign hospitals and governments are heavily invested in serving the US population with healthcare. They also understand that the publicity associated with even one bad outcome could quickly end the growing flow of US patients.

Caution: Blood Clots in the Veins

Air travel after surgery may put you at risk of deep vein thrombosis (DVT), a term that describes the formation of a clot, or thrombus, in one of the deep veins, usually in the lower leg. The immobility of long flights increases the risk, as does recent surgery. The symptoms of DVT may include pain and redness of the skin over a vein or swelling and tenderness in the ankle, foot, or thigh. More serious symptoms include chest pain and shortness of breath.

You can take preventive measures to reduce your risk of DVT. Wear compression stockings and move about frequently while on planes and trains. Ask your doctor about how soon after surgery you can undertake a long, sedentary trip.

OTHER WAYS TO REDUCE DVT RISK

Before you travel:

✦ Stop smoking.

✦ Lose weight if you need to.

✦ Get enough exercise to be at least minimally fit before your surgery and your travel.

✦ Discuss stopping birth control pills and hormone replacement therapy with your doctor.

✦ Travel on an airline that provides sufficient leg room.

✦ Wear loose clothing.

✦ Reserve an aisle seat on the airplane so you can get up and move around easily.

✦ Ask your surgeon about using a pneumatic compression device during and after surgery.

✦ Before your return flight home, ask your surgeon if you need an anticoagulant.

✦ Walk briskly for at least half an hour before takeoff.

On the plane:

✦ Don't stow your carry-on luggage under your seat if it restricts your movement.

✦ Flex your calves and rotate your ankles every 20–30 minutes.

✦ Walk up and down the aisle every two hours or less.

✦ Sleep only for short periods.

✦ Do not take sleeping pills.

✦ Drink lots of water to avoid dehydration.

✦ Avoid alcohol, caffeine, and diet soda.

✦ Wear elastic flight socks or support stockings.

✦ Don't let your stockings or clothing roll up or constrict your legs.

✦ Take deep breaths frequently throughout your flight.

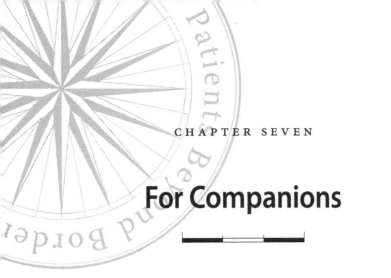

For Companions

"Hold a true friend in both your hands."
— Nigerian proverb

Joining a friend, family member, or other loved one on a medical journey is truly a gift, but the rewards are many. Some companions simply appreciate the opportunity to travel. Others enjoy the chance to spend one-on-one time with a person who is important to them, perhaps to deepen a relationship. With most companions, there's an element of "being in this together" — working through a unique experience and its inevitable surprises, then heading home with great stories to tell!

First Things First: Are You Up for the Job?

Before you overthink that question, here's some succinct advice: go with your first instincts.

✦ If you've already agreed to be a companion health traveler and you've not been bribed, railroaded, or otherwise coerced

---

into the job, then chances are your first impressions were correct. While the journey won't always be a cakewalk, most memorable and worthwhile experiences are less than easy, and they're the stuff of profound and lasting memories.

✦ If you've been asked to be a companion and are having strong reservations about it for any reason, then either talk it out or politely decline.

✦ If you're on the fence about being a companion, you might want to flip through Chapter Two, "Planning Your Health Travel Journey," where you'll find important criteria for a successful companion-patient relationship. In brief, if you're reliable, organized, and like to have some fun, chances are good you and your partner will be enriched by the experience, despite — and often because of — the rough patches you'll inevitably encounter.

Know there are no magic formulas, although a good dose of common sense mixed with empathy and attentiveness are the main initial requirements. Each patient is different, as is each relationship between patient and companion. Use the sections below to get an idea of the broad requirements and the journey's milestones, and the rest will follow.

Before the Trip

The devil of any medical trip is in the details. The more of them you and your partner nail down before boarding the plane, the more successful the trip and treatment will be. Patients are often distracted prior to the trip, not only by the usual family and professional concerns, but also by perfectly understandable worries about their upcoming treatment and travel. A good companion can help keep heads together, maintain calm in the household, and expedite trip planning greatly.

Use the checklist below to make sure that either you or your partner has addressed each important preparation:

✦ **Passports and visas.** At least a month prior to your departure, check to see that you and your partner have them and that they're on order. Just before your departure, make sure both of you carry them on your person. Don't leave them on the dining room table.

✦ **Medical documentation.** Make sure the health traveler has packed all written diagnoses, treatment recommendations, cost estimates, x-rays, lab reports, blood test results, and any other information related to the treatment. Your partner's in-country physician and staff will appreciate having these documents, and taking them will save time and money.

> The devil of any medical trip is in the details. The more of them you and your partner nail down before boarding the plane, the more successful your trip and treatment will be.

✦ **Kids, cats, and newspaper delivery.** Work with your partner to make sure all the family living arrangements are in order, and ask frequently how you can help. Examples of services you might provide include finding a pet sitter, making sure bills are paid in advance, and suspending newspaper delivery.

✦ *Confirm and reconfirm appointments and reservations.* A couple of days prior to departure, call or email the physician and treatment center to reconfirm all appointments and scheduled treatments. Do the same for your flight reservations, lodging, and any local transportation you've booked.

✦ *Read up on your destination.* If you can spare the time, become acquainted with your travel destination. Check your local library for travel guides, skim them for content, make notes, and then buy the one you and your partner like best. Or do an Internet search for the city and country where you'll be staying, print what interests you, and toss the printout into your travel bag.

> If you learn some facts about the culture and history, the local people will invariably appreciate your interest.

Although you need not be fluent in the language, at least one of you should know a little something about the local customs, protocol, transportation, restaurants, and historic sites. If you learn some facts about the culture and history, the local people will invariably appreciate your interest. That goes double if you take time to learn even a few words of the language.

✦ *Prescriptions and other essentials.* While you can purchase just about anything abroad that you might have forgotten to pack, some things are more easily replaced than others, especially on a medical trip. Don't worry about a comb or shampoo, but make sure you and your partner have packed important medications and prescriptions, an extra set of eyeglasses if you wear them, plus special creams, medicinal soaps, hard-to-find ointments, and the like. Thoroughly check the medicine cabinet and bathroom counter to make sure you've packed all the creature comforts and necessities that might be difficult to purchase abroad. In these days of tight airport security, it's best to pack liquids and gels in checked luggage, but keep prescription medicines (in their original containers) in your carry-on bag.

✦ **Finances.** Sometimes even the best of friends can encounter misunderstandings about who is to pay for what. Avoid damaging your relationship by addressing financial questions early. Spell out expectations. For example, who's paying for the airfare? Lodging and meals? Sightseeing and tours? Generally, with the more expensive surgeries (e.g., cardiovascular and orthopedic), the cost of a companion is factored into the overall savings of the procedure. However, a tooth cleaning and whitening that's more vacation than medical journey might entail a different set of financial parameters and expectations. In any event, get it straight before the trip, and you'll both breathe easier.

> Spell out expectations. For example, who's paying for the airfare? Lodging and meals? Sightseeing and tours?

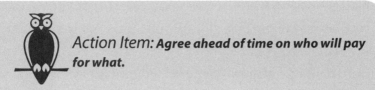

*Action Item: **Agree ahead of time on who will pay for what.***

While You're There

Once you've landed, a zillion challenges large and small will confront you, and they can be disconcerting, especially if you're not accustomed to traveling. That is where travel partners are either at their best or at their worst with each other. Keep your cool. Take a deep breath. Seasoned travelers know to "go with the flow" and have faith that all will turn out well. It usually does.

At the airport. Even if you are a seasoned international traveler, touchdown at your in-country destination is likely to be the most challenging part of your trip. You've just arrived in a strange land, full of oddly dressed people who are moving about with a lot more confidence than you are. The simplest of signs are a linguistic mystery: "Does *damas* mean restroom?" You're exhausted and grimy from the trip; the only things on your mind are a shower and a bed. But you have things you must do first. Keep your wits, snag some local currency from the airport money exchange, suffer your way through immigration and customs, gather *all* your luggage, find your transportation, and make a beeline for your hotel or treatment center. After that, the worst is behind you.

Hospital check-in. As in the US, hospitals and clinics can be chaotic, bewildering places until you learn your way around. Two sets of eyes — and vocal cords — are better than one. Most often, you'll be surprised by the level of attention and care given to international health travelers. In the unlikely event that you're not getting the service you need, gently, but firmly, find the right personnel and make sure you're noticed and served. If not, contact your physician or health travel agent directly.

Pre-Treatment. Once checked into the hospital or hotel, companions can turn their attention to providing emotional support, easing pre-treatment jitters, and doing little things to help the health traveler settle comfortably into unfamiliar surroundings and circumstances. Order flowers for the room? Draw a relaxing bath?

Probably more than any other time spent in-country, the period between the hospital check-in and the procedure itself requires the greatest vigilance and the largest number of quick decisions. During this brief time, both you and the patient will be meeting with doctors and staff, becoming acquainted with the facilities, and deriving a mutual understanding about what to expect in the coming days and weeks.

During this period, it's not uncommon for health travelers to experience doubts and second thoughts. It's natural to wonder if a huge life mistake has been made, particularly when far from the comforts of home and family.

Generally, if the surroundings are clean, the staff attentive, and the physicians and surgeons communicative, you and your partner have little to worry about. You'll find that your misgiv-

> Generally, if the surroundings are clean, the staff attentive, and the physicians and surgeons communicative, you and your partner have little to worry about.

ings are like passing storms — turbulent and upsetting, and then followed by calm and bright light. However, if you and your partner have persistent concerns, particularly about hospital hygiene, staff competence, or treatment outcomes, voice them immediately. Or, if you feel that important facts have been misrepresented (such as physician credentials, hospital accreditation, or surgery success rates), arrange additional consultations until you've resolved the problem. No patient should venture into treatment until reasonable trust has been established with the physician and other healthcare providers.

Post-Treatment. Even after the least invasive procedures, patients experience discomfort, even pain. Your partner will also probably experience disorientation from medications, particularly if painkillers are involved. This is a time to be extremely sympathetic and attentive. During the first few days after treatment, patients often experience discouragement, irritability, and sometimes unnerving mood swings. This is normal for any treatment and more so when recuperating far from the comforts of home.

This phase passes. The trauma and discomfort of the treatment becomes more familiar and manageable, the pain recedes, and you both become more comfortable in your surroundings. During those initial days post-treatment, a little positive thinking goes a long way.

Here's how you can help in the days immediately following treatment:

Have big ears. Listen carefully to advice and directives given by physicians and staff, and then follow them. Your partner may be unable to retain it all. You might need to head out and fill a prescription or two. Or maybe the respiratory therapist didn't show up, and you need to find out why. Or the doctor gave orders for two days of ice-pack treatment, but the ice hasn't materialized. Medical directives in a hospital or clinic are often verbal. The more of them that you remember and act upon, the better the patient's prognosis.

Help stay in touch. Just when loved ones at home are most concerned about the outcomes, your partner may not yet feel up to talking on the phone or sitting at a computer and tapping out a reassuring email. When you have a good grasp of how things are going, ask your partner if it's all right for you to get in touch with family and friends. Often, just a call or two will reassure the folks back home, who will appreciate hearing news from afar.

> During the first few days after treatment, patients often experience discouragement, irritability, and sometimes unnerving mood swings. This is normal for any treatment and more so when recuperating far from the comforts of home.

Get away. As helpful and needed as you are, you're not super-human. You, too, require time for yourself—so take it! Find an hour or an afternoon to get away from the hospital or hotel. With a little research, you'll quickly find that most destinations offer a rich array of nearby, easily accessible excursions. If you're in India or Thailand, temples abound. They are wonderful refuges of beauty where you can usually find a quiet, contemplative corner. If in San José, Costa Rica, jump in a taxi and visit the Jade Museum. In Kuala Lumpur, Malaysia, a stroll through one of the many parks, plazas, or markets will be relaxing and richly rewarding. These little sojourns will help rejuvenate you, and you'll return home with some colorful memories of your visit.

> As helpful and needed as you are, you're not super-human. You, too, require time for yourself — so take it!

Back Home

Be in contact often. If you're a spouse or close family member who's gone along as a health traveler's companion, then you may resume living under the same roof when you return home, and maintaining contact won't be a problem. But friends who act as travel companions may need to make more effort. As life at home quickly gives way to daily routine, it's comforting for the patient to hear the travel companion's voice or see that friendly, reassuring face occasionally. So check in from time to time, ask if there's anything you can do, and simply be a friend. Recoveries are often lonely periods for a patient, who, despite all other indications, isn't quite ready yet to rejoin the real world.

Help promote compliance. Good post-treatment compliance is the best way to prevent complications and ensure a fast, full recovery. As the companion who lived and breathed the patient's experience and heard the doctor's orders first-hand, you're best equipped to prod your partner into maximal compliance with every part of the post-treatment program.

Encourage family members and friends to participate. Even if you live under the same roof with the patient, you can't do it all. So, encourage those closest to your partner to participate. Spread out the work by assigning specific tasks, such as bathing, bandage changing, or transport to post-treatment consultations and physical therapy appointments. Sometimes friends and family want to be helpful, but they don't know what they can do. Your insider's understanding of the patient's needs can be crucial during the important first weeks after the trip.

Help your partner stay physically, mentally, and socially active. After treatment, some patients lapse into relative isolation and inactivity, particularly if they weren't athletic or social in the first place. Get your partner up and out for a walk around the block, offer gentle reminders about church or school events, and do everything you can to keep the recovering health traveler functional and alert.

Action Item: **Help your partner stay mentally and physically active during the recovery period.**

A Note to Patients about Your Companion

A person who joins you on a medical trip is the best friend you have in the world. Respect the gift. Both of you will be in a new land, trying to process a bewildering range of new experiences, while facing serious concerns about your health and your immediate future. During those challenging moments that confront every health traveler, take it easy on one another and keep the faith that all will turn out well.

When you have specific wants or needs, express them to your companion as clearly as you can. Take the time to verbalize your appreciation for your partner's presence. He or she made a big effort to join you — gave a large and true gift of love. Be as gentle and patient as possible with one another, and the deepened kinship fashioned from your travel experience will be its own reward.

CHAPTER EIGHT

Dos and Don'ts
for the Smart Health Traveler

Much of the advice in this chapter is covered in greater detail elsewhere in this book. Consider this a capsule summary of essential information, sprinkled with practical advice that will help reduce the number of inevitable "gotchas" that health travelers encounter. You may want your travel companion and family members to read this chapter, along with the Introduction to Part One, so they better understand medical travel. They can use this information as a gateway to the more in-depth sections of this book.

✔ *Do* Plan Ahead

Particularly if you'll be traveling at peak tourist season, the further in advance you plan, the more likely you are to get the best doctors, the lowest airfares, and the best availability and rates on lodging. Remember, you'll be competing for treatment with other health travelers. You'll also be competing with other tourists for hotels and amenities. If possible, begin planning at least three months prior to your expected departure date. If you're concerned about having to change plans, *do* be sure to confirm cancellation policies with airlines, hotels, and travel agents. For more information, see Chapter Two, "Planning Your Health Travel Journey."

✔ *Do* Be Sure about Your Diagnosis and Treatment Preference

The more you know about the treatment you're seeking, the easier your search for a physician will be. For example, if you're seeking dental work, you should know specifically whether you want implants or bridgework. If the former, then you'll be narrowing your search to accredited implantologists. *Do* work closely with your US doctor or medical specialist, and make sure you obtain exact recommendations — in writing, if possible. If you are unsure of your needs or not confident of your doctor's diagnosis, seek a second opinion. Then, when you know your specific course of action, learn as much as you can about your procedure using textbooks, medical references, and reliable sites on the Internet. (For more information on recommended health research sites, see Part Three, "Resources and References," in the back of the book.)

✔ *Do* Research Your In-Country Doctor Thoroughly

This is the most important step of all. By following a few basics, you'll see the process is not daunting. When you've narrowed your search to two or three physicians, invest time and money in personal telephone interviews, either directly with your doctor or through your health travel planning agency. *Don't* be afraid to ask questions — lots of them — until you arrive at a comfort level with a competent physician. For more information, see Chapter Two.

✗ *Don't* Rely Completely on the Internet for Your Research

While the online world has matured over the last few years, searching for information isn't yet on automatic pilot. Deeper digging — and more effort on your part — are usually required. While it's okay to use the Web for your initial research, *don't* assume that Web sites offer complete and accurate information. Cross-check your online findings with referrals, articles in leading newspapers and magazines, word of mouth, and your health travel agent. You'll begin to find the same names of clinics and physicians popping up. Narrow your search from there.

✔ *Do* Engage a Good Health Travel Planner

Most countries featured in this book are now served by at least one qualified health travel agent. Even the most intrepid, adventurous medical traveler is well served by the knowledge, experience, and in-country support these professionals can bring to any health journey. *Do* thoroughly research an agent before plunking down your deposit. Contact references, including clinics and former patients. Check for recommendations from hospitals and read articles from the local media. For more information, see Chapter Four, "Choosing and Working with a Health Travel Planner."

✔ *Do* Get It in Writing

Cost estimates, appointments, recommendations, opinions, second opinions, air and hotel accommodations — get as much as you can in writing, and *do* be sure to take all documentation with you on the plane. Email is fine, as long as you've retained a written record of your key transactions. If you prefer to use the telephone, confirm your conversation(s) with a follow-up email: "As we discussed, it's my understanding that the cost for my treatment, including an extraction and two implants, will be 1,250 US dollars. Is that correct? Could you please confirm that in a letter or email?" The more you get in writing, the less the chance of a misunderstanding, particularly when confronting language and cultural barriers.

✔ *Do* Insist on English

As much as many of us would like to have a better command of another language, the time to brush up on your Spanish is most definitely *not* when negotiating that new set of porcelain-on-titanium crowns in Costa Rica!

As you begin your research into a medical trip, consider the language barrier as an early warning sign in your screening process. If a clinic, physician, or health travel service that claims to serve international patients doesn't have a good grasp of English, then politely apologize for your lack of language skills and move on. There are plenty of English-speaking options in the global healthcare arena, and establishing a comfortable, reliable rapport with your key contacts is paramount to your success as a health traveler.

✗ *Don't* Schedule Your Trip Too Tightly

Most veteran health travelers admit that one of their biggest surprises was the efficiency of medical service they received while abroad. Staff-to-patient ratios are generally lower than in US cities, and the level of personal commitment is often better. Yet, it's best not to plan your trip with military precision. A missed consultation or an unanticipated extra two days of recovery overseas can mean rescheduling that nonrefundable $1,300 airfare, with penalties. More important, scheduling a little leeway lets everyone breathe more easily and gives you the flexibility of adapting seamlessly when things don't go precisely as planned.

A good rule of thumb is to add one more day for every five days you've already scheduled for consultation, treatment, and recovery. If you're planning a facelift and tummy tuck, consultation and surgery might require three days, with a recommended recovery of ten days (totaling 13 days). Thus, you should add two or three more days to your travel schedule to allow for weather-related delays, missed appointments, additional tests, and other unexpected events.

✗ *Don't* Forget to Alert Your Bank and Credit Card Company

The consumer fraud units of banks and credit card institutions have recently deployed hair-trigger monitoring for unusual spending activity. Thus, overseas travelers — just when they need their credit cards and ATM cards the most — often find their accounts canceled immediately after using them in-country. Then the fun begins, as you try to connect with your bank's voice-activated customer service line, using your new overseas cell phone!

The easy fix is to contact your bank and credit card company (or companies) *prior to your trip.* Inform them of your travel dates, and tell them where you will be. If you plan to use your credit card for large amounts, alert the company in advance. Also, if you plan to use your credit card to pay for expensive treatments, this might be a good time to reconfirm your credit limits.

✔ *Do* Learn a Little about Your Destination

Once you've settled on your health travel destination, spend a little time getting to know something about the country you're visiting. You'll find a little knowledge goes a long way: the locals will differentiate you from less caring travelers and express sincere appreciation for your interest. *Do* buy or borrow a couple of travel guides, learn a little history, and practice a few basic phrases (such as hello, goodbye, please, thank you, and excuse me). When in-country, pick up an English-language newspaper, which will get you up to speed on current events, happenings around town, and local gossip.

✔ *Do* Inform Your Local Doctors Before You Leave

Telling your doctor you're planning to travel overseas for treatment is a little like calling your auto mechanic to say you're taking your business to a competitor down the road. However, although you may never again see your former car mechanic, you *do* want to preserve a good working relationship with your family physician and local specialists.

Although they may not particularly like your decision, most doctors will respect your desire to travel overseas for medical care. Even if they privately question your judgment, they will appreciate learning about your plans *prior* to your trip. The pre-trip notification will pay off for you, too. When you return, you won't have to make an awkward call just when you most need a prescription refilled. If your physician attempts to dissuade you, *do* be attentive and polite, but stay firm in your resolve if you've done your homework and made your choice. For more on this topic, see Chapter Two.

✗ *Don't* Scrimp on Lodging

Unless your finances absolutely demand it, avoid hotels and other accommodations in the "budget" category. In foreign lands, particularly Asia and Central and South America, there's often a world of difference between "moderate" and "no-frills." The latter can land you in unsavory parts of town, with cold-water showers and shared bathrooms of questionable cleanliness. On the other hand, hospitals and travel agents tend to recommend deluxe hotels that charge astronomical rates even by US standards.

Press your health travel contacts to recommend a good, moderately priced hotel in the $125-per-night range. While such affordability may not be possible or desirable in certain cities — some in India, for example — there's often a huge price difference at the four-star or three-star levels just below deluxe, where a range of perfectly comfortable, service-rich accommodations can be found.

✗ *Don't* Stay Too Far from Your Treatment Center

When booking hotel accommodations for you and your companion, make sure the hospital or doctor's office is nearby. This is doubly true in large cities. While in-town transportation costs are usually low, traffic and noise levels can be horrendous, and long, stop-and-start cross-town trips can be as stressful as a 24-hour flight. Check with your doctor, hospital, treatment center, or health travel planner for appropriately located lodging.

✔ *Do* Befriend Staff

Nurses, nurse's aides, paramedics, receptionists, clerks, and even maintenance people — consider each of them a vital member of your health team! Often overlooked and always overworked, these professionals are omnipresent in the day-to-day operation of a hospital or clinic, and they wield a good deal of quiet power. You and your companion might find you need one of these folks most in the wee hours when no one else is around. Invariably, it will be the second-floor lobby clerk who knows how to get in touch with your doctor or the nightshift nurse's assistant who fetches a clean bedsheet.

You and your companion should take the time to chat with medical staff members, learn their names, inquire about their families, and proffer any small gifts you might have brought. Above all, treat staff with deference and respect. When you're ready to leave the hospital, a heartfelt thank-you note and a modest cash tip makes a great farewell.

✔ *Do* Comply with Doctor's Orders

One of the best ways to help assure a successful medical travel journey — and to avoid unnecessary complications — is to follow the pre- and post-procedure program set forth by your in-country and local MD. It's easy to return home and go lax on your physical therapy program, or fail to refill your prescription, or less-than-diligently manage your surgical wounds. To ensure a successful recovery, redouble your efforts to rigorously follow *all of your* doctor's orders.

✘ *Don't* Return Home Too Soon

After a long flight to a foreign land, multiple consultations with physicians and staff, and a painful and disorienting medical procedure, most folks feel ready to jump on the first flight home. That's understandable but not advisable. Your body needs time to recuperate, and your physician needs to track your recovery progress. As you plan your trip, ask your physician how much recovery time is advised for your particular treatment. Then add a few extra days, just to be on the safe side.

✘ *Don't* Be Too Adventurous with Local Cuisine

Chicken vindaloo in Bangalore! Spicy prawn soup in Bangkok! Grilled snapper picante in Puerto Vallarta! Yes, it's true that most health travel destinations also have robust, tasty cuisine, with a variety of local culinary fare to tempt nearly any palate. But one sure way to get your treatment off to a bad start is to enter your clinic with a rising case of traveler's diarrhea or even a mild stomach upset due to local water or food intolerance.

So, when hunger calls, go easy with your food choices. Prior to treatment, avoid rich, spicy foods, exotic drinks (no ice!), and eat only cooked foods. If you can't survive without fresh fruits and vegetables, follow the international travel rule: "Boil it, cook it, peel it (yourself), or forget it!"

If you're staying in the hospital as an inpatient, don't be afraid to ask the dietician for a menu that's easy on your digestion.

Use only bottled water, even when brushing your teeth. *Insist* on bottled water in developing countries throughout Asia, Central and South America, and even in most parts of Europe. Make sure the seal is intact.

Finally, find out about food interactions for any pharmaceuticals you're taking before or after your procedure. Some drugs don't work — or become downright risky — if certain foods are consumed. In short, play it safe on your medical trip; your digestive tract will thank you.

✔ *Do* Set Aside Some of Your Medical Travel Savings for a Vacation

You and your companion deserve it! If you're not able to take leisure time during your trip abroad, then set aside the extra dollars for some time off after you return home, even if only for a weekend getaway. You've demonstrated great courage and perseverance in making a difficult trip abroad, and you've earned some downtime with your cost savings.

✔ *Don't* Ever Settle for Second Best in Treatment Options

While you can cut corners on airfare, lodging, and transportation, always, always insist on the very best healthcare your money can buy. Go the extra mile to find that best physician or surgeon. Although everyone likes a bargain, the best treatment doesn't always come from the lowest bidder. Focus on quality, not just price.

✔ *Do* Get All Your Paperwork Before Leaving the Country

Understandably, after you've undergone a treatment — whether a simple root canal or a hip replacement — you're eager to get home, or go on vacation, or just get your life back. Too often and in too much of a hurry to leave, patients exit their treatment center lacking instructions, prescriptions, and other essential paperwork. Get copies of everything. For more information, see Chapter Two.

✔ *Do* Trust Your Intuition

Your courage and good judgment have brought you this far. Continue to rely on your sixth sense throughout your trip. If, for example, you feel uncomfortable with your in-country consultation, switch doctors. If you get a queasy feeling about extra or uncharted costs, don't be afraid to question them. Thousands of health travelers have beaten a successful path abroad, using good information and common sense. If you've come this far, chances are good you'll join their ranks.

Safe travels!

PART TWO

The Most-Traveled
Health Destinations

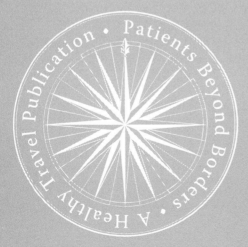

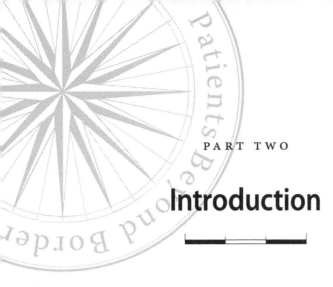

Introduction

Having read Part One, you now have a fair idea of what it takes to be a smart and informed health traveler. If you're reading this section of the book, chances are you've already reached a decision about your course of treatment, and you may even have narrowed your search to several countries or a particular region.

Part Two, "The Most-Traveled Health Destinations," gives an overview of 37 destinations in 21 countries and includes important information about accreditation, leading hospitals and clinics, health travel agents, recommended accommodations, and cultural considerations.

To help you navigate this section, we've provided a quick-reference "Treatment and Country Finder." Consult that chart to locate the treatment you're seeking, and you'll quickly discover which countries specialize in your area of interest. Then hunker down and explore the destinations on the following pages. As you read, consider the following:

Things change. While *Patients Beyond Borders* is the cumulative result of literally thousands of hours of research, keep in mind that contemporary medical travel is undergoing rapid changes. New hospitals gain accreditation by the month, and entire countries are on the verge of emerging as leading medical travel centers. Moreover, travel and treatment prices fluctuate, countries become more or less stable, and exchange rates move the US dollar in and out of favor. And, depending upon current events, even our domestic attitudes vary toward health travel—and travel in general.

If you stay informed, shop wisely, and always keep high-quality, reliable treatment at the top of your priority list, you'll be on a firm path to success as a global health traveler. If you've reached a decision to travel abroad for treatment, we hope you'll continue to look to us for guidance. For updates and additional services, visit our Web site at www.patientsbeyondborders.com.

A Note about Prices

In the "Destinations" entries in Part Two of *Patients Beyond Borders*, you'll find estimates of costs for some frequently performed procedures. For some destinations, you'll find only a few typical costs on the list. For other destinations, the lists are more complete. In either case, you may find that cost estimates vary greatly.

Why such a wide range? During the long and winding course of our research, we often received widely varying cost estimates from hospitals in the same country, sometimes in the same city. Perhaps those cost differentials are real—so it pays to shop around, because there are bargains to be had. However, some of the cost variation results from different service providers' including different items in their total cost estimates. For example, you may find that a lower estimate might not include your hospital stay, anesthetist's charges, operating room expenses, or even doctors' fees. A higher estimate, on the other hand, might include most, if not all, of a procedure's costs. Thus, we advise you to use our "typical costs" only to arrive at a general idea of what to expect. When doing your research, make sure your quote contains specifics, in writing, about all the included fees, as well as any extra costs. In health travel, the old Latin adage applies doubly: *Caveat emptor.* Let the buyer beware!

Customer service. Hospitals and clinics are busy places, and as much as these organizations would like to cater to medical travelers, truth is they're in the healthcare business, not the travel business. Thus, don't be surprised if some hospitals are slow to respond; and, despite their excellent reputation, accreditation, and references, some may not respond at all.

If you experience poor customer service in your initial contacts with a hospital or clinic, try working through one of the health travel agents listed in this book. You may have learned about an agency or planner from a friend or a Web search. Many agents have partnerships with hospitals, clinics, hotels, and airlines. All of the better agents have good contacts with the best physicians in a given treatment area. Unlike hospitals and other treatment centers, a health travel planner's job is to do exactly that—plan health travel.

Accreditation. You may notice that for some countries we did not provide full information on all JCI-accredited hospitals. There are good reasons. For example, although Brazil boasts a high number of JCI-accredited hospitals, the country generally does not cater to North

American health travelers. Web sites of Brazilian hospitals are generally not in English, and we found the customer service to be poor to nonexistent. Similarly, if a hospital in a given country did not respond within a reasonable amount of time to our inquiries and requests for information, we excluded it from our list.

While JCI accreditation is a benchmark of quality and an indicator that patients should seriously consider when making their healthcare choices, it is not the only measure of quality. All the countries featured in this section impose internal accreditation standards on their hospitals and clinics. Requirements and oversight vary with each country: Mexico's standards and enforcement, for example, are far lower than Thailand's or Malaysia's, and there's no international organization that rates accreditation standards by country or region.

If you're considering a hospital or clinic that's not JCI-accredited, double and redouble your research efforts for that facility. Has your hospital met its country's accreditation requirements? How many patients does your hospital see annually? How many surgeries of your specific procedure have been performed there? What are the hospital's morbidity and success rates?

Medical jargon. *Patients Beyond Borders* was written as a consumer book for you, the layperson, not as a formal medical reference. Thus, while we've taken great pains to ensure medical accuracy throughout these pages, we often use lay terminology interchangeably with medical terminology, particularly when treatment names themselves tend to be used interchangeably by physicians. For example, you might see "tummy tuck" instead of the tongue-twisting "abdominoplasty" and "gum disease treatment" in place of "periodontics." If you need clarification on a medical term, please consult the Glossary in the back of this book. There we've listed and defined the medical terms most frequently used in *Patients Beyond Borders*. For more information on terms not covered in the Glossary, consult a good medical dictionary or your physician.

Passports, visas, immunizations. Information listed on the following pages applies to US citizens. If you live outside the US, please check appropriate sources for requirements in your country.

A Note about Immunizations

The Centers for Disease Control and Prevention (CDC) recommends that all travelers stay up-to-date with routine immunizations, which include influenza, chickenpox (or varicella), polio, measles/mumps/rubella (MMR), and diphtheria/pertussis/tetanus (DPT). Although childhood diseases, such as measles, rarely occur in the US today, they are not uncommon in many parts of the world. A traveler who is not vaccinated is at risk for infection.

The CDC also recommends that medical travelers be immunized against hepatitis B. This vaccine is recommended for all travelers who might be exposed to blood or other body fluids through medical treatment.

The specific immunizations listed for each of the countries in Part Two are in addition to the hepatitis B vaccine and the other routine vaccines noted above.

To learn more, look up your destination country on the CDC's Web site, www.cdc.gov/travel/destinationList.aspx, or check with your local or state health department. You can also search for a travel medicine physician or clinic at the Web site of the International Society of Travel Medicine, www.istm.org.

Safety in numbers. As you read this section, you'll see numerous references to specific numbers of procedures, surgeries, specialties, and superspecialties. As any medical professional will tell you, one of the best ways to gauge the success of a hospital or clinic is by learning the number of procedures performed there. This statistic, combined with the success rate *of a specific procedure,* tells as much or more about a hospital's practices as any other number. Thus, a hospital that claims 2,700 angioplasties with a success rate of 98.4 percent should inspire you with more confidence than one that has performed 65 and cannot furnish a success rate. You'll get an even better picture if you can find out the number of procedures performed by your specific physician or surgeon.

Old school, new school. The date a hospital was established is often a good clue to its appearance, but looks aren't the health traveler's most important consideration. Some hospitals have been operating for decades in what has become an old building, but they offer excellent physicians and state-of-the-art equipment. Other newly opened facilities may boast shiny marble lobbies and five-star accommodations yet lack a track record you can use in assessing the quality of care you can expect there. For new hospitals, you may need to dig deep in your research to make sure your physicians and surgeons gained ample experience at other institutions.

Data. The information in the following pages was gleaned from a long and exhaustive research process, including hospital surveys, hospital site visits, interviews with hospital administrators and patients, and research on the Web. Despite the thoroughness of our research, please know that it's impossible for us to audit hospitals' records or authenticate their statements. While we believe that our information is correct, it's up to you, the patient—whether seeking treatment across the water or across the street—to validate information about accreditation, physicians' credentials, numbers of surgeries, success rates, and more. Once you've zeroed in on your hospital of choice, take the extra step of revalidating and cross-checking the information found in these pages.

Completeness. With all the changes occurring in the medical travel sector, this edition of *Patients Beyond Borders* cannot possibly include every excellent dental clinic, cosmetic surgery center, or specialty hospital that is out there. But we add new entries with every edition, and we are constantly updating our Web site. Did you have a successful treatment at a place we haven't yet mentioned? If so, we hope you'll visit our Web site (www.patientsbeyondborders.com) and let us know about it, so that we may further research your findings and broaden the base of information for our readership. You can remain anonymous, and any information you provide will remain completely confidential.

■ MAP OF THE MOST-TRAVELED HEALTH DESTINATIONS

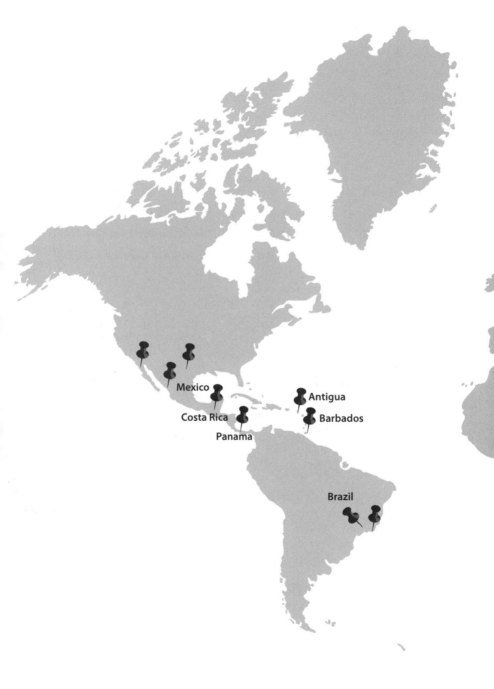

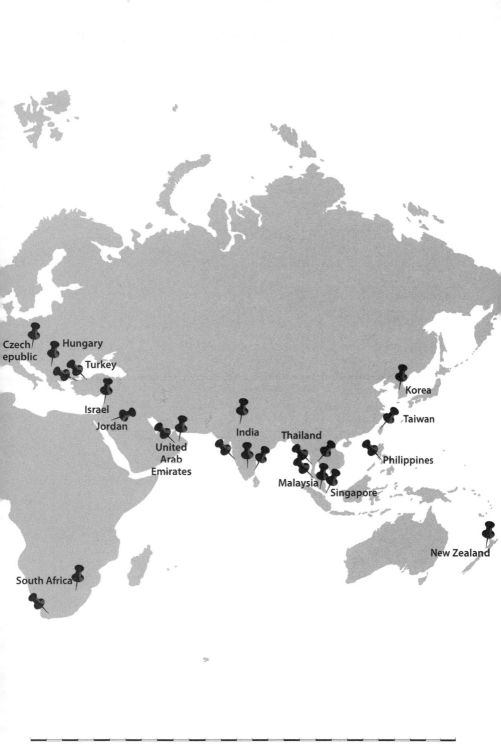

Czech
Republic

Hungary

Turkey

Israel

Jordan

United
Arab
Emirates

India

Thailand

Malaysia

Singapore

Korea

Taiwan

Philippines

New Zealand

South Africa

TREATMENT	Brazil	Caribbean	Costa Rica	Czech Republic	Hungary	India
Cardiovascular			■			■
Cosmetic & Plastic Surgery	■		■	■	■	
Dentistry	■		■	■	■	■
Fertility & Reproductive	■					■
Neurology and Spine						■
Orthopedic (all)			■			■
Total Hip Replacement						■
Birmingham Hip Resurfacing						■
Oncology			■			■
Stem Cell Research						
Sex Change & Cosmetic	■					
Weight Treatment (Bariatric)	■		■			■
Wellness/Alternative		■			■	■

■ **Primary destination for health travelers**

■ **Secondary destination for health travelers**

Israel	Jordan	Korea	Malaysia	Mexico	New Zealand	Panama	Philippines

(continued)

TREATMENT	Singapore	South Africa	Taiwan	Thailand	Turkey	UAE
Cardiovascular	■	■	■	■	■	■
Cosmetic & Plastic Surgery	■			■	■	
Dentistry	■	■		■		
Fertility & Reproductive	■	■		■		
Neurology and Spine	■			■		
Orthopedic (all)	■			■	■	■
Total Hip Replacement	■			■		■
Birmingham Hip Resurfacing	■			■		
Oncology	■	■		■		■
Stem Cell Research	■		■	■		
Sex Change & Cosmetic	■	■		■		
Weight Treatment (Bariatric)	■	■	■	■		
Wellness/Alternative	■	■	■	■		

ANTIGUA AND BARBADOS

■ **AT A GLANCE**

St. John's, Antigua; Christ Church, Barbados

Language:	English
Time Zone:	GMT -4
Country Dialing Code:	*Antigua:* 268; *Barbados:* 246
Electricity:	*Antigua:* 230V, Plug types A & B; *Barbados:* 115V, Plug types A & B
Currency:	*Antigua:* East Caribbean dollars (XCD); *Barbados:* Barbadian dollars (BD)
Visa Required?	Not for stays shorter than 90 days
Recommended Immunizations:	Hepatitis A; Typhoid Booster
Treatment Specialties:	Addiction Recovery, Fertility/Reproductive Health
Leading Hospitals and Clinics:	*Antigua:* Holberton Hospital, Adelin Clinic, Crossroads Clinic; *Barbados:* Barbados Fertility Centre, BayView Hospital, Queen Elizabeth Hospital
JCI-Accredited Hospitals:	Barbados Fertility Centre
Standards and Accreditation:	National Association of Addiction Treatment Providers (NAATP), Association for Addiction Professionals, European Association for the Treatment of Addiction, American Society of Addiction Medicine, Human Fertilisation and Embryology Authority (UK), American Society of Reproductive Medicine, JCI

■ TREATMENT BRIEF

The West Indies islands are located in the western Atlantic Ocean, east of the Caribbean Sea and relatively close to South America. It takes only a few hours to fly from Miami to Antigua. From there, it's a short airplane ride to Barbados. While *Patients Beyond Borders* generally places health considerations before vacations and leisure, it's easy to let one's guard down when thinking about these two destinations. Picture miles of white sandy beaches, year-round mild temperatures, and balmy winds. The isolation and discretion offered by these two islands make Antigua and Barbados tailor-made for recovery and stress-free treatment. Thus, it's no wonder people with substance abuse challenges seek help there in recovering from addictions, or that couples find the setting ideal for addressing stressful, emotionally charged fertility issues.

Barbados has two main hospitals: Queen Elizabeth Hospital (QEH) and Bay-View Hospital. QEH is a 600-bed acute-care hospital that's been operating since 1964. Recently, the hospital has been undergoing major renovation, with a $25 million upgrade of its medical equipment in the works. QEH's newly renovated and relocated gastrointestinal unit opened in 2006. The hospital has also modernized its library, computer, and voice recording communication systems.

BayView Hospital is located on the outskirts of Bridgetown. This privately owned facility began operating in 1989. It's tiny, with only seven private rooms and four semi-private rooms—so personal care is emphasized. BayView's specialties include ear-nose-throat surgery, reconstructive surgery, urology, neurology, and orthopedics.

Antigua also has two main hospitals. Holberton Hospital in St. John's has departments for maternity, radiology, pathology, intensive care, surgery, and pediatrics. Adelin Clinic, also in St. John's, is privately owned. It offers emergency care, minor surgeries, plastic and reconstructive surgery, and other services.

But the real specialties of these islands are addiction recovery and fertility treatments. Contemporary music icon Eric Clapton founded the Crossroads Centre in Antigua. It opened its doors in 1998, its mission to help people cope with their personal addictions. Soon the world heard about the clinic's success, and it wasn't long before the center's integrated 12-step program and serene environment started attracting clients from Europe and North America. The Barbados Fertility Centre earned JCI accreditation in 2007. The center serves couples from the Caribbean, UK, US, Canada, and Europe with a full range of fertility services in a relaxed, vacation environment.

■ TYPICAL TREATMENTS AND COSTS

Addiction Recovery:

Residential Dependency Program at Crossroads (29-day live-in): $21,500

Fertility/Reproductive Health:

IVF: $6,000
IVF with ICSI: $7,000
IUI: $375

■ HOSPITALS AND CLINICS

ANTIGUA

Crossroads Centre, Antigua
Willoughby Bay, St. Phillip's Parish
P.O. Box 3592
St. John's, Antigua, WEST INDIES
Tel: 1 888 452.0091 (US and Canada toll-free); 011 268 562.0035
Fax: 011 268 562.3278
Email: info@crossroadsantigua.org
Web: www.crossroadsantigua.org

Opened by Eric Clapton in 1998, the 32-bed Crossroads Centre (CC) is a nonprofit international center of excellence for the treatment of alcohol or drug addiction and other addictive disorders. The center's mission is to help people and their families make the changes necessary to find new health, a new sense of well-being, and a new life of recovery. The center deploys the "whole-person approach" to healing and recovery by assisting each client in improving the quality of his or her relationships, career, and social, emotional, physical, and spiritual well-being.

CC specializes in medical detoxification, rehabilitation services, and discharge and aftercare planning. The 29-day residential chemical dependency program includes medical detoxification services, 12-step meetings and groups, individual and group therapy, individual assignments, nutritional counseling, and recovery lectures. English is the only language spoken among the 52 full-time staff members.

Additional services are provided as part of the package to enhance recovery: yoga, auricular acupuncture, spiritual counseling, fitness training, experiential therapy,

and therapeutic massage. Included in the total cost is a four-day family outpatient program. Trained staff members help families understand the disease of addiction, improve family relationships, and support the recovery process. In 2006, 87 percent of the clients visiting Crossroads were international patients, with 73 percent from the US and Canada. Free transportation is provided to and from the airport, and patients and families are met at the airport by a staff member. Family members attending the family outpatient program stay at one of several (pricey) local hotels approximately 30 minutes from the center, which is a boost for confidentiality.

Aftercare is an important part of the recovery program at Crossroads, where "alumni services" have their own coordinator to help former patients sustain and strengthen their recovery experiences. Alumni groups meet regularly in New York and Florida, with other chapters soon to be added. The center offers five- to six-day renewal programs for people in recovery, in which patients can reconnect with the program and receive help for problems they may be encountering.

CC is affiliated with The Sanctuary in Delray Beach, Florida, a transitional living home for men in recovery (see "Recovery Accommodations," below).

BARBADOS

Barbados Fertility Centre, Inc.
Seaston House, Hastings
Christ Church
Barbados, WEST INDIES BB15154
Tel: 011 246 435.7467
Fax: 011 246 436.7467
Email: info@barbadosivf.org
Web: www.barbadosivf.org

Although in vitro fertilization (IVF) is a serious issue for couples, the Barbados Fertility Centre (BFC) emphasizes that it needn't be a stressful experience. The more relaxed resort environment of Barbados plays a major role in keeping couples focused on the positive. To reduce the stress even further, only a limited number of patients is accepted each month so that BFC is always able to provide individualized and personalized care. Couples stay an average of 14 nights at nearby hotels and have their choice of comfort, luxury, premium, or elite packages. The staff of ten includes a consultant gynecologist. All staff members speak English.

BFC received its JCI accreditation in 2007. The center has treated hundreds of local and international couples since becoming a full-time IVF unit in 2004. Approximately 80 percent of the clinic's patients are from other Caribbean countries, the US, Canada, and the UK. Approximately 30 US and Canadian couples are treated each year, and the numbers are growing.

Because the male factor is often significant in infertility, many of BFC's clients require an intracytoplasmic sperm injection (ICSI), which is an injection of sperm into the egg. A high standard of care, relaxing atmosphere, and flexible embryo culture system (which permits blastocyst culture)

all contribute to high success rates, which continue to improve each year.

In women 37 years and younger, BFC's success rate is 54 percent compared to the average US rate of 41 percent and the average UK rate of 25 percent. The center's success is in part due to an individualized treatment program tailored to each patient's needs.

Annually, the center performs the following procedures: 350–400 IVF and ICSI, and 1,500 intrauterine inseminations (IUI). BFC boasts cutting-edge technology in reproduction, and the center strives for the best personalized medical care.

IVF costs are substantial, and the procedure is usually not covered by health insurance. IVF costs include medical consultations, private hospital fees, anesthesia, theater fees, laboratory services, scans, and blood tests. Medications are a separate cost. BFC ensures that financial coordinators are available to assist in making payment arrangements to suit all needs. The center offers accommodations packages in a variety of price ranges.

■ RECOVERY ACCOMMODATIONS

The Sanctuary
P.O. Box 8463
Delray Beach, FL 33483
Tel: 1 561 843.2797
Fax: 1 561 278.2292
Email: tgentry@sanctuarydelraybeach.com
Web: www.sanctuarydelraybeach.com

Located in Delray Beach, Florida, The Sanctuary is now a subsidiary of Crossroads Centre. This accommodation brings men's transitional living to new standards. The three-house, 15-bed unit offers the highest quality of service and best possible start to a new life. The 24-hour staff supervision provides needed consistency and account-ability in addition to random drug screen-ing. The Sanctuary is located near 12-step clubs at which patients can integrate safely back into social settings. Patients accepted into The Sanctuary must make at least a three-month commitment to recovery.

■ HOTELS: DELUXE

Crossroads Centre provides accommoda-tions for patients. The Barbados Fertility Centre's treatment packages include hous-ing, and couples can choose from a range of prices.

ANTIGUA

Grand Pineapple Beach Resort
P.O. Box 2000
Long Bay
St. John's, Antigua, WEST INDIES
Tel: 1 877 846.3290 (US toll-free); 011 268 463.2006
Fax: 011 268 463.2452
Web: www.grandpineapplebeachresort .com

The Inn at English Harbour
P.O. Box 187
English Harbour
St. John's, Antigua, WEST INDIES
Tel: 1 800 970.2123 (US toll-free); 011 268 460.1014
Fax: 011 268 460.1603
Email: theinn@candw.ag
Web: www.theinn.ag

BARBADOS

The House
Paynes Bay, St. James
Barbados, WEST INDIES
Tel: 1 800 467.4519 (US toll-free); 011 246 432.5525
Web: www.thehousebarbados.com

■ HOTELS: MODERATE

ANTIGUA
Trade Winds Hotel
P.O. Box 1390
Dickenson Bay
St. John's, Antigua, WEST INDIES
Tel: 011 268 462.1223
Fax: 011 268 462.5007
Web: www.twhantigua.com

BARBADOS

Allamanda Beach Hotel
Hastings
Christ Church, Bridgetown
Barbados, WEST INDIES
Tel: 1 888 790.5264 (US toll-free); 011 246 438.1000
Fax: 011 246 435.9211
Email: vacation@allamandabeach.com
Web: www.allamandabeach.com

■ **AT A GLANCE**

Rio de Janeiro and São Paulo

Language:	Portuguese (some English)
Time Zone:	GMT -3
Country Dialing Code:	55
Electricity:	127V & 220V (Brazil's electricity is notoriously nonstandard); check your specific destination for plug type
Currency:	Real
Visa Required?	Yes
Recommended Immunizations:	Yellow Fever; Hepatitis A; Typhoid Booster
Treatment Specialties:	Cosmetic, Dental, Ophthalmology, Weight Loss
Leading Hospitals and Clinics:	Ivo Pitanguy Clinic, Hospital da Plástica, Hospital do Coração, Hospital Israelita Albert Einstein (Albert Einstein Jewish Hospital), Hospital Samaritano
JCI-Accredited Hospitals:	*Rio de Janeiro:* AMIL Total Care (3); PRONEP; Hospital de Traumato; Instituto Estadual de Hematologia–Hemorio; *São Paulo:* AMIL Total Care; PRONEP; Hospital do Coração; Hospital Israelita Albert Einstein (Albert Einstein Jewish Hospital); Hospital Samaritano; *Porto Alegre:* Hospital Moinhos de Vento
Standards and Accreditation:	Brazilian Society of Plastic Surgery, International Society of Aesthetic Plastic Surgeons, Brazilian Society of Aesthetic Dentistry, JCI

■ TREATMENT BRIEF

Brazilians take beauty seriously, perhaps to a fault. If, for example, you'd like perkier ears on Snoozie, your family schnauzer, Dr. Edgado Brito, a São Paulo veterinarian of 20 years, has performed thousands of cosmetic alterations on pets worldwide—undoubtedly an extreme spillover from one of the world's most body-conscious countries.

Brazil boasts more than 4,500 licensed cosmetic surgeons, with the highest per capita number of practicing cosmetic physicians in the world. Most international patients head to São Paulo and Rio de Janeiro, Brazil's two largest cities. Smaller, cozier destinations, such as Porto Alegre and Santos, are also popular.

Prices vary widely. While the celebrity "surgeons-to-the-stars" command fees comparable to the highest found in the US, dozens of excellent, lesser-known clinics serve patients from all regions and income brackets. Brazil is home to the internationally revered Ivo Pitanguy, the world's most renowned plastic surgeon. The clinic and institute bearing his name were established in 1963, and more than 4,000 surgeons have visited there for training, workshops, and continuing education. Pitanguy and his protégés have set a standard for cosmetic and aesthetic surgery higher than anywhere else in the world.

Yet, for all its notoriety, Brazil lacks the medical travel infrastructure found in some smaller, less developed nations, such as Costa Rica. The Brazilian government has chosen not to follow the rise in international medical interest with corresponding investment, unlike many governments in Europe and Asia. In fact, Brazilian doctors are not allowed to advertise, and any commercialization of medical services is frowned upon by peers. Thus, Brazil's medical community has largely kept to itself, content to serve the apparently limitless local need for body beautification.

To further muddy the health travel waters, the language barrier looms large. While it's comforting to know that Brazil boasts 11 JCI-accredited treatment centers, only three of them post Web pages in English. All other sites are in Portuguese. It's one of medical travel's great mysteries that a hospital would endure all the expense and hardship of obtaining JCI accreditation, only to serve English-speaking clientele inadequately.

Nonetheless, health travel services are gradually gaining ground, with the numbers of conscientious, reliable agents, recovery accommodations, and travel support services growing. Health travelers intent on Brazil should redouble their efforts to work from a base of reliable information or through a trustworthy third-party agent.

Prices vary widely, and travelers will find cosmetic surgery in Brazil to be generally more expensive than in Costa Rica, India, or Southeast Asia. The best-known treatment centers cater to high-profile clients, driving prices to nearly US levels. Thus, when considering Brazil, savings will likely take a backseat to a vacation or retreat.

Note: If you're planning to go to Rio, you may want to see—or perhaps avoid—the annual Carnival (*Carnaval* in Portuguese) festival. This *grande dame* of all street fairs occurs in late February or early March, and it makes our Mardi Gras look like a needle-point convention. If you wish to avoid the chaos, steer clear of those dates. If you wish to enjoy the revelry, make sure you reserve air travel and lodging well in advance.

■ TYPICAL TREATMENTS AND COSTS

Cosmetic:
Breast Augmentation: $4,500-$5,100
Breast Lift/Reduction: $3,425-$4,025
Facelift: $3,450-$4,830
Liposuction (one region): $650
Tummy Tuck: $3,450-$4,250

Dental:
Crown (all porcelain): $230
Porcelain Veneer: $230
Implant: $460
Extraction (surgical, per tooth): $50-$100
Root Canal: $85

Vision:
Glaucoma: $1,725
LASIK (per eye): $345-$460

■ HEALTH TRAVEL AGENTS

CosmeticVacations
Rua Mexico, 119 – Sala 204
Centro, Rio de Janeiro, RJ, BRAZIL
Tel: 1 877 627.2556 (US toll-free); 1 305
   433.8377 (Florida); 1 212 537.8377
   (New York)
Fax: 1 954 565.8052
Email: mb@cosmeticvacations.com
Web: www.cosmeticvacations.com

Although CosmeticVacations offers services out of Florida and New York, the agency is headquartered in Rio de Janeiro, the "World Capital of Plastic Surgery." More plastic and cosmetic surgeries are performed in metropolitan Rio de Janeiro than anywhere else in the world. The in-country offices of this agency lie in the heart of Rio's business district, close to the surgeons, hospitals, and the agency's medical travelers. Ninety percent of the clients of CosmeticVacations are from the US. The company's international representatives work closely with clients to help them organize their trip, including flights and hotel accommodations.

Although Rio de Janeiro is known for its high-quality plastic surgery, its innovations in the field, and its surgical safety, it is not the cheapest place in the world to receive plastic surgery. Nevertheless, Cosmetic-Vacations says its clients can expect to achieve a 30–40 percent savings over comparable costs in the US.

All CosmeticVacations' physicians and surgeons are members of the Brazilian Society of Plastic Surgery, the national equivalent of the American Society of Plastic Surgeons and the largest organization of its kind in Latin America. For dentistry, all CosmeticVacations' surgeons are members of the Brazilian Society of Aesthetic Dentistry. All staff members and partner surgeons of CosmeticVacations speak English.

MedNetBrazil Concierge Services, Inc.
Offices in Florida, California, and Texas
Tel: 1 877 963.3638 (US toll-free)
Fax: 1 801 998.0133
Email: concierge@mednetbrazil.com
Web: www.mednetbrazil.com

Christi deMoraes, Brazilian-American owner and president of MedNetBrazil (MNB), was once morbidly obese. Bypass surgery and a move to Brazil eventually translated into a healthy lifestyle and a new career.

MedNetBrazil was founded in late 2002, after friends were encouraged by Christi's transformation through plastic surgery in Brazil. MNB now serves nearly 200 patients from the US and Canada each year.

Christi recommends only physicians who speak English. All Brazilian staff members, including Christi, speak English and Portuguese, in addition to some Spanish and French. All healthcare arrangements are made by the agency, although patients are free to call doctors and treatment centers on their own.

In addition to medical fees, MNB charges $300 per week for its medical concierge support system. Services include airport and doctor's office transportation, blood tests, five lymphatic drainage massages, a private nurse for the first 24 hours after treatment, daily home healthcare in your hotel room, and cell phone use, plus a pre-operative spa date to prepare the skin.

Patients using MNB receive healthcare at one of two São Paulo hospitals in the Santos municipality: Hospital Frei Galvao or Santos Day Hospital. Afterwards, they recover in comfortable flats or apartments, which have a small kitchenette, living room, and bedroom.

MedRetreat
2042 Laurel Valley Drive
Vernon Hills, IL 60061
Tel: 1 877 876.3373 (US toll-free)
Fax: 1 847 680.0484
Email: customerservice@medretreat.com
Web: www.medretreat.com

For more information on MedRetreat, see Malaysia.

Perfect Plastic Surgery
Avenida Paulo Faccini, 1829, Jd. Maia
Guarulhos, São Paulo, BRAZIL 07111-000
Tel: 011 55 11 9490.9441
Email: atendimento@perfect.com.br
Web: www.perfect.com.br

Serving Brazil's bustling city of São Paulo, Perfect Plastic Surgery caters mostly to Brazilian and European clientele, but most of its staff members and partner physicians speak English. If you don't speak Portuguese, insist on English up front.

Perfect Plastic Surgery has positioned its facilities for comfort, with offices, lodging, and partner clinics all within ten minutes of the São Paolo airport, South America's largest. That's a good strategy, for São Paulo is a sprawling, largely commercial, somewhat impersonal megalopolis; patients interested only in healthcare can focus on the conveniences offered by Perfect Plastic Surgery.

Those choosing Perfect Plastic Surgery's full package receive lodging in a deluxe room near the clinic; free transportation to and from airport, hotel, and hospital; post-operative escort services between hotel and hospital; post-operative medications; and a post-operative massage, in addition to referrals, consultations, and surgeries. Its most frequently performed procedures are breast augmentations, liposuctions, and tummy tucks.

■ HOSPITALS AND CLINICS

Of Brazil's 11 JCI-accredited hospitals, only three offer a Web site in English, and callers into these hospitals usually face a formidable language barrier. The same holds true for the renowned Hospital da Plástica in Rio. Patients who have selected Brazil as a destination should seek personal references, media references, or the services of a health travel planner.

RIO DE JANEIRO

Ivo Pitanguy Clinic

Rua Dona Mariana, 65
Botafogo, Rio de Janeiro, BRAZIL 22280-020
Tel: 011 55 21 2266.9500
Fax: 011 55 21 2539.0314
Web: www.pitanguy.com.br

Dr. Ivo Pitanguy, considered a founding father of plastic surgery, established his world-famous clinic in 1963 after first studying in the US and England. The clinic also houses the **Pitanguy Institute,** where plastic surgeons from 40 countries learn Pitanguy's techniques during a three-year master-apprentice study program.

In Brazil, 80 percent of all plastic surgery is cosmetic. In a country with a surplus of plastic surgeons, Pitanguy stands out. The clinic specializes in cosmetic/aesthetic surgeries, including those of the face, nose, and ears, in addition to body contouring and hair transplants. Reconstructive surgeries include scar revision, as well as skin grafts, skin expansion, and breast reconstruction.

The Pitanguy Clinic is the only known center where two patients receive surgery (even different procedures) simultaneously in the same operating room. Despite this, infection rates are low. Only local and regional anesthetics are used, and it is not uncommon for patients to converse during their surgeries.

It is a paradox that the most prominent treatment center in Latin America, serving celebrity patients, is situated in one of the largest and poorest shantytowns in Brazil. The crime rate is high in Rio de Janeiro, and the Pitanguy Clinic is located in a dangerous neighborhood.

Hospital da Plástica

Rua Sorocaba, 552
Botafogo, Rio de Janeiro, BRAZIL
Tel: 011 55 21 2539.5599
Fax: 011 55 21 2527.1469
Web: www.hospitaldaplastica.com.br

In 2006 Hospital da Plástica celebrated its thirty-fifth anniversary, having grown from a small clinic to today's 12 operating rooms and 21 suites. It also has recovery and intensive care facilities. It is dedicated exclusively to plastic surgery. Since the hospital's founding, 35,000 patients have had reconstructive and cosmetic procedures there, and the hospital boasts not a single reported infection. Hospital da Plástica has earned the Quality Award from the Brazilian Society of Plastic Surgeons. Recovery accommodations are provided through partnerships with the Ipanema Tower, Parthenon Arpoador, and Parthenon Sorocaba Hotels. (See "Hotels: Deluxe: Rio de Janeiro," below.)

SÃO PAULO

Hospital do Coração
Rua Desembargador Eliseu Guilherme, 147
Paraíso, São Paulo, BRAZIL
Tel: 011 55 11 3053.6611
Email: hcor@hcor.com.br
Web: www.hcor.com.br/index.asp

Hospital do Coração translates as "Hospital for the Heart," and that's exactly what this treatment center is. Since its founding three decades ago, it has operated as a philanthropic institution providing cardiac care to needy infants and children. Its future plans call for expansion to become a major center for the treatment of cardiovascular illnesses in Latin America. It earned JCI accreditation in 2006.

Cardiology is not the only specialty on offer at Hospital do Coração. Located in the Paraíso neighborhood of São Paulo, the hospital offers treatment in 37 medical specialties, including orthopedics, oncology, neurology, urology, gastroenterology, and general surgery. More than 700 physicians practice there. Hospital do Coração was a pioneer in the performance of cardiac transplants and the first in Brazil to perform a cardiopulmonary transplant (1985).

Hospital Israelita Albert Einstein (Albert Einstein Jewish Hospital)
Avenida Albert Einstein, 627/701
Morumbi, São Paulo, BRAZIL 05651-901
Tel: 011 55 11 3747.1301
Fax: 011 55 11 3747.1041
Email: atendimentocomercial@einstein.br
Web: www.einstein.br/ingles

JCI-accredited Hospital Israelita Albert Einstein opened its doors in 1971 as a nonprofit diagnostic and treatment center, and today it boasts more than 5,000 employees including 500 full-time physicians. Its specialties include integrated cardiology, neurology, and oncology diagnosis and treatment, as well as organ transplantation, orthopedics, dermatology, gastroenterology, hematology, ophthalmology, plastic surgery, and urology. Einstein also has a **Diagnostic and Preventive Medicine Center** that offers numerous tests. **Einstein's Bariatric Surgery Excellence Center** opened in 2007.

Einstein prides itself on personalized care for its patients, employing state-of-the-art protocols, procedures, and technologies. Recent equipment acquisitions include a 64-row computed tomography (CT) scanner, image-guided radiation therapy (IGRT), three-dimensional transthoracic echocardiograph, high-resolution electrocardiogram (HRECG), cardiac event monitoring, Da Vinci surgical system (a robotic technology designed to extend the benefits of minimally invasive surgery), and One-Stop Clinic for Assessment of Risk (OSCAR), one of the most advanced prenatal screening tools available.

Einstein is Latin America's largest liver transplant center, performing some 200 transplants annually. In 2006 the Einstein Transplant System passed the 1,000-transplant mark. The hospital boasts a consistent liver transplant success rate of 90 percent, on par with the best US and European hospitals.

The bilingual staff of the hospital's **Commercial Service Center** works with international patients on price-checking and negotiation with insurance companies. The hospitality and concierge departments can assist with travel plans, local accommodations, and more.

Hospital Samaritano

Rua Conselheiro Brotero, 1486
Higienópolis, São Paulo, BRAZIL 01232-010
Tel: 011 55 11 3821.5300
Email: international@samaritano.org.br
Web: www.samaritano.com.br

Hospital Samaritano has been in business for more than a century, but it hasn't lagged behind the times. It has expanded and modernized across many decades, consistently investing in new equipment, technology, and professional education for its medical and support staffs. Specialties include orthopedic surgery, neonatology, pediatrics, cardiology, oncology, neurology, and video-assisted surgeries. Samaritano is recognized as a reference center for bariatric surgery, epileptic surgery, cosmetic and reconstructive plastic surgery, and cochlear implants.

■ RECOVERY ACCOMMODATIONS

Independent recovery lodging is not yet available in Rio or São Paolo. Ask your hospital or health travel agent about recovery options. Most agents offer information on post-operative services and accommodations.

■ HOTELS: DELUXE

We found that many hotel Web sites are in Portuguese, not English. If you are persistent, the hotels will connect you with a staff member who speaks English.

RIO DE JANEIRO

Ipanema Tower Apart Hotel

Rua Prudente de Moraes, 1008
Ipanema, Rio de Janeiro, BRAZIL
Tel: 011 55 21 2247.7033
Web: www.riodejaneiroguide.com/hotel/ tower

Parthenon Arpoador

Rua Francisco Otaviano, 61
Arpoador, Rio de Janeiro, BRAZIL 2208-004
Tel: 011 55 21 3222.9603
Email: reservasarpoador@accorhotels .com.br
Web: www.accorhotels.com.br

Parthenon Sorocaba

Endereço: Rua Sorocaba, 305
Botafogo, Rio de Janeiro, BRAZIL
Tel: 011 55 21 2266.9200
Fax: 011 55 21 2266.9240
Email: reservasarpoador@accorhotels .com.br
Web: www.accorhotels.com.br

Excelsior Copacabana Hotel

Avenida Atlantica, 1800
Copacabana, Rio de Janeiro, BRAZIL 22021-001
Tel: 011 55 21 2545.6000
Web: http://travel.ian.com

SÃO PAULO

Caesar Park São Paulo Faria Lima

Rua das Olimpiadas, 205
São Paulo, Cidade São Paulo, BRAZIL 04551-000
Tel: 011 55 11 3049.6666
Web: www.caesarpark.com.br

Marriott Renaissance São Paulo
Alameda Santos, 2233
São Paulo, BRAZIL 01419-002
Tel: 011 55 11 3069.2233
Fax: 011 55 11 3064.3344
Web: www.marriott.com

Parque Balneário
Avenida Ana Costa, 555
Gonzaga, Santos
São Paulo, BRAZIL
Tel: 011 55 13 3289.5700
Fax: 011 55 13 3284.0475
Web: www.parquebalneario.com.br

Ibis Guarulhos
Rua General Osorio
19 Centro Guarulhos
Guarulhos, São Paulo, BRAZIL 07024-000
Tel: 011 55 11 6463.5400
Fax: 011 55 11 6463.5422
Web: www.Ibishotel.com

■ HOTELS: MODERATE

RIO DE JANEIRO

Hotel Promenade Visconti
Rua Prudente de Moraes, 1050
Ipanema, Rio de Janeiro, BRAZIL 22420-042
Tel: 011 55 21 2111.8600
Web: www.promenade.com.br

Copa Sul
Avenida Nossa Senhora de Copacabana,
1284
Rio de Janeiro, RJ, BRAZIL
Tel: 011 55 21 3202.9450
Fax: 011 55 21 2287.7497
Email: copasul@copasul.com.br
Web: www.copasul.com.br

SÃO PAULO

Comfort Hotel Downtown
Rua Araujo, 141 Consolacao
São Paulo, BRAZIL 01220-020
Tel: 011 55 11 2137.4600
Fax: 011 55 11 2137.4601
Email: hotelhelp@choicehotels.com
Web: www.choicehotels.com

Hilton São Paulo Morumbi
Avenida das Nacoes Unidas, 12901
São Paulo, BRAZIL 04578-000
Tel: 011 55 11 6845.0000
Fax: 011 55 11 6845.0001
Email: saomohifom@hilton.com
Web: www.hilton.com

Mendes Plaza Hotel
Avenida Marechal Floriano Peixoto, 42
Gonzaga, Santos
São Paulo, BRAZIL 11060-300
Tel: 011 55 13 3208.6500
Fax: 011 55 13 5082.1530
Web: www.mendesplaza.com.br

Tryp Higienópolis Hotel
Rua Maranhao, 371 Higienópolis
São Paulo, BRAZIL 01402-002
Tel: 011 55 11 3665.8200
Fax: 011 55 11 3665.8201
Email: tryp.higienopolis@solmelia.com
Web: www.solmelia.com

DESTINATION: **COSTA RICA**

■ **AT A GLANCE**

San José and Escazú

Language:	Spanish (English widely spoken)
Time Zone:	GMT -6
Country Dialing Code:	506
Electricity:	120V, Plug type A
Currency:	Colon
Visa Required?	No
Recommended Immunizations:	Hepatitis A; Typhoid Booster
Treatment Specialties:	Cosmetic, Dental, Ophthalmology, Orthopedics, Weight Loss
Leading Hospitals and Clinics:	CIMA Hospital San José, Hospital Clínica Bíblica, Santa María Hospital and Clinic, Hospital Clínica Católica, Rosenstock-Lieberman Center for Cosmetic Plastic Surgery, Prisma Dental Center, Meza Dental Care
JCI-Accredited Hospitals:	Hospital Clínica Bíblica
Standards and Accreditation:	Ministry of Health, Costa Rica; American Academy of Cosmetic Dentistry (AACD); American Academy of Implant Dentistry (AAID)

■ TREATMENT BRIEF

With so many Americans vacationing in, traveling to, or buying real estate in Costa Rica, many "Ticans" wonder if their country won't soon become the US's fifty-first state. Health travel is huge as well: some 15 percent of Costa Rica's international tourists visit this small, lush country to take advantage of its medical services, mostly cosmetic surgery and dental care. Costa Rica is one of the top five countries most visited by Americans for medical treatment.

Three hospitals—CIMA/San José, Clínica Católica, and Clínica Bíblica—are striving to modernize and attract international patients. Clínica Bíblica was the first in the country to achieve JCI accreditation, and more are hoping to join the ranks. Yet, some facilities in Costa Rica are slow in addressing the needs of health travelers: some hospital Web sites are still in Spanish only, and most physicians and staff are not yet "ready for prime time" with English-speaking patients. Lobbies are often overcrowded, with few international patient services facilities compared to the best hospitals in India, Malaysia, Singapore, and Thailand. Thus, health travelers to Costa Rica should focus more upon the many fine private clinics, which can be found in the capital city of San José and its Americanized suburb, Escazú.

Costa Rica boasts hundreds of board-certified physicians, surgeons, and dentists, mostly practicing in or near San José. Capitalizing on its success in cosmetic and dental surgery, Costa Rica's international medical offerings have expanded to include eye surgery and other elective procedures, such as bariatric surgery (for weight loss) and orthopedics.

One of Costa Rica's health travel specialties is the "recovery retreat," a hotel or ranch-style accommodation that serves recovering patients exclusively. Situated close to clinics, these retreats have all the amenities of a normal hotel, but they are staffed with nurses and interns who attend to the special needs of recovering patients. Transportation to and from the airport is usually included with the cost, as is transport to clinics for consultation and treatment. Guests in these retreats chat at breakfast and dinner about their latest treatment, and a snapshot of the clientele at any point in time is usually a portrait of recovery's progress—from the bruises of yesterday's facelift procedure to the confident smile and gait of the patient heading home.

With its emphasis on ecotourism and its long history of relative political tranquility, Costa Rica can hardly be classified as a third-world nation. Perhaps no other country offers the recovering health traveler such easy access to leisure activities. Breathtaking national parks of volcanoes and cloud forests are less than an hour's drive from San José, and both the Pacific and Caribbean coasts are easily accessible, with plenty of local and westernized accommodations. For those planning minimally invasive procedures, Costa Rica's proximity to the US and reputation as a tourist destination offer the best of both worlds to the medical traveler.

■ TYPICAL TREATMENTS AND COSTS

Cardiovascular:
Coronary Artery Bypass Graft: $24,100
Bypass + Valve Replacement (single):
    $30,000
Pacemaker (single-chambered): $7,700
Pacemaker (double-chambered): $10,700

Orthopedic:
Birmingham Hip Resurfacing: $9,500
Joint Replacement:
    Knee: $8,000-$10,700
    Hip: $8,000-$11,400
    Shoulder: $9,000

Cosmetic:
Breast Augmentation: $1,000-$3,200
Breast Lift/Reduction: $2,200-$3,400
Rhinoplasty (nose): $850
Facelift: $1,350-$4,900
Liposuction (stomach, hips, and waist):
    $1,000-$5,000
Tummy Tuck: $2,000-$4,200

Dental:
Porcelain Veneer: $350
Crown (all porcelain): $400
Inlays and Onlays: $350
Implant (titanium with crown): $650-$800
Extraction (surgical, per tooth): $90-$300

Weight Loss:
LAP-BAND System: $3,500-$10,500

Other:
Gall Bladder Removal: $3,500-$4,200
Prostate Surgery (TURP): $2,000-$2,700

■ HEALTH TRAVEL AGENTS

BridgeHealth International, Inc.
(also Medical Tours International)
5299 DTC Boulevard, Suite 800
Greenwood Village, CO 80111
Tel: 1 800 680.1366 (US toll-free); 1 303
    457.5745
Fax: 1 303 779.0366
Email: info@bridgehealthintl.com
Web: www.bridgehealthintl.com

In 2008 BridgeHealth International (BHI) acquired Medical Tours International (MTI; see below). Together, these companies now send patients to Argentina, Brazil, China, India, Korea, Panama, Singapore, South Africa, Thailand, and Turkey. Serving the business and insurance markets as well as individual consumers, the BHI/MTI staff is composed entirely of RNs and medical care coordinators.

Before accepting a client, BHI screens for health and "travelability." Clients pay no facilitation fees; the fees are paid by BHI's approved list of physicians, clinics, and hospitals. BHI refers patients only to JCI-accredited or equivalent hospitals. Services include passport and visa assistance, air reservations, medical consultations, medical records transfer assistance, pre-operative and post-operative counseling, follow-up care arrangements, and full in-country concierge services. BHI coordinates a full range of care from cosmetic, dental, bariatric, and stem cell procedures to orthopedic surgery, neurosurgery, cardiovascular surgery, and organ transplants.

Global MD

269 South Beverly Drive, Suite 622
Beverly Hills, CA 90212
Tel: 1 800 903.5690 (US toll-free);
 1 310 746.5932
Fax: 1 310 274.7588
Email: info@yourglobalmd.com
Web: www.yourglobalmd.com

This agency opened in 2007 with service to Costa Rica, and attorneys/owners Amanda Hayes and Natasha Bellroth have plans to expand their contacts in Mexico, Panama, Barbados, Singapore, and Thailand. Global MD organizes a teleconference between patient and physicians and offers loans for financing treatments, in addition to case management, flight bookings, recovery arrangements, and passport and visa assistance. The agency digitizes medical records and aids clients in decision-making by providing extensive information on service providers. In Costa Rica, the agency often sends patients to Hospital Clínica Bíblica (see "Hospitals and Clinics," below) and the Peralta Cosmetic Surgery Clinic.

Healthbase Online, Inc.

287 Auburn Street
Newton, MA 02466
Tel: 1 888 691.4584 (US toll-free); 1 617
 418.3436
Fax: 1 800 986.9230 (US toll-free)
Email: info.hb@healthbase.com
Web: www.healthbase.com

For more information on Healthbase, see India: Chennai.

Medical Tourism of Costa Rica

Costa Rica Office
Apartado Postal 459-1260
Escazú, COSTA RICA
Tel: 011 506 353.7176
Email: info@medicaltourismofcostarica
 .com
Web: www.medicaltourismofcostarica.com

and

US Office

42 Riverview Drive West, #202
Memphis, TN 38103
Tel: 1 267 886.3888
Email: info@medicaltourismofcostarica
 .com
Web: www.medicaltourismofcostarica.com

Established in 2005, Medical Tourism of Costa Rica was founded by Richard Feldman, who spent most of his career as a hospital administrator in the US and as the director of operations of CIMA Hospital in San José (see "Hospitals and Clinics," below). Serving around 20 patients a month, this agency boasts the usual health travel amenities, including assistance with airlines, hotels, tours, medical treatment, and surgical aftercare. A $300 concierge fee covers these services, as well as 24/7 extras while the patient is in-country, including airport and in-town transportation, restaurant reservations, sightseeing tours, rental cars, cell phones, and travel insurance.

According to Feldman, Medical Tourism of Costa Rica has sent more than 400 patients—mostly from the US—to Costa Rica for medical and dental care since it opened its doors. Feldman and his team are at the forefront of expanding their Costa Rican treatment offerings to include general surgery, bariatric (weight-loss) surgery, ophthalmology, orthopedics, and wellness/ preventive care.

Partnerships with the Intercontinental Hotels and Resorts and the Barceló Hotels and Resorts offer discounted rates and special amenities for this agency's clients (see "Hotels: Deluxe," below).

Medical Tours International

6 Forge Gate Drive, G-7
Cold Spring, NY 10516
Tel: 1 845 809.5254
Fax: 1 845 496.0350
Email: info@medicaltoursinternational.com
Web: www.medicaltoursinternational.com

Established in 2002, Medical Tours International (MTI) initially opened its doors serving only Costa Rica. Since its recent acquisition by BridgeHealth International (see above), the agency has since expanded into several other countries, including Argentina, Brazil, South Africa, and Thailand. Founder Stephanie Sulger is a registered nurse of over 30 years' experience, and her staff is composed entirely of RNs. Before accepting any client, MTI screens the potential patient for health and "travelability."

MTI clients pay no additional fees; the agency's fees are paid by MTI's approved short-list physicians and clinics. MTI refers patients only to accredited clinics and board-certified physicians and surgeons. Services include booking air reservations, medical consultations, and in-country accommodations; assistance shipping medical records; and pre-operative and post-operative counseling.

Med Journeys

2020 Broadway, Suite 4C
New York, NY 10023
Tel: 1 888 633.5769 (US toll-free); 1 212 931.0557
Fax: 1 212 656.1134
Email: sonnyk@medjourneys.com
Web: www.medjourneys.com

For more information on Med Journeys, see India: Delhi.

MedRetreat

2042 Laurel Valley Drive
Vernon Hills, IL 60061
Tel: 1 877 876.3373 (US toll-free)
Fax: 1 847 680.0484
Email: customerservice@medretreat.com
Web: www.medretreat.com

For more information on MedRetreat, see Malaysia.

Planet Hospital

23679 Calabasas Road, Suite 150
Calabasas, CA 91302
Tel: 1 800 243.0172 (US toll-free); 1 818 665.4801
Fax: 1 818 665.4810
Email: rudy@planethospital.com
Web: www.planethospital.com

For more information on Planet Hospital, see Singapore.

■ HOSPITALS AND CLINICS

CIMA Hospital San José

500 metros oeste del Peaje a Santa Ana
Escazú, COSTA RICA
Tel: 011 506 208.1068
Fax: 011 506 208.1107
Email: cima@hospitalcima.com
Web: www.hospitalsanjose.net

The 62-bed CIMA Hospital San José was the first Costa Rican hospital to be accredited by the Costa Rica Ministry of Health and is the only hospital in Central America accredited by the US Department of Veterans Affairs. It boasts more than 500 physicians representing over 60 specialties; a complete imaging department, including open magnetic resonance imaging (MRI), computed tomography (CT), x-ray, ultrasound, and endoscopy; a full-service laboratory; and a 24-hour pharmacy. Its specialties include orthopedics, cosmetic and reconstructive surgery, laparoscopic surgery, urology, and otolaryngology (ear, nose, and throat). Health travelers most often visit CIMA for cosmetic, eye, hip, and knee surgery, for which it reports some of the lowest prices in the country. Surgeons at CIMA perform nearly 400 breast augmentations annually, and more than 500 arthroscopic procedures. The hospital's **International Insurance Claims Department** has a staff specially trained to assist Americans. CIMA patients may recuperate in the ten-room Kalexma Hotel, which caters to CIMA patients (see "Hotels: Moderate," below).

Hospital Clínica Bíblica

1st & 2nd Streets, 14th & 16th Avenues
P.O. Box 1307-1000
San José, COSTA RICA
Tel: 1 800 503.5358 (US toll-free); 011 506 522.1414
Fax: 011 506 257.7307
Email: international@clinicabiblica.com
Web: www.clinicabiblica.com

In 2008 Hospital Clínica Bíblica became the first in Costa Rica and only the second in Latin America to receive JCI accreditation. While it's been around since 1929, don't expect anything old-fashioned about its facilities or services. Clínica Bíblica boasts a $50-million infrastructure (including a new $35-million hospital building) for 200 physicians who specialize in cardiology, cosmetic and reconstructive surgery, ophthalmology, orthopedics, and preventive medicine. Doctors there also perform a large number of minimally invasive laparoscopic procedures, such as bariatric surgery, arthroscopy, hernia repair, prostatectomy, gall bladder removal, hernia repair, and colonoscopy. Many of the physicians are bilingual and US- or European-trained. More than 20 percent of Clínica Bíblica's patients are international travelers.

Clínica Bíblica's **International Department** assists patients with all aspects of treatment planning. Each patient is assigned a personal Health Care Assistant (HCA) who works one-on-one to coordinate doctor contact, pre-procedure consultations, and surgical procedures; paperwork and price quotes; hospital admittance and bedside follow-up and assistance; contacts with family via phone or email post-surgery; VIP concierge services (superior-class lodging, transfers, and sightseeing tours); airport pickup/dropoff and assistance through immigration; recovery retreat and hotel accommodations; regular visits by a qualified nurse and staff; and patient follow-up back home.

Patients at Clínica Bíblica can expect to save as much as 70 percent of a surgical cost compared to the US or Canada. For example, a knee replacement at a US hospital costs approximately $40,000; at Clínica Bíblica, the procedure (using the same equipment and techniques) costs $10,700.

Hospital Clínica Católica

San Antonio de Guadalupe al Costado sur
de los Tribunales de Justicia
Guadalupe, San José, COSTA RICA
Tel: 011 506 246.3000
Fax: 011 506 283.6171
Email: info@clinicacatolica.com
Web: www.hospitallacatolica.com/eng/
files/servicios.html

Hospital Clínica Católica was founded in 1963 by the Franciscan Sisters. Since then the hospital has grown and changed. In 2002 its new, expanded facilities opened, housing emergency and observation services. Clínica Católica is affiliated with Our Lady of the Lake Regional Medical Center in Baton Rouge, Louisiana. The hospital provides all the usual departments for services and surgical procedures; it employs a variety of technologies for diagnosis and treatment, including a hyperbaric oxygen chamber, neuroelectric diagnostics, and an 18-channel electroencephalogram. Special units provide pain treatment, coronary care, digestive endoscopy, and pulmonary function testing.

Santa María Hospital and Clinic

Avenida 8 - Calle 14
San José, COSTA RICA
Tel: 011 506 523.6000
Fax: 011 506 523.6060
Web: www.hospitalcsantamaria.com

Santa María offers a full range of specialties and services, including outpatient surgery, minimally invasive surgery (laparoscopic and arthroscopic), osteosynthesis, scanning and imaging services, endoscopy, colonoscopy, and cardiovascular diagnosis and surgery. The hospital boasts modern and comfortable facilities, up-to-date surgery rooms, general and coronary intensive care units, and a recovery area for post-surgical care. Patient rooms have telephone, cable TV, air-conditioning, and Internet. Waiting rooms and guest beds are available for relatives and companions. Pharmacy and lab services operate 24 hours.

Rosenstock-Lieberman Center for Cosmetic Plastic Surgery

28th Street & 2nd Avenue
San José, COSTA RICA
Tel: 011 506 223.9933
Fax: 011 506 223.9171
Email: info@cosmetic-cr.com
Web: www.cosmetic-cr.com

Founded in 1982 by Drs. Noe Rosenstock and Clara Lieberman (both still practicing!), the Rosenstock-Lieberman Center focuses on cosmetic surgeries. All its surgeons are members of the American Society of Aesthetic Plastic Surgery, the American Academy of Cosmetic Surgery, the American Academy of Liposuction, or the International Society of Cosmetic Surgery.

Since 1997 the Rosenstock-Lieberman

Center has been offering courses on cosmetic surgery to selected physicians worldwide under the sponsorship of the American Academy of Cosmetic Surgery.

Rosenstock-Lieberman offers a variety of procedures, including hair transplant, facelift, blepharoplasty (eyelid surgery), otoplasty (ear surgery), rhinoplasty (nose surgery), fat transfer, lip embellishment, necklift, brachioplasty (arm lift), neck aug-mentation, breast augmentation, breast reduction/lift, liposuction, thigh lift, lower body lift, and tummy tuck.

Because most procedures at the center are done on an ambulatory basis, patients should plan to stay in one of the nearby recovery retreats or hotels (see "Recovery Accommodations," below).

Dental Implant Costa Rica
P.O. Box 1475-2150
San José, COSTA RICA
Tel: 011 506 823.0986
Fax: 011 506 289.6984
Email: lobando@dentalimplantcr.com
Web: www.dentalimplantcr.com

Over the past two decades, the use of dental implants has grown in favor over traditional bridges and crowns, so much so that an entire dental subspecialty—dental implantology—has made a huge mark on contemporary prosthetic dentistry. While general dental practitioners can—and often do—provide implantology services, the complexity of the practice and variety of implants warrant the services of a certi-

Case Study: Betty P., Illinois

I am a registered nurse with specialties (board certification) in infection control and gerontology. I have been to Costa Rica on five occasions for surgeries. In June of 2001, I had a tummy tuck, chin/face lift, upper and lower eyelifts, and arm lifts. I had lost nearly 100 pounds and needed a lot of loose skin/fat removed.

I went again in March 2002 and had my thighs and breasts lifted. I also had a lot of liposuction done. Then I returned the first week of May of 2003 for revisions of some of the previous work. When you lose as much body fat as I did, it takes a series of vis-its to attain good results. In November of 2003, I returned and had a hair transplant and more lipo done. In May of 2004, I returned for a medial T-incision thigh lift.

I cannot say enough wonderful things about the care and skill of the doctors I saw in Costa Rica. I have trusted them with my life several times, and each time I have had only more respect for them both personally and professionally. I am extremely happy with my results from all my trips.

While in Costa Rica, I stayed at a recovery resort, where I was treated very well. The owners of the resort gave me specialized care and transportation to and from the airport and clinic visits. Since I am not a world traveler and do not speak Spanish, I found it a very comforting experience to be in their care.

fied implantology specialist. After several years of practice in two Costa Rican general dental clinics, Dr. Luis Obando decided to specialize in implantology. His services include dental implants, bone grafting, bone expansion, sinus lifts, single tooth implants, crowns and bridges (using implants as the base), and implant-supported dentures. Dr. Obando reports that Dental Implant Costa Rica has no fixed street address. He works in clinics throughout the city, he says; his secretary will arrange a treatment site near the patient's hotel.

Note: Traditional implantology requires a two-stage procedure. The metal implant is first set into the lower or upper jawbone. In three to six months, after new bone has set around the implant, the patient must return for a post, crown, and finish work. While the newer "immediate load" implant technique offers a one-step process, its application is still debated and is also limited by the patient's dental profile. Thus, Dr. Obando advises his patients to budget the time and expense for at least two trips.

Prisma Dental Clinic

Rhomoser Boulevard, Prisma Building,
   3rd Floor
San José, COSTA RICA
Tel: 011 506 291.5151
Fax: 011 506 291.5454
Email: dental@cosmetics-dentistry.com
Web: www.cosmetics-dentistry.com

Founded more than 20 years ago, the highly publicized Prisma Dental Clinic is the crème de la crème of Costa Rican dentistry. Spacious quarters and a large staff cater to busy Americans and Canadians, who now make up most of Prisma's clientele. Its in-house

laboratory, offering panoramic x-rays and fully digitized imagery, saves on outside trips to the radiologist.

Prisma's founders, Drs. Thelma Rubenstein and Josef Cardero, received their advanced training in Switzerland and Montreal and at the University of Miami. Both are members of the International Congress of Oral Implantologists (US). Nearly every type of dental procedure is performed at Prisma, including recent techniques in Invisalign bracing (clear removable braces), gingivoplasty (gum surgery), porcelain veneers, and inlays.

While Prisma's fees are still far less expensive than US prices, patients will nonetheless pay a comparative premium for the range of services offered by Prisma, as well for its extensive advertising and marketing campaigns.

Meza Dental Care Clinic

Condominium Torres del Campo
Barrio Tournon
San José, COSTA RICA
Tel: 1 877 337.6392 (US toll-free); 011 506
   258.6392
Email: info@mezadentalcare.com
Web: www.mezadentalcare.com

Founded in 1995 by Dr. Alberto Meza, this full-service clinic now employs seven dentists, surgeons, endodontists, periodontists, and implantologists. Dr. Meza is a member of the American Academy of Cosmetic Dentistry. He and his staff members engage in a continuing education program at UCLA Dental School. Meza Dental Care offers a full range of dental procedures and services. The clinic specializes in cosmetic dentistry and related services, including full-mouth restoration, porcelain veneers, full porcelain crowns, dental implants, root canal therapies, gum surgeries, and more. Meza Dental works with an agency to help patients with travel arrangements and lodging.

■ RECOVERY ACCOMMODATIONS

Chetica Medical Recovery Ranch
San Jeronimo de Moravia
San José, COSTA RICA
Tel: 011 506 268.6133
Fax: 011 506 268.6133
Email: chetica@racsa.co.cr
Web: www.cheticaranch.com

Twenty minutes northeast of San José and Escazú, this 80-acre ranch was established in 1996, making it Costa Rica's longest-running recovery retreat. Since they opened the doors, hosts Ruben and Lorena Martin have served more than 2,000 international patients. Their guest register and associated patient kudos are truly impressive.

Medical and related services offered at Chetica include bathing and showering assistance, bandage changing, experienced injection care, dressing assistance, transportation to and from clinic and pharmacy, and patient monitoring (including blood pressure and temperature readings). A full-time nurse lives on the premises and, should complications arise, doctors visit the retreat regularly for patient checkups.

Paradise Cosmetic Inn
P.O. Box 644
Escazú, San José, COSTA RICA
Tel: 1 786 228.9148 (US); 011 506 252.3530
Fax: 011 506 252.2392
Email: info@paradisecosmeticinn.com
Web: http://paradisecosmeticinn.com

Paradise Cosmetic Inn is located on top of San Antonio, Escazú's famous mountains, 20 minutes from the San José International Airport. Its five-acre facility is close to all ten major hospitals and clinics. Recovery rooms have hospital beds and hand rails in the bathrooms. Paradise offers free local transportation to and from the airport and the doctor's office, 24-hour nursing services, unlimited direct calls to the US and Canada, wireless Internet, laundry services, and spa services. There's also a dental office on the premises.

Villa Le Mas
Tel: 011 506 289.8881
Fax: 011 506 289.3767
Email: le_mas@racsa.co.cr
Web: www.plasticsurgerycostaricaafter carefacility.com

This American-owned and American-operated retreat specializes in recovery after plastic surgery and dentistry. Located in the city of Escazú, it lies less than 20 minutes from hospitals, clinics, and doctors. Guests at Villa Le Mas enjoy the facility's many acres of protected rainforest, and the views of Pico Blanco during the day and the lights of the city at night are spectacular.

■ HOTELS: DELUXE

Hotel Camino Real Intercontinental
Multiplaza Road, Prospero Fernandez
    Highway
San José, COSTA RICA
Tel: 1 800 980.6429 (US toll-free);
    011 506 208.2100
Fax: 011 506 208.2101
Email: sanjose@interconti.com
Web: www.ichotelsgroup.com

Hotel Parque del Lago
Baceocolon Avenue & 14th Street
San José, COSTA RICA
Tel: 011 506 257.8787
Email: info@parquedellago.com
Web: www.parquedellago.com

Barceló San José Palacio
Residencial El Robledal, La Uruca
San José, COSTA RICA
Tel: 011 506 220.2034
Fax: 011 506 220.2036
Email: san.jose.palacio@barcelo.com
Web: www.barcelosanjosepalacio.com

■ HOTELS: MODERATE

Marriott Courtyard San Jose
Prospero Fernandez Highway
Calle Marginal N Plaza Itskatzu
San José, COSTA RICA
Tel: 011 506 208.3000
Fax: 011 506 298.0033
Web: www.marriott.com

Kalexma Hotel
P.O. Box 6833-1000
San José, COSTA RICA
Tel: 011 506 232.0115
Fax: 011 506 231.0638
Email: frontdesk@kalexma.com
Web: http://kalexma.com

Apartotel La Sabana
Sabana Norte, del Restaurante Rostipollos
    150 metros norte
Apartado Postal 658-1200 Pavas
San José, COSTA RICA
Tel: 1 877 722.2621 (US toll-free); 011 506
    220.2422
Fax: 011 506 231.7386
Email: info@apartotel-lasabana.com
Web: www.apartotel-lasabana.com

Hotel El Rodeo Country Inn
San Antonio de Belén
San José, COSTA RICA
Tel: 011 506 293.3909
Fax: 011 506 239.3464
Email: info@elrodeohotel.com
Web: www.elrodeohotel.com

DESTINATION: CZECH REPUBLIC

■ AT A GLANCE

Prague

Language:	Czech (English not widely spoken)
Time Zone:	GMT +1
Country Dialing Code:	420
Electricity:	230V, Plug type E
Currency:	Koruny
Visa Required?	No
Recommended Immunizations:	Hepatitis A; Typhoid Booster
Treatment Specialties:	Cosmetic, Dental
Leading Hospitals and Clinics:	Na Homolce Hospital, Esthé Clinic, Esthesia Clinic, MyClinic Prague
JCI-Accredited Hospitals:	Na Homolce Hospital
Standards and Accreditation:	Czech Medical Chamber; Czech Dental Chamber; Czech Society of Aesthetic Plastic Surgery; Czech Plastic Surgery Association; Czech Society of Burn Plastic Surgery; International Societies of Plastic, Reconstructive and Aesthetic Surgery; European Societies of Plastic, Reconstructive and Aesthetic Surgery

■ TREATMENT BRIEF

One of the most popular American tourist destinations in Eastern Europe is the Czech Republic's capital city, Prague, where health travelers will find most of the country's best clinics. Health travelers generally head to Prague for either cosmetic surgery or dental care. Over the past decade, several privately funded clinics have opened that cater mostly to international patients from Western Europe and the UK. Staff and physicians speak English and provide care based on western-style models. Prague has also recently seen a great increase in western-trained doctors opening private practices.

That said, the Czech Republic's healthcare system is in transition. The Czech Republic enjoys long-standing healthcare oversight and stringent requirements for physicians and surgeons. Cosmetic surgery is strictly regulated by the government and by the Czech Medical Chamber. Three years' study are required to become a general surgeon and six to become a cosmetic surgeon. Yet, in a country where many physicians in the public sector earn less money than office workers, health travelers must double their research to ensure quality of service.

Patients who travel for medical care cite Prague as a favorite sightseeing destination. They factor extra travel time into their trips, taking advantage of less invasive procedures and shorter recovery times to enjoy vacations, weekend getaways, or Prague's endless urban activities.

Fees vary widely. Quoted prices usually include all pre-operative tests, examinations, surgery, medications, overnight stays, post-operative treatments, and an extra $200 for a friend or partner to accompany the patient. Health tourism packages often include bike tours through the wine country, mountain exploration, hiking, horseback tours, and art and heritage festivals.

For those concerned about antibiotic-resistant infections, the Czech Republic is reputed to have one of the lowest methicillin-resistant *Staphylococcus aureus* (MRSA) rates in Europe (meaning that unlike in the US, most staph infections in the Czech Republic can still be treated effectively with certain antibiotics).

■ TYPICAL TREATMENTS AND COSTS

Cosmetic:
Breast Augmentation: $4,025-$5,750
Breast Lift/Reduction: $3,680-$4,600
Facelift: $2,900-$4,450
Liposuction (stomach, hips, and waist):
   $3,100-$4,025
Tummy Tuck with Liposuction: $5,200

Dental:
Porcelain Veneer: $540-$630
Crown (all porcelain): $460-$540
Inlays and Onlays: $330-$430
Implant: $750-$1,150
Extraction (surgical, per tooth): $35-$115

■ HEALTH TRAVEL AGENTS

Beauty in Prague
Truhlarska 24
Prague, CZECH REPUBLIC 110 00
Tel: 011 420 222 314.198
Email: beauty@beautyinprague.com
Web: www.beautyinprague.com

Founded in 2005 by Tamara Zdinakova, this Prague-based agency caters mostly to a European crowd taking advantage of low-cost healthcare in a great urban vacation setting. However, more North Americans began visiting after an article featuring Zdinakova and Beauty in Prague appeared in a 2006 issue of *Business Week*. All staff members speak English, as do all the physicians, surgeons, and dentists engaged by the agency.

Beauty in Prague's standard package includes full consultation with a plastic surgeon, pre-operative blood and electrocardiography (EKG) tests, full examination by an internist, surgery, all medications, up to five nights in the clinic, and free transportation between lodging and the clinic. Personal services include airport pickup (although the client must pay a $30 fare) and arrangements for shopping and sightseeing.

Beauty in Prague lodges patients in apartments near Prague's trendy Old Town, a five-minute walk from some of the city's best restaurants and shopping. Apartments are equipped with high-speed Internet access. For families, Beauty in Prague offers babysitting and full day and night care.

■ HOSPITALS AND CLINICS

Na Homolce Hospital
Roentgenova 2 150 30
Prague, CZECH REPUBLIC 5
Tel: 011 420 2 5727.3036
Fax: 011 420 2 5727.3097
Email: vladimir.dbaly@homolka.cz
Web: www.homolka.cz/en/index.php

The first building of what is now Na Homolce Hospital was constructed between 1984 and 1989 as a medical facility for top communist functionaries. At that time it was known as the "State Institute of National Health" and more commonly referred to as "Sanopz." It opened in 1989 as a "luxury facility" with an outpatient unit, rehabilitation unit, and wards in internal medicine, cardiology, and neurology. Within months, it reopened to the general public under the new name of Na Homolce Hospital (from Homolka Hill on which it stands).

Today, the full range of services is available, and the hospital's specialties are grouped into three priority clinical programs, in which all the individual departments participate: the **Cardiovascular Program**, **Neuroprogram**, and **General Medical Care Program.** JCI accreditation came in June 2005. Na Homolce has 357 beds. Annually Na Homolce's physicians and surgeons treat nearly 18,000 inpatients, perform more than 14,000 surgeries, and examine more than 1 million outpatients.

Esthé Clinic
Na Příkopě 17, 110 00
Prague, CZECH REPUBLIC 1
Tel: 011 420 222 868.811 (Plastic Surgery); 011 420 222 868.831 (Laser Center)
Email: esthe@esthe.cz; laser@esthe.cz
Web: www.esthe.cz

Founded in 1996, Esthé Clinic has two centers, one devoted to cosmetic surgery and the other to laser resurfacing. Esthé's six plastic surgeons and four laser and dermatology specialists form one of Eastern Europe's largest cosmetic surgery centers. The **Plastic Surgery Center** performs breast, eyelid, facial, nose, and outer-ear surgeries; lip enlargement; liposuction; and tummy tucks, often using endoscopic procedures. The **Laser Center** has amassed an impressive arsenal of the latest laser machines and instrumentation, including many of Candela Laser Corporation's high-end devices. Treatments include

■ *Wrinkle removal and lip enlargement:* Acne scars, facial wrinkles, and other irregularities in facial contours can be corrected by skin implant injections, which are applied into the upper layers of skin with ultra-thin needles. The volume of the injections and subsequent water retention smooth the skin's uneven surface and diminish wrinkles. The injections are most frequently used to fill nose-mouth lines and fine lip lines or to correct deeper forehead, cheek, and chin wrinkles.

- *Spider veins:* Esthé uses a high-performance V-beam laser to treat spider veins on the face, thighs, and lower legs. The vascular laser is also helpful in removing warts and other dermal outgrowths.

- *Pigmentation and tattoo treatments:* Tired of that "Robert Still Loves Me" tattoo? The Alexandrite laser focuses a 750-nm beam that pulverizes unsightly pigment into small segments, which are then washed away by the cellular system. Pigmentations resulting from age or sun, birthmarks, freckles, permanent make-up, scars, tattoos, and other hyper-pigmentations are treated using this technique.

- *Depilation:* Permanent removal of unwanted hair from face, thighs, underarms, and other parts of the body is carried out with the Candela GentleLase laser.

- *Acne treatment:* Esthé uses Candela's SmoothBeam laser to interrupt the cycle of acne scarring caused by hardening of the upper layer of skin around plugged pores (which become inflamed and then produce even more pore-clogging oil). This noninvasive procedure is used to treat ongoing acne, as well as old acne scars. Up to three sessions are usually required, combined with chemical peeling.

Laderma Klinik

22 Rumunska Street (4th Floor) 120 00
Prague, CZECH REPUBLIC 2
Tel: 011 420 775 118.005
Email: info@laderma.com
Web: www.laderma.com

You'll find the full range of cosmetic, aesthetic, and reconstructive procedures available at Laderma Klinik, including eyelid surgery (blepharoplasty), ear surgery (otoplasty), nose surgery (rhinoplasty), chin augmentation, facelift, breast enlargement, breast lift/reduction, tummy tuck, liposuction, Botox, and more.

More than 70 percent of Laderma's clientele comes from the UK, Germany, Austria, Switzerland, Canada, and the US. Laderma's cosmetic surgeons boast training in the US and Europe. The chief surgeon, Dr. Zuzana Cerna, is certified to perform operations in the Czech Republic, Austria, and the UK.

MyClinic Prague

Panská 5, 110 00
Prague, CZECH REPUBLIC 1
Tel: 011 420 296 827.530
Fax: 011 420 296 827.532
Email: info@myclinic.cz
Web: www.myclinic.cz

Highly specialized, MyClinic Prague deploys injectables to reduce skin's signs of aging. Procedures help to diminish skin irregularities and coarseness, increase skin tone, reduce the depth of wrinkle lines or the size of pores, and unify the color of irregular skin pigmentations. Other treatments help to diminish minor acne scars and improve acne-prone skin conditions.

The favored treatment is the highly

touted Botox/Dysport, used mostly to relax facial expression lines. Other injectables and treatments include

■ *Bio-Alcamid:* implants for cosmetic corrections, deep wrinkles, and folds.

■ *Restylane:* a naturally occurring acid, used for smoothing wrinkles and furrows and improving the contours of the lips.

■ *Silicon oil/PMS:* implants applied by injection, used for fuller lips and filling minor wrinkles.

■ *Beautical:* temporary implant to correct deeper wrinkles, furrows, and reduced skin volume.

■ *Chemical peeling:* application of fruit acids to improve skin tone and elasticity.

MyClinic is entirely outpatient; a typical visit lasts two to three hours, including consultation, "before" and "after" photos, and treatment. MyClinic employs two full-time staff physicians, both certified by the Czech Medical Chamber.

Prices are generally about half what you would expect to pay for similar treatments in the US or Canada. It may not be worth a trip to Eastern Europe solely for a Restylane fix, but while in Prague....

Esthesia Clinic
Opletalova 59
Prague, CZECH REPUBLIC 1
Tel: 011 420 284 680.530
Email: info@esthesia.cz
Web: www.esthesia.cz

Four doctors and a staff of six run this small clinic in the heart of Prague. Esthesia Clinic is one of the few clinics in Prague affiliated with the Czech Dental Chamber, Czech

Orthodontic Society, and Czech Society for Pediatric Dentistry. The clinic offers extractions, including wisdom teeth; implants; pediatric and adult orthodontics; periodontics; prosthetics, including ceramic veneer, crowns, bridgework, and dentures; restorative dentistry; and root canals.

Dentaktiv Clinic
Lumírova 21, 128 00
Prague, CZECH REPUBLIC 2
Tel: 011 420 224 938.389
Email: info@dentaktiv.cz
Web: www.dentaktiv.cz

Dentaktiv Clinic's six doctors and surgeons handle the usual gamut of dental services, including bridges, cosmetic dentistry, crowns, dentures, fillings, implants, pediatric dentistry, periodontics, root canals, and tooth whitening. Dentaktiv also specializes in diagnoses and treatment of temporomandibular joint syndrome (TMJ), the troublesome jaw disorder often caused by trauma or stress.

European Dental Clinic
Vaclavske Square 33, 2nd Floor
Prague, CZECH REPUBLIC 1
Tel: 011 420 224 229.984
Email: edc@quick.cz
Web: www.edcdental.cz

Can you imagine a dental clinic that's open until 11 P.M.? This one, run by a Russian émigré, offers late-evening service for the owls, but with no loss of morning service for the larks, as it opens at 8 A.M. European Dental Clinic offers the full range of services, including implants, cosmetic dentistry, fillings and restorations, crowns, bridges, dentures, oral surgery, orthodontics, treatment of periodontal disease, and root canals. The setting is upscale with high ceilings, parquet floors, and the best paintings and photographs on the walls. There is no shortage of modern equipment either, with digital x-ray that reduces radiation exposure and a laser scanner that makes impressions a thing of the past. European Dental gives you a computer file to take to your dentist back home. Expect higher prices here, but the service may be worth the expense.

■ HOTELS: DELUXE

Hotel Constans
Břetislavova 309
118 00 Malá Strana
Prague, CZECH REPUBLIC 1
Tel: 011 420 234 091.818
Fax: 011 420 234 091.860
Email: hotel@hotelconstans.cz
Web: www.hotelconstans.cz

Hilton Prague
Pobrezni 1
Prague, CZECH REPUBLIC 18 600
Tel: 011 420 224 841.111
Fax: 011 420 224 842.378
Email: guestcentre.prague@hilton.com
Web: www.hilton.com

Hotel U Prince
Staroměstské Náměstí 9 11000
Prague, CZECH REPUBLIC 1
Tel-**Fax:** 011 420 224 213.807
Email: info@hoteluprince.com
Web: www.hoteluprince.com

■ HOTELS: MODERATE

Golden Tulip Hotel
Hybernská 42
Prague, CZECH REPUBLIC 11 000
Tel: 011 420 224 100.100
Fax: 011 420 224 100.180
Email: info@tulipinnterminus.com
Web: www.tulipinnterminus.com

Hotel Anna
Budecska 17 12000
Prague, CZECH REPUBLIC 2
Tel: 011 420 222 513.111
Fax: 011 420 222 515.158
Email: sales@hotelanna.cz
Web: www.hotelanna.cz

DESTINATION: **HUNGARY**

■ **AT A GLANCE**

Budapest and Northwestern Hungary (Győr, Mosonmagyaróvár, Héviz, and Szombathely)

Language:	Hungarian (little English spoken)
Time Zone:	GMT +1
Country Dialing Code:	36
Electricity:	220V, Plug type B
Currency:	Forint (HUF)
Visa Required?	Not for stays shorter than 90 days
Recommended Immunizations:	Hepatitis A; Typhoid Booster
Treatment Specialties:	Dental
Leading Hospitals and Clinics:	*Budapest:* Villányi Dent, Marident-Vár, Marident Csalogány; *Mosonmagyaróvár:* Eurodent Aquadental Dental Clinic; *Héviz:* Gelenscér Dental Clinic; *Szombathely:* Isis Dental Clinic; *Győr:* Smile-Zentrum Dental Clinic and Implantation Centre (Smile Centre)
JCI-Accredited Hospitals:	None
Standards and Accreditation:	Hungarian Accreditation Council, Association of Hungarian Medical Societies, Hungarian Medical Chamber, Hungarian Dental Association

■ **TREATMENT BRIEF**

Hungary is no stranger to health tourism; for centuries the well heeled have been flocking to its restorative mineral springs, lakes, baths, and spas.

German and Swiss patients head to Hungary—literally by the busload—for inexpensive, high-quality dental work, and patients from the US and Canada are beginning to catch on as well. Hungary boasts more dentists per capita than any other country, and post–Cold War Hungarian dentists pride themselves on their state-of-the-art equipment. Since the country's admission to the European Union in 2004, travel and communications have grown easier, and Hungary has begun to upgrade accreditation and care standards to match those of Western Europe.

Hungary's cosmopolitan capital, Budapest, boasts the country's largest number of dental clinics—although they tend to be the region's most expensive. Dental travel agents also offer trips to smaller, sleepier (and more economical) towns, such as Mosonmagyaróvár and Győr, both near the Austrian border. Although a small town of 30,000 inhabitants, Mosonmagyaróvár is home to an incredible 160 dental offices!

While it's economical for Europeans to travel to Hungary for a dental checkup or a cleaning, most American patients traveling to Hungary are seeking more extensive care, including cosmetic oral surgeries, full-mouth restorations, and implants. Such work can be had at less than half the US price, including travel and accommodations.

Hungarian dentists must complete five years of dental training. In order to practice, a dentist must be registered with the Hungarian Medical Chamber. Accreditation and standards are set by the State National Health Commission and Medical Service, Hungarian Medical Chamber, and International Society of Aesthetic Plastic Surgeons. All that said, compliance to standards varies widely in Hungary, and health travelers should rely doubly on trusted sources, such as referrals or a reputable health travel agent.

As in so many other Eastern European countries that have suffered decades of repression, the infrastructure remains spotty. The healthcare sector is no exception, so be sure to do your homework. Either engage the services of a health travel planner or check references carefully.

■ TYPICAL TREATMENTS AND COSTS

Dental:

Porcelain Veneer: $620

Crown (porcelain fused to gold): $500-$680

Inlays and Onlays: $500

Implant (titanium with crown): $1,220-$1,500

Root Canal: $110-$130

Full Denture (per jaw): $740

Extraction (surgical, per tooth): $200-$330

■ HEALTH TRAVEL AGENTS

Dental-Offer (formerly Dental-Value)

Scheuer és Társa BT

Halász Utca 10

Máriakálnok, HUNGARY H-9231

Tel: 011 36 70 586.9600

Fax: 011 36 96 224.300

Email: info@dental-offer.com

Web: www.dental-offer.com

Based in Hungary and operated by founder and CEO Florian Scheuer, Dental-Offer serves US and Canadian patients in partnership with Posh Journeys of Reno, Nevada (see below). All staff members speak English and all clients are from either the US or Canada. Dental-Offer representatives promise to take care of international patients and their travel to Eastern Europe from America, providing top accommodation and selecting the best dental clinics.

Healthbase Online, Inc.

287 Auburn Street

Newton, MA 02466

Tel: 1 888 691.4584 (US toll-free); 1 617 418.3436

Fax: 1 800 986.9230 (US toll-free)
Email: info.hb@healthbase.com
Web: www.healthbase.com

For more information on Healthbase, see India: Chennai.

Posh Journeys
530 East Patriot Boulevard
Reno, NV 89511
Tel: 1 775 852.5105
Fax: 1 775 852.5105
Email: contact@poshjourneys.com
Web: www.poshjourneys.com

This Reno-based travel company, run by Jack and Helga van Horn, has been con-ducting international tours since 1987. Following their own positive dental treatment experience in Hungary, the couple has been arranging dental travel to Hungary for their clients since 2001.

Posh Journeys works with their Hungary-based partner, Florian Scheuer of Dental-Offer (www.dental-offer.com; see above), to arrange cost estimates, make dental appointments, arrange interviews with dentists, and suggest the best dentist for a patient's procedure. The agency also arranges airline tickets, airport transfers, lodging, and sightseeing. Posh Journeys offers a wide range of accommodation options,

Case Study: Brenda B., Minnesota

Brenda B. received the antibiotic tetracycline as a child, so her teeth were tinted yellow. She dreamed of an attractive smile, but the costs of having her teeth capped in the US were too high for her budget. So she started investigating the dental tourism industry.

"Hungary was my country of choice," says Brenda, "because of the large number of highly qualified dentists offering services at competitive prices. I also liked the fact that it is in Europe and I could visit capitals in surrounding countries."

"I chose the city of Mosonmagyaróvár for several reasons. I liked the idea of relaxing in the thermal spa pool after a long session in the dental chair. Mosonmagyaróvár turned out to be a charming little town with an old-European feel to it. There were quaint bakeries and coffee shops to enjoy along its cobblestone streets and avenues. The people were friendly, and I felt extremely safe walking the streets alone (even at night). From Mosonmagyaróvár, I took day trips to Bratislava (capital of Slovakia), Budapest, and Vienna."

Brenda was happy with the dental services she received. Her dentist took care to avoid the pain Brenda had previously experienced from her sensitive teeth. After doing tests that confirmed Brenda's allergy to the metals cobalt and nickel, her dentist removed amalgam from her mouth and used gold to make her new crowns.

"Now I have a pretty smile, and my teeth aren't overly sensitive," Brenda says. "Much appreciation and gratitude goes to my heath travel agent and my dental team for enabling me to fulfill this dream."

from full-service spa hotels complete with hot springs to condominiums with kitchens, where patients can cook their own meals from food bought at a local market.

Posh Journeys arranges health journeys to Mosonmagyaróvár (40 miles southeast of Vienna), Budapest, and Bratislava in Slovakia, where one of the most modern dental clinics in Europe is located.

■ HOSPITALS AND CLINICS

Note: Dental clinics literally line the streets in northwestern Hungarian towns, such as Héviz, Mosonmagyaróvár, and Győr, with wide variations in service and expertise. Even the top clinics can vary in the amount of English spoken and the level of customer service provided. The clinics below represent the best Hungary has to offer. Travelers to Hungary should make an extra effort to attain the highest comfort level with their clinic and doctor beforehand. The services of a good health travel agent are recommended.

BUDAPEST

Villányi Dent

6 Villányi Street, Room 1, First Floor
Budapest, HUNGARY H-1114
Tel: 011 36 1 279.1184
Web: www.Villányident.hu

Established in 1999, Villányi Dent is located in the heart of Budapest. With seven practicing dentists and surgeons, this clinic's warm surroundings near the banks of the Danube are a plus for visitors. All dentists speak English.

Dental services include cosmetic, crowns and bridges, extractions, fillings, implants, inlays and onlays, orthodontics, and veneers.

The clinic conducts extensive pre-visit consultations and works closely with the highly regarded Hübi-Labi Technical Laboratory for all its imagery and lab work.

Marident-Vár

1014 Bp., Szentháromság Tér 7
Budapest, HUNGARY
Tel-Fax: 011 36 1 487.0518
Email: info@marident.com
Web: www.marident.com

and

Marident-Csalogány

1027 Bp., Csalogány Utca 3/c
Budapest, HUNGARY
Tel-Fax: 011 36 1 212.2103
Email: info@marident.com
Web: www.marident.com

Marident has two facilities in Budapest, both specializing in cosmetic dentistry, although the full range of diagnostic and restorative services is available. In business since 1995, these clinics offer tooth-whitening, filling, prosthetics, oral hygiene, oral surgery, and supplementary services, in addition to crowns, bridges, prosthodontics, implants, root canals, bone grafting, sinus lifts, and more. Marident's six dentists all speak English. Only metal-free biocompatible materials are used, and all work is guaranteed.

NORTHWESTERN HUNGARY

Eurodent Aquadental Dental Clinic

Györi Kapu Utca 7
Mosonmagyaróvár, HUNGARY H-9200
Tel: 011 36 96 578.250
Fax: 011 36 96 217.200
Email: eurodent@eurodent.hu
Web: www.eurodent.hu

Established in 1993, Eurodent Aquadental Dental Clinic's six dentists and staff of 20 serve mostly Europeans seeking to combine Viennese vacations with dental checkups and cleanings. Vienna is less than 90 minutes away, and border crossings have become much easier for tourists.

Treatments at Eurodent include closed sinus elevations; cosmetic and preservative fillings, inlays, and veneers; laser therapies; oral surgery (extractions, root canals); prosthetics (crown and bridge removal and a variety of metal and nonmetal crowns, including zirconium); and restorations.

Gelenscér Dental Clinic

Vörösmarty Street 75
Héviz, HUNGARY H-8380
Tel: 011 36 83 340.183
Fax: 011 36 83 540.253
Email: info@gelencserdental.hu
Web: www.gelencserdental.hu

Nine dentists, eight technicians, and a total staff of 22 make up one of Héviz's largest dental clinics. Established more than 30 years ago, Gelenscér Dental Clinic boasts its own lab, where most of the bridges, crowns, and other dental items are made onsite. Bone grafting and implants are specialties. All dentists speak English.

Isis Dental Clinic

Thököly Utca 16
Szombathely, HUNGARY H-9700
Tel: 011 36 94 339.155
Fax: 011 36 94 510.892
Email: isisdental@isisdental.hu
Web: www.isisdental.hu

Located at the foot of the Alps in Szombathely (one of Hungary's oldest towns, established in 43 AD by the Roman Emperor Claudius), Isis Dental Clinic offers the full range of diagnoses, treatments, and surgeries. An onsite laboratory helps shorten wait periods for crowns, dentures, and implants. Implantologists at Isis boast the use of products from Oraltronics and Nobel Biocare, two well-known European dental manufacturers. Other aesthetic services include permanent bleaching with the Brite Smile system and a wide range of tooth jewelries.

Isis offers three-, six-, and nine-day "Dental Week" packages that include consultations, various treatments, and free pickup and dropoff to and from Vienna (50 minutes) or Graz (40 minutes). For those patients planning annual visits, the clinic offers a five-year guarantee on all prosthetic work with annual checkups.

Smile-Zentrum Dental Clinic and Implantation Centre (Smile Centre)

Bálint Mihály Utca 121
Győr, HUNGARY H-9025
Tel: 011 36 96 528.910
Fax: 011 36 96 528.909
Email: info@smile-zentrum.hu
Web: www.smilezentrum.hu

Győr offers the tourist some elegant old architecture and charming shopping streets, but at the same time, it's a fast-developing industrial town, where you'll find factories for Audi, Leier, Wolf, Philips, and more. So, if you are traveling on business, maybe there's time to get your teeth fixed while you're there. At the Smile Centre, you'll find the full range of dental services, including radiography (panoramic or small-size), ultrasound scaling of tooth film, mycoderm treatment, groove closing, bleaching, fillings, prostheses, inlays/onlays of gold and ceramics, ceramic caps, crowns, dentures, oral surgery, implants (Titan), root canals, extractions, and more.

■ RECOVERY ACCOMMODATIONS

We found most recovery accommodations in northwestern Hungary to be drab, offering uninspired service. You're better off staying in hotels, many of which offer transportation, special diets, and other amenities to health travelers. Alternatively, Dental-Offer can arrange self-catering apartments in northwestern Hungary. Check with that agency concerning the quality of the facilities.

■ HOTELS: DELUXE

BUDAPEST

Four Seasons Hotel
Gresham Palace
Roosevelt Tér 5-6
Budapest, HUNGARY H-1051
Tel: 011 36 1 268.6000
Fax: 011 36 1 268.5000
Web: www.fourseasons.com/budapest

Kempinski Hotel Corvinus Budapest
Erzsébet Tér 7-8
Budapest, HUNGARY H-1051
Tel: 011 36 1 429.3777
Fax: 011 36 1 429.4777
Email: hotel.corvinus@kempinski.com
Web: www.kempinski-budapest.com

NORTHWESTERN HUNGARY

Naturmet Hotel Carbona
Attila Utca 1
Héviz, HUNGARY H-8380
Tel: 011 36 83 501.500
Fax: 011 36 83 340.468
Email: hotel@carbona.hu
Web: www.carbona.hu

Hotel Lajta Park
Vízpart Utca 6
Mosonmagyaróvár, HUNGARY H-9200
Tel: 011 36 20 460.2134
Fax: 011 36 1 288.7061
Email: lajtapark@ohb.hu
Web: www.ohb.hu/lajtapark

■ HOTELS: MODERATE

BUDAPEST

Danubius Hotel Flamenco
Tas Vezér Utca 3-7
Budapest, HUNGARY H-1113
Tel: 011 36 1 889.5600
Fax: 011 36 1 889.5651
Email: flamenco.reservations@
  danubiusgroup.com
Web: www.danubiushotels.com/flamenco

City Hotel Mátyás
Március 15, Tér 7-8
Budapest, HUNGARY H-1056
Tel: 011 36 20 460.2134
Fax: 011 36 1 288.7061
Email: matyas@mail.ohb.hu
Web: www.ohb.hu/matyas

NORTHWESTERN HUNGARY

Arany Szarvas Hotel
Rado Setany 1
Györ, HUNGARY H-9025
Tel: 011 36 96 517.452
Fax: 011 36 96 517.454
Email: salidus.aranyszarvas@t-online.hu
Web: www.aranyszarvas-gyor.hu

Thermal-Hotel Mosonmagyaróvár
Kolbai Karoly, Utca 10
Mosonmagyaróvár, HUNGARY
Tel: 011 36 96 206.871
Fax: 011 36 96 206.872
Email: thermhot@axelero.hu
Web: www.thermal-movar.hu

DESTINATION: INDIA: DELHI

■ **AT A GLANCE**

Delhi

Language:	Hindi (English widely spoken)
Time Zone:	GMT +5:30
Country Dialing Code:	91
Electricity:	220V, Plug types B & E
Currency:	Rupee
Visa Required?	Yes
Recommended Immunizations:	Hepatitis A; Boosters for Typhoid and Polio; Antimalarial Drugs
Treatment Specialties:	Cardiovascular, Cosmetic, Dental, General Surgery, Ophthalmology, Orthopedics, Transplants, Weight Loss
Leading Hospitals and Clinics:	Indraprastha Apollo Hospital, Escorts Heart Institute and Research Center, Max Super-Specialty Hospital, Artemis Health Institute
JCI-Accredited Hospitals:	Indraprastha Apollo Hospital
Standards and Accreditation:	Ministry of Health and Family Welfare, Indian Medical Association, Indian Health Care Federation, British Medical Association (BMA), General Medical Council (GMC), JCI

■ TREATMENT BRIEF

Note: This section serves as an introduction to India's medical services, as well as an overview of Delhi. Readers interested in the three other Indian destinations featured in this section (Bangalore, Chennai, and Mumbai) will find the information below of interest as well.

India Overview

Who could have guessed ten years ago that India would grow into one of the world's most popular destinations for health travelers? Driven by a surging economy, a surplus of well-trained healthcare practitioners, and a proven national penchant for international outsourcing of customer service, India now aims to be the leader in health travel. Serving more than 150,000 international patients annually, it's off to a good start.

India's official national health policy encourages medical travel as part of its economy's "export" activities, even though the services are performed within India. The government uses revenues generated from medical travel to increase its holdings in foreign currency. With government and corporate investment solidly behind its healthcare system, more hospitals and superspecialty centers are opening every year.

Unlike its Asian counterparts, which have traditionally encouraged medical travel by aggressively recruiting top-of-the-line physicians from other countries, India produces some of the world's finest physicians and surgeons internally, with excellent in-country teaching hospitals and research centers. (Many Indian physicians have joined American hospitals. At last count some 35,000 Indian specialists practice in the US—and more than one in six surgeons practicing in the US are of Indian descent!)

India clearly has a two-tier health delivery system. Because of the country's widespread poverty, the Indian public healthcare system offers medical care to the poor at little or no cost. Few in India can afford cosmetic surgery and other elective treatments that attract foreign patients. The good news is that large, private hospitals are plowing profits from their international business into improved healthcare services for the indigent.

Currently, India's medical travel industry is clipping along at a 30 percent growth rate annually. Recently, those gains have come from increasing numbers of Americans, Canadians, and Europeans seeking treatment, particularly the more expensive cardiac and orthopedic surgeries, for which health travelers can save tens of thousands of dollars compared to the cost of treatment at home. Cardiac care has become a specialty in India, with centers such as Wockhardt (Mumbai), Apollo (New Delhi and Chennai), and the Institute of Cardiovascular Diseases (Chennai) leading the way. Success and morbidity rates are on par with those found in the US and Europe, with major surgeries at 15–50 percent the cost. More Americans travel to India for cardiac and orthopedic procedures than for all other treatments combined.

Most patients traveling to India stay in one of the larger cities, such as Bangalore, Delhi, Chennai, or Mumbai, where the best private hospitals are located. For more information, see those city entries.

Delhi

Most health travelers heading to India go to Delhi for superspecialty cardiovascular or orthopedic treatment. The city has more than its share of 200+-bed hospitals, including the JCI-accredited Indraprastha Apollo Hospital, Max Healthcare, and the acclaimed Escorts Heart Institute and Research Center. Apollo, India's largest healthcare provider, owns 41 hospitals with 8,000 beds. In Delhi, cardiac patients are often treated at the Escorts Heart Institute, which is headquartered there (with eight additional centers throughout the subcontinent). Max Healthcare has several superspecialty centers, all located in New Delhi.

Health travelers willing to undergo the long flight and endure the bustling capital city will find nearly every treatment specialty available, including knee replacement, cosmetic surgery, heart bypass surgery, valve replacement, prostate surgery, spinal rehabilitation, dental care, cataract removal, bone marrow transplant, neurosurgery, radiotherapy for brain tumors, hair restoration, and preventive healthcare checks.

New Delhi is sprawling, busy, noisy, and, as the name implies, relatively new. Although startling cultural and economic contrasts exist, travelers are likely to find themselves more at home in Delhi than in other Indian cities, such as Mumbai or Chennai. Delhi is the nearest medical center and point of departure for those patients willing and able to visit India's star tourist attraction, the Taj Mahal in Agra (about 200 kilometers, or 120 miles, away).

■ TYPICAL TREATMENTS AND COSTS

Cardiovascular:
Coronary Artery Bypass Graft: $8,800
Pacemaker (single-chambered): $6,500
Pacemaker (double-chambered): $9,000

Orthopedic:
Birmingham Hip Resurfacing: $9,900
Joint Replacement:
Knee: $8,400
Hip: $9,500
Ankle: $7,100
Shoulder: $8,400

Cosmetic:
Breast Augmentation: $3,300-$5,300
Breast Lift/Reduction: $3,300-$5,050
Facelift: $5,700
Liposuction (stomach, hips, and waist):
$1,000-$2,650

Dental:
Porcelain Veneer: $420
Crown (all porcelain): $360
Inlays and Onlays: $600-$1,100
Implant (titanium with crown): $1,100

Vision:
Glaucoma: $1,050
LASIK (per eye): $810

Weight Loss:
LAP-BAND System: $6,600
Gastric Bypass: $7,200

■ HEALTH TRAVEL AGENTS

Global Med Network
5823 Middlebelt Road
Garden City, MI 48135
Tel: 1 877 GMN.NETWORK (US toll-free);
   1 734 421.6388
Fax: 1 734 421.9954
Email: akambhatla@globalmednetwork.
   com
Web: www.globalmednetwork.com

For more information on Global Med
Network, see India: Bangalore.

Healthbase Online, Inc.
287 Auburn Street
Newton, MA 02466
Tel: 1 888 691.4584 (US toll-free); 1 617
   418.3436
Fax: 1 800 986.9230 (US toll-free)
Email: info.hb@healthbase.com
Web: www.healthbase.com

For more information on Healthbase
Online, see India: Chennai.

India America Global Solutions, Ltd.
333 South Allison Parkway, Suite #205
Lakewood, CO 80226
Tel: 1 800 466.9502 (US toll-free);
   1 303 987.2220
Fax: 1 303 987.1010
Email: tom@iagsolutions.com
Web: www.iagsolutions.com

India America Global Solutions (IAG) started
operation in 2005. Its founder's first-hand
experience undergoing open-heart surgery and mitral valve replacement in Delhi
prompted its creation. The agency started
with heart care, then expanded into orthopedic treatments with a focus on hip resur-

facing; it currently sends patients to India,
Thailand, and Belgium. IAG selects doctors
to match the patient's condition, processes
visas, transfers medical records, and coordinates travel schedules. It frequently sends
patients to Escorts Heart Institute, Max
Healthcare, Wockhardt, Fortis, and Apollo
Hospital in Delhi (see "Hospitals and Clinics," below).

IndUSHealth
7413 Six Forks Road, #362
Raleigh, NC 27615
Tel: 1 800 779.1314 (US toll-free)
Fax: 1 888 627.6492 (US toll-free)
Email: info@indushealth.com
Web: www.indushealth.com

Founded in 2005, this US-based firm has
established leadership in helping its clients
obtain medical treatments at leading facilities in India, including Bangalore, Chennai,
Delhi, and Mumbai.

   Focusing on major medical procedures,
including orthopedic, cardiovascular, bariatric, oncological, and spinal treatments,
IndUSHealth has forged strong ties with
superspecialty centers, such as Apollo Hospitals, Fortis Escorts Hospitals, Max Hospitals, and Wockhardt Hospitals.

   IndUSHealth's case managers are experienced registered nurses who educate
and guide patients through the process of
pursuing medical treatment overseas. They
help patients evaluate the viability and cost
of their treatment, and they explain the
potential risks and follow-up needs. They
are also equipped to coordinate care with
local doctors and medical centers when
required.

   IndUSHealth's services include telecon-
ferences with physicians, medical records

conversion and transfer, travel reservations
and ticketing, travel insurance, ground
transportation, cell phone for use in-
country, expedited passport/visa processing, and financing assistance, if required.
In addition to serving individual patients,
IndUSHealth works with US employers large
and small to offer comprehensive medical
travel programs to employees.

Med Journeys
2020 Broadway, Suite 4C
New York, NY 10023
Tel: 1 888 633.5769 (US toll-free);
  1 212 931.0557
Fax: 1 212 656.1134
Email: sonnyk@medjourneys.com
Web: www.medjourneys.com

This agency sends most of its clients to
India, Thailand, Costa Rica, and Mexico, but
it has also cemented relationships with hospitals in other countries, including Singapore, Malaysia, Turkey, and Poland. Since its
establishment in 2005, Med Journeys has
sent more than 350 patients abroad, and
the numbers are growing. Med Journeys'
standard package includes the medical procedure, accommodations during recuperation (including three meals daily), airfare,
private transportation in the host country,
and premium concierge services. Extra fees
are generally charged for optional tours,
companions, extended stays, and added
medical procedures. Med Journeys encourages clients to contact physicians directly
to check references or ask questions about
medical procedures. Med Journeys staff
members speak Spanish, Hindi, and Thai.

MedRetreat
2042 Laurel Valley Drive
Vernon Hills, IL 60061
Tel: 1 877 876.3373 (US toll-free)
Fax: 1 847 680.0484
Email: customerservice@medretreat.com
Web: www.medretreat.com

For more information on MedRetreat,
see Malaysia.

Planet Hospital
23679 Calabasas Road, Suite 150
Calabasas, CA 91302
Tel: 1 800 243.0172 (US toll-free); 1 818
  665.4801
Fax: 1 818 665.4810
Email: rudy@planethospital.com
Web: www.planethospital.com

For more information on Planet Hospital,
see Singapore.

Recover Discover Healthcare
G 47, Sector 6, Noida
Uttar Pradesh, INDIA
Tel: 011 91 120 435.9281
Fax: 011 91 120 425.8281
Email: contactus@recoverdiscover.com
Web: www.recoverdiscover.com

Recover Discover Healthcare was established in 2005; it served 22 US and Canadian
clients in its first two years. The agency
arranges teleconsultations, local transportation, tests, medications, hotel stays,
comprehensive medical reports, air travel.
It also sets up a system for daily emails for
the patient's family and referring physician.
It most often sends patients to Apollo Hospital in New Delhi or Wockhardt Hospital in
Mumbai.

The Taj Medical Group, Limited
The TechnoCentre, Coventry University
  Technology Park
Puma Way
Coventry, UNITED KINGDOM CV1 2TT
Tel: 1 877 799.9797 (US toll-free); 011 44
  2476 466.118
Fax: 011 44 2476 466.118
Email: info@tajmedical.com
Web: www.tajmedical.com

and

US Office - NYC
The Taj Medical Group
408 West 57th Street, Suite 9N
New York, NY 10019
Tel: 1 877 799.9797 (US toll-free)
Email: info@tajmedical.com
Web: www.tajmedical.com

and

US Office - VA
The Taj Medical Group
9513 Brant Lane
Glen Allen, VA 23060
Tel: 1 877 799.9797 (US toll-free)
Email: info@tajmedical.com
Web: www.tajmedical.com

Based in the UK with offices in India, Singapore, the US, and Canada, Taj Medical Group cofounders Jag and Dipa Jethwa have sent more than 1,000 patients to India over the past four years, mostly from Canada, Great Britain, and other parts of Europe. Taj's new US offices in New York City and Virginia were opened in 2007 to facilitate the needs of American health travelers.

All Taj staffers speak fluent English, and Taj insists that all their recommended physicians and surgeons be highly experienced and internationally qualified (often UK-trained or US board-certified). All the doctors speak English, too. Taj charges no up-front fees, and the agency provides all pre-travel planning, pre-operative consultation, and post-operative consultation and checkups, along with full, personal, in-country concierge service.

Taj has long-standing formal partnerships with many hospitals in India, including Escorts Heart Institute, Apollo Hospitals Group, Wockhardt Hospitals, and Max Healthcare. Taj has recently expanded its hospital partnerships and now sends clients to JCI-accredited hospitals in the UK, Germany, India, Singapore, Malaysia, Korea, Thailand, and South America. Taj uses its extensive physician contacts to match each patient's requirements with the best physician, procedure, provider, and price.

WorldMed Assist
1230 Mountain Side Court
Concord, CA 94521
Tel: 1 866 999.3848 (US toll-free)
Fax: 1 925 905.5898
Email: whoeber@worldmedassist.com
Web: www.worldmedassist.com

For more information on WorldMed Assist, see India: Bangalore.

■ HOSPITALS AND CLINICS

Max Super-Specialty Hospital

1 Press Enclave Road
Saket, New Delhi, INDIA 110017
Tel: 011 91 11 2651.5050
Fax: 011 91 11 2651.0050
Email: info@maxhealthcare.in
Web: www.maxhealthcare.in

Six specialty clinics with more than 700 beds and 500 doctors make Max Healthcare Delhi's largest hospital network and one of the country's most influential health centers. International health travelers usually visit one of Max's two superspecialty centers, mostly for cardiac and orthopedic surgeries.

The **Max Heart and Vascular Institute** (also called the **Max Devki Devi Heart and Vascular Institute)** offers noninvasive heart surgery, nuclear medicine, cardiac imaging, interventional cardiology cardiac pacing, and electrophysiology. The **Max Institute of Orthopaedics and Joint Replacement Surgery** is a state-of-the-art facility located in South Delhi. It is a tertiary-care center that prides itself on infection control and specialized physiotherapy and support services for all its patients.

Max's **International Patients Services** department offers initial screening and diagnosis, telemedicine evaluation and recommendations, travel arrangements to Delhi (including visa, ticketing, airport pickup, money transfer and exchange, and ATM withdrawals), interpreters, lodging assistance, special return journey arrangements, and an exclusive help-desk and dedicated relationship manager to ensure quality service.

Max also boasts a new vision clinic, **Max Eyecare,** which offers the full range of ophthalmologic specialties and procedures. Its **Institute of Neurosciences** focuses on brain tumors, aneurysms, stroke, infectious diseases of the brain, spinal tumors and infections, and chronic spinal pain. Max also has an **Institute of Aesthetic and Reconstructive Plastic Surgery,** where surgeons correct birth defects and perform the usual range of cosmetic procedures.

Indraprastha Apollo Hospital

Sarita Vihar
Delhi Mathura Road
Delhi, INDIA 110 076
Tel: 011 91 11 2692.5858
Fax: 011 91 11 2682.5709
Email: helpdesk_delhi@apollohospitals.com
Web: www.apollohospdelhi.com

Indraprastha Apollo Hospital, with 560 beds and 14 operating theaters, treats more than 12,000 international patients annually. This Apollo hospital was the first in India to receive JCI accreditation. As a result of the ensuing media coverage, American and Canadian patients are now more frequently seen, interspersed with princes, sheiks, and other VIPs in Apollo's international waiting lounge.

Indraprastha Apollo's treatment specialties include cardiology and cardiac surgery, pediatrics, orthopedics, neurology, oncology, and transplantation. Apollo is particularly proud of the latter, with more than 800 kidney transplants and 90 liver transplants to its credit. On the cardiac front, Indraprastha Apollo has performed thousands of angiograms, angioplasties, and mitral balloon valvoplasties. Cardiac surgeries carry a 98.5 percent success rate across Apollo, higher than most brand-name US hospitals. A recently acquired 64-slice computed tomography (CT) scanner enables instantaneous, noninvasive angiography procedures at about half the cost of a similar procedure in the US.

Orthopedics is also huge here, and Apollo has pioneered procedures like total hip and knee replacements and the Birmingham hip resurfacing technique. While the Birmingham procedure was only recently approved in the US, Apollo's specialist surgeons have performed hundreds over the past decade, with a 98+ percent success rates.

Escorts Heart Institute and Research Center

Okhla Road
New Delhi, INDIA 110 025
Tel: 011 91 11 2682.5000
Fax: 011 91 11 2682.5013
Email: contact@ehirc.com
Web: www.ehirc.com

Headquartered in New Delhi, with 20 centers and associated hospitals throughout India, Escorts Heart Institute and Research Center now manages nearly 900 beds. The 326-bed New Delhi institute has nine operating rooms and carries out 5,000 open-heart surgeries, 5,000 angioplasties, and 15,000 angiographies annually. Cardiac specialties include standard and specialty coronary bypass surgery, transmyocardial laser revascularization (TMLR), heart port surgery, robotic surgery for aortic aneurysms and dissections, carotid endarterectomy, valve surgery, and treatment of peripheral vascular disease. Escorts emphasizes preventive cardiology with a fully developed program of monitored exercise, yoga, meditation, and lifestyle management.

The institute's latest addition is its **Car-**diac Scan Centre,** where state-of-the-art magnetic resonance imaging (MRI) and computed tomography (CT) scans are used to diagnose coronary artery disease at its earliest stages. Escorts' **International Services Department** offers airport pickup and dropoff, travel arrangements, an interpreter, currency exchange, customized in-hospital cuisine, and sightseeing.

Note: The entire Escorts chain of hospitals was recently acquired by Fortis Healthcare (now India's second largest healthcare and hospital network). Fortis has recently established a network-wide **International Patients Service Centre,** which serves Escorts in New Delhi as well as other Escorts and Fortis facilities throughout India. For information on Fortis's numerous healthcare packages, contact:

Fortis Healthcare

International Patients Service Centre
Piccadilly House
275-276, Capt Gaur Marg
Sriniwas Puri, New Delhi, INDIA 110 065
Tel: 011 91 11 4229.5222
Fax: 011 91 11 4180.2121
Email: fipsc@fortishealthcare.com
Web: www.fortishealthcare.com/intl_
patients/fipsc.html

Artemis Health Institute

Sector 51, Gurgaon
Haryana, Delhi, INDIA 122 001
Tel: 011 91 12 4676.7999
Email: anas@artemishealthsciences.com
Web: www.artemishospital.in

Artemis Health Institute (AHI) is a 500-bed, superspecialty flagship hospital established by Artemis Health Sciences (AHS), a healthcare venture launched by one of India's biggest tire companies. Artemis specializes in cardiology, oncology, orthopedics, minimally invasive surgery, and bariatric surgery; it runs specialized clinics for breast cancer, chronic pain, and asthma.

The institute is equipped with the latest technology in predictive, diagnostic, and therapeutic imaging as well as specialty equipment for inpatient monitoring. AHI employs a paperless and filmless hospital information system. Artemis was the first healthcare facility in India to offer functional magnetic resonance imaging (MRI) scanning using noncontrast imaging for cancers, MRI-PET fusion technology, and 3-D dynamic road-mapping for reconstructive imaging.

The hospital offers a range of services for international patients, including teleconsulting with specialists, travel arrangements, airport pickups and hospital transfers, international cuisines, lodging for companions, and a wi-fi environment within the hospital. After a patient's discharge, Artemis offers sightseeing tours of Delhi, facilitation of return-home travel, and teleconsultation between Artemis doctors and physicians back home.

Case Study: Nancy K., Colorado

Like many Americans, I was unable to qualify for health insurance due to a preexisting condition (prolapsed mitral valve and atrial septal defect). Traveling for the care I needed started out solely as a financial consideration, but as I learned more, I realized that I would feel more confident about getting high-quality care overseas than I would here. So I traveled to Delhi, India, with my husband. I did research on the Internet, and I chose a treatment center that I thought was right for me.

My diagnosis was that I needed to replace the mitral valve and repair the hole between the chambers of my heart. An extraordinary team performed my surgery. Their English was flawless, because most Indian doctors have been trained in either the UK or US. My key surgeon is internationally known for his skill in the technique he used for my surgery.

I was in the hospital for four weeks. I had no problems there, but my trip home was very difficult, naturally, because the journey was so long and I didn't have a lot of energy.

I have had lung issues since my return to the states. I live at an altitude of 7,500 feet, and the thin air here has taken a toll on me. My follow-up care is the same as if I had had my surgery at home, because my personal cardiologist looks after me, not the surgeon.

My total costs (including travel) were about 10 percent of what I would have paid here. I would absolutely travel abroad again for healthcare. The high level of care and supreme cleanliness cannot be found in most of the sadly understaffed hospitals in this country. The main thing for anyone considering healthcare in another country is *do your research!*

■ RECOVERY ACCOMMODATIONS

Recover Discover Healthcare recommends several recovery accommodations. One of them is the Stay Inn.

The Stay Inn
Tel: 011 91 11 2953.2619
Fax: 011 91 11 2648.8237
Email: info@thestay-inn.com
Web: www.thestay-inn.com

■ HOTELS: DELUXE

Note: Good, safe, reliable, full-service hotels in India aren't cheap, and budget hotels are often lacking in the amenities that help any recovering patient feel more at ease. Deluxe hotels such as those listed here are frequently in the $300+ range, and "moderate" hotels are often in the $200–$300 range. A breakfast buffet is usually included. Rates can vary significantly based on season and availability.

Health travel planners, as well as hospitals' international patient centers, often offer hotel discounts through their partnerships. Check with your agent or clinic before paying full freight.

Hotel Intercontinental Nehru Place
Nehru Place
New Delhi, INDIA 110 019
Tel: 1 888 424.6835 (US toll-free);
   011 91 11 4122.3344
Fax: 011 91 11 2622.4288
Web: www.ichotelsgroup.com

Crowne Plaza New Delhi
New Friends Colony
New Delhi, INDIA 110 025
Tel: 011 91 11 2683.5070
Fax: 011 91 11 2683.7758
Email: crowneplaza@crowneplazadelhi.com
Web: www.ichotelsgroup.com

The Oberoi Hotel
Dr. Zakir Hussein Marg
New Delhi, INDIA 110 003
Tel: 011 91 11 2436.3030
Fax: 011 91 11 2436.0484
Email: devendra@oberoidel.com
Web: www.oberoidelhi.com

■ HOTELS: MODERATE

Hotel Savoia
Friends Colony, Mathura Road
Delhi, INDIA
Tel: 011 91 22 2404.2211
Fax: 011 91 22 2404.2242
Email: savoia@nivalink.com
Web: www.nivalink.com/savoia

Centrum Hotel
D-984, New Friends Colony
New Delhi, INDIA 110 065
Tel: 011 91 22 2807.9270
Fax: 011 91 22 2806.5818
Email: travel@indiatravelite.com
Web: www.indiatravelite.com

Hotel Rockland
C-30, Panchsheel Enclave
New Delhi, INDIA 110 017
Tel: 011 91 26 499.780
Fax: 011 91 26 495.004
Email: info@rocklandinn.com
Web: www.rocklandinn.com

DESTINATION: INDIA: BANGALORE

■ AT A GLANCE

Bangalore

Language:	Hindi (English widely spoken)
Time Zone:	GMT +5:30
Country Dialing Code:	91
Electricity:	220V, Plug types B & E
Currency:	Rupee
Visa Required?	Yes
Recommended Immunizations:	Hepatitis A; Boosters for Typhoid and Polio; Antimalarial Drugs
Treatment Specialties:	Cardiovascular, Cosmetic, Dental, General Surgery, Neurology, Ophthalmology, Orthopedics, Stem Cell, Weight Loss
Leading Hospitals and Clinics:	Manipal Hospital Bangalore, Wockhardt Hospital
JCI-Accredited Hospitals:	Wockhardt Hospital and Heart Institute
Standards and Accreditation:	Ministry of Health and Family Welfare, Indian Medical Association, Indian Health Care Federation, British Medical Association (BMA), General Medical Council (GMC)

■ TREATMENT BRIEF

Situated in southern India midway between the Arabian Sea and the Indian Ocean, this capital of the state of Karnataka has 6 million inhabitants. It is India's fifth largest and fastest growing city.

Bangalore has so many nicknames that one might suspect a public relations agency was working overtime. Its many local parks and abundant flora have earned it the name the "Garden City." As India's center for software production and outsourcing, Bangalore also qualifies as "India's Silicon Valley." Its rich array of produce, including grapes, mangoes, and guavas, has tagged Bangalore as the "Fruit Market of the South." Bangalore is also known as the "Stone City" for its abundant granite deposits.

To this list one might add "Healthcare City," as Bangalore boasts the largest number of World Health Organization-approved systems of medicine in a single city. Patients will find here a broad array of established treatment centers, including Manipal Hospital Bangalore and Wockhardt Hospital's Center of Cardiovascular Surgery. Over the past five years, the average success rate for cardiac surgeries performed in Bangalore's eight cardiac-care hospitals was 99.3 percent, on par with hospitals in US cities.

Bangalore is also India's unofficial seat of alternative treatments, where patients seeking help off the beaten medical path will find a multitude of choices, including ultramodern allopathy, Ayurvedic medicine, holistic naturopathy, spa-based rejuvenation, yoga, and more.

■ TYPICAL TREATMENTS AND COSTS

Cardiovascular:
Coronary Artery Bypass Graft: $8,800
Pacemaker (single-chambered): $6,500
Pacemaker (double-chambered): $9,000

Orthopedic:
Birmingham Hip Resurfacing: $9,900
Joint Replacement:
Knee: $8,400
Hip: $9,500
Ankle: $7,100
Shoulder: $8,400

Cosmetic:
Breast Augmentation: $3,300-$5,300
Breast Lift/Reduction: $3,300-$5,050
Facelift: $5,700
Liposuction (stomach, hips, and waist):
$1,000-$2,650

Dental:
Porcelain Veneer: $420
Crown (all porcelain): $360
Inlays and Onlays: $600-$1,100
Implant (titanium with crown): $1,100

Vision:
Glaucoma: $1,050
LASIK (per eye): $810

Weight Loss:
LAP-BAND System: $6,600
Gastric Bypass: $7,200

■ HEALTH TRAVEL AGENTS

Global Med Network
5823 Middlebelt Road
Garden City, MI 48135
Tel: 1 877 GMN.NETWORK (US toll-free);
1 734 421.6388
Fax: 1 734 421.9954
Email: akambhatla@globalmednetwork
.com
Web: www.globalmednetwork.com

This agency began operation in 2006 and sent 70 clients to India for medical care in its first year. Its services include reviewing medical requirements, processing medical records, and coordinating surgery, air travel, visa services, in-country transportation, and post-operative care. Global Med Network arranges care at Wockhardt and Apollo Hospitals in Bangalore (see "Hospitals and Clinics," below) and Delhi as well as other sites.

Health Tourism Bangalore
64 2nd Main, 1st Block, Koramangala
Bangalore, INDIA 560 034
Tel: 001 91 802 553.5137
Email: healthtourismbangalore@gmail.com
Web: www.healthtourismbangalore.com

A husband-and-wife team started Health Tourism Bangalore in 2003. Since then they've arranged medical travel for more than 100 clients, about 40 percent from the US and Canada. The agency often refers patients to Bangalore's Hosmat Hospital and Sparsh Hospital. Clients are encouraged to speak directly with physicians.

IndUSHealth
7413 Six Forks Road, #362
Raleigh, NC 27615
Tel: 1 800 779.1314 (US toll-free)
Fax: 1 888 627.6492 (US toll-free)
Email: info@indushealth.com
Web: www.indushealth.com

For more information on IndUSHealth, see India: Delhi.

Med Journeys
2020 Broadway, Suite 4C
New York, NY 10023
Tel: 1 888 633.5769 (US toll-free); 1 212 931.0557
Fax: 1 212 656.1134
Email: sonnyk@medjourneys.com
Web: www.medjourneys.com

For more information on Med Journeys, see India: Delhi.

MedRetreat
2042 Laurel Valley Drive
Vernon Hills, IL 60061
Tel: 1 877 876.3373 (US toll-free)
Fax: 1 847 680.0484
Email: customerservice@medretreat.com
Web: www.medretreat.com

For more information on MedRetreat, see Malaysia.

The Taj Medical Group, Limited
408 West 57th Street, Suite 9N
New York, NY 10019
Tel: 1 877 799.9797 (US toll-free)
Email: info@tajmedical.com
Web: www.tajmedical.com

For more information on Taj Medical Group, see India: Delhi.

WorldMed Assist
1230 Mountain Side Court
Concord, CA 94521
Tel: 1 866 999.3848 (US toll-free)
Fax: 1 925 905.5898
Email: whoeber@worldmedassist.com
Web: www.worldmedassist.com

This agency started in 2006 and has established partnerships with the Apollo Hospitals in Delhi, Chennai, Hyderabad, and other Indian cities; Wockhardt in Mumbai and Bangalore (see "Hospitals and Clinics," below); Anadolu Medical Center in Istanbul, Turkey; ANCA in Gent, Belgium; and Hospital Angeles in Tijuana, Mexico. WorldMed Assist arranged the first liver transplant for an American in India in the summer of 2007, and several high-profile cases followed. The agency and its patients have been featured on BBC, ABC News, and NPR's *All Things Considered*. WorldMed facilitates interaction between patients and their physicians abroad through emails and conference calls. The agency advertises its highly competitive rates with no markups on surgeries and conducts negotiations on behalf of the client with its ongoing partners. Staff members speak English, Spanish, and Dutch.

■ HOSPITALS AND CLINICS

Manipal Hospital Bangalore
98, Airport Road
Bangalore, INDIA 560017
Tel: 011 91 80 2502.4444
Fax: 011 91 80 2526.6757
Email: info@manipalhospital.org
Web: www.manipalhospital.org

Launched in 1990, this hospital is owned by a giant healthcare management company, the Manipal Group. With 11 hospitals, 1,250 physicians, and 4,250 beds, the Manipal Group is one of Asia's largest and most respected hospital networks. Manipal Hospital Bangalore is huge in its own right, with 600 beds and 39 specialties. Centers of excellence include

■ **Manipal Heart Foundation,** which performs 15 heart surgeries and 30 other cardiac procedures per day. The center specializes in patients with congenital heart diseases, such as atrial septal defect, ventricular septal defect, and patent ductus arteriosus. More than 14,000 cardiac surgeries have been performed in the past five years.

■ **Manipal Institute of Neurological Disorders,** which has 100 beds reserved for neurosurgery and neurology and four fully loaded operation theaters. It is one of India's largest centers for the diagnosis and treatment of brain-related maladies. The institute conducts around 1,000 major neurological operations annually, including surgery to treat brain hemorrhages and tumors, epilepsy, head injury, Parkinson's disease, spinal injury and tumors, stroke, and congenital anomalies. Specialties include pediatric neurosurgery, neurovascular surgery, functional and stereotactic surgery, and neuron endoscopy, in addition to craniofacial, skull-base, carotid, peripheral nerve, and spinal procedures.

■ **Manipal International Institute of Dental Medicine (MIIDM),** which boasts a wide range of general and surgical dentistry. The institute also specializes in dentofacial orthopedics, in which facial deformities are surgically corrected. MIIDM is equipped to treat patients who have multiple chronic diseases and complicated medical and drug histories. The center provides periodontics, oral surgery, and dental treatment for medically compromised and physically handicapped individuals.

■ **Manipal Orthopedics Center,** which averages 160 surgeries a month. Its surgeons have conducted 350 knee replacements, 250 total hip replacements, 1,500 interlocking nailings, 1,000 arthroscopies, and 200 spinal instrumentation procedures. The center reserves one operation theater exclusively for joint replacement procedures. Success rates average 98+ percent.

Wockhardt Superspecialty Hospital
154/9, Bannerghatta Road
Opp. IIM-B
Bangalore, INDIA 560 076
Tel: 1 800 730.6373 (US and Canada toll-
free); 011 91 80 6621.4444
Email: pthukral@wockhardtin.com
Web: www.wockhardthospitals.net

After 18 years of pioneering clinical achieve-
ments at its first heart hospital on Bangalore's Cunningham Road, Wockhardt's
opened the doors to its new state-of-the-art,
400-bed superspecialty hospital in August
2006. In 2008, JCI accreditation was announced. This hospital's specialties include
cardiovascular surgery, cardiology, orthopedics, neurosciences, minimal access surgery,
and women's and children's services.

Wockhardt Hospital at Bangalore was
designed in consultation with Harvard
Medical International (HMI), the global
arm of Harvard Medical School. HMI works
with selected healthcare providers across
the globe to improve excellence in clinical
medicine, medical education, and biomedical research.

Wockhardt's medical services include
the following:

■ **Adult Cardiology and Cardiac Surgery
Center,** which specializes in closed-heart
surgeries such as a Blalock-Taussig (BT)
shunt; simple open-heart surgeries such as
septal defect repairs; and complex open-
heart surgeries. Superspecialties include
interventional cardiology (coronary
angiography, angioplasty, and stenting);
angiography and angioplasty of arteries in
the neck, leg, arm, and kidney; permanent
pacemaker (single- and double-chamber);

heart failure device implantation; and
endovascular aneurysm repair.

■ **Cardiothoracic and Vascular Surgery:** off-pump bypass surgeries, valve
surgeries and repairs, and left ventricle
size restoration surgery. (Nearly all of
Wockhardt's bypass surgeries are now
done off-pump.)

■ **Wockhardt's Center for Bone and Joint
Care** provides up-to-date diagnosis and
treatment in orthopedics, joint replacement surgeries, hip resurfacing, and
musculoskeletal problems ranging from
minimally invasive arthroscopic surgeries to complex trauma services. Other
services include pediatric orthopedics,
orthopedic oncology (including custom-
made prosthetics), and sports medicine.

The center employs the minimal access
surgery approach for fractures, which until
recently have required more invasive surgeries. Superspecialties include

■ *Total Knee Replacement:* unicondylar
knee replacement (which requires only a
small incision to promote rapid recovery);
failed, infected, or revision joint replacements; extracorporeal irradiation; and
total joint replacement.

■ *Total Hip Replacement:* cementless total
hip replacement (which is less complicated in the fixation of prosthesis);
hip resurfacing/surface replacement
artroplasty; cementless bipolar/partial
hip replacement in elderly with fractures;
shoulder replacement; and revision joint
replacement (for patients whose earlier
replacements have failed).

The **Neurology and Neurosurgery Superspecialty Center** addresses head trauma, complex brain and spinal surgeries, and other conditions. The **Brain and Spine Center** uses advanced microsurgical techniques to conduct precision-driven complex microsurgeries. Endoscopic techniques are being developed for complex brain and spinal surgeries, along with the most recent minimally invasive procedures.

Operative services include

■ *Microsurgery for Brain Tumors:* endoscopic brain surgery, skull-base surgery, and surgery for brain trauma and congenital cranial deformity; brain surgery for abnormal blood vessels, epilepsy, and removal of blood clots; pre-operative embolization of spinal lesions.

■ *Slipped Disc in the Neck or Lower Back:* microscopic lumbar discectomy or decompression, microscopic anterior cervical discectomy, and endoscopic discectomy.

■ *Degenerative Disc Disease:* minimally invasive spinal fusion, total disc replacement surgery, corrections of spinal deformities (congenital and acquired), and treatment of osteoporosis.

For those who desire alternatives to the "big knife," Wockhardt's specialists are particularly proud of their **Center for Minimal Access Surgery.** The center is dedicated to performing surgical procedures using the latest minimal access techniques, allowing patients to enjoy faster recovery and fewer post-surgical complications. The procedures minimize surgical trauma, pain, and blood loss. The center has recruited leading surgeons in the fields of laparoscopic, endo-

scopic, and robotically assisted surgeries in a wide range of superspecialties, including

■ *Laparoscopic Surgery:* appendectomy, gall bladder removal, hernia, spleen, colorectal surgery, adrenalectomy, pancreatic surgery, and bariatric surgery.

■ *Other Minimal Access Surgeries:* TURP (transurethral resection of prostate), PCNL (percutaneous nephrolithotripsy), laparoscopic urology, thoracoscopic surgery, and minimal access cardiac surgeries.

■ **Wockhardt's International Patient Service Center** offers airport pickup and dropoff, travel arrangements, coordination of all appointments, arrangements for accommodating companions and family, locker facilities for valuables, and cuisine tailored to suit individual palates.

Wockhardt offers a credit card payment gateway on its Web site, a toll-free phone helpline in the US and the UK, and a 24-hour contact center for international patients.

■ RECOVERY ACCOMMODATIONS

Ginger Bangalore
128, EPIP Phase II
Opp. KTPO and SAP Labs
Whitefield
Bangalore, INDIA 560 066
Tel: 011 91 80 6666.3333
Fax: 011 91 80 6666.3366
Email: reservations.bangalore@
gingerhotels.com
Web: www.gingerhotels.com

■ HOTELS: DELUXE

Note: Good, safe, reliable, full-service hotels in India aren't cheap, and budget hotels are often lacking in the amenities that help any recovering patient feel more at ease. Deluxe hotels such as those listed here are frequently in the $300+ range, and "moderate" hotels are often in the $200–$300 range. A breakfast buffet is usually included. Rates can vary significantly based on season and availability.

Health travel planners, as well as hospitals' international patient centers, often offer hotel discounts through their partnerships. Check with your agent or clinic before paying full freight.

Royal Orchid Hotel
1, Golf Avenue
Bangalore, INDIA 560 051
Tel: 011 91 80 2520.5566
Email: rooms@royalorchidhotels.com
Web: www.royalorchidhotels.com

The Leela Palace Kempinski
23, Airport Road
Bangalore, INDIA 560 008
Tel: 011 91 80 2521.1234
Fax: 011 91 80 2521.7234
Email: reservations.bangalore@theleela
.com
Web: www.theleela.com/hotel-bangalore
.html

■ HOTELS: MODERATE

Buena Vista Guest House
1A, 1st Floor
Wilo Crisa Apartment
#14, Rest House Crescent Road, Church
Street
Bangalore, INDIA 560 001
Tel: 011 91 80 4112.2757
Email: info@bangaloreresidency.com
Web: www.bangaloreguesthouses.com

Hotel Bangalore International
2A-2B, Crescent Road, High Ground
Bangalore, INDIA 560 001
Tel: 011 91 80 226.8011
Fax: 011 91 80 226.3191
Email: nahbi@blr.vsnl.net.in
Web: www.nalapad.com

DESTINATION: INDIA: CHENNAI

■ **AT A GLANCE**

Chennai

Language:	Hindi (English widely spoken)
Time Zone:	GMT +5:30
Country Dialing Code:	91
Electricity:	220V, Plug types B & E
Currency:	Rupee
Visa Required?	Yes
Recommended Immunizations:	Hepatitis A; Boosters for Typhoid and Polio; Antimalarial Drugs
Treatment Specialties:	Cardiovascular, Cosmetic, Dental, General Surgery, Ophthalmology, Orthopedics, Transplants, Weight Loss
Leading Hospitals and Clinics:	Apollo Hospital/Chennai (Corporate Headquarters), Apollo Dental Centre, Institute of Cardiovascular Diseases, Sankara Nethralaya Eye Hospital
JCI-Accredited Hospitals:	Apollo Hospital/Chennai
Standards and Accreditation:	Ministry of Health and Family Welfare, Indian Medical Association, Indian Health Care Federation, British Medical Association (BMA), General Medical Council (GMC), JCI

■ TREATMENT BRIEF

Located on India's southeastern Bay of Bengal coast, Chennai (formerly Madras) is the capital city of the state of Tamil Nadu and the fourth largest city in India. Known for its numerous temples and classical Indian dances, Chennai is also home to the corporate headquarters of Apollo Hospitals, India's largest hospital network. Much medical activity has grown around Apollo, and Chennai is now one of India's most important medical centers. Apollo has more than 8,000 beds in 41 locations, and its broader network includes nursing and hospital management colleges, pharmacies, diagnostic clinics, and a dental center also located in Chennai.

In Chennai a host of specialty clinics and research centers have followed Apollo's example, and standards are steadily rising. In 2006 Apollo/Chennai became the second hospital in the Apollo network to receive JCI accreditation. According to hospital officials, Americans use its services mostly for cardiovascular and orthopedic procedures.

As with most other Asian destinations, larger surgeries are the focus for international patients. Cardiac specialties and orthopedics abound, particularly knee and hip replacements. More talked about is the popular Birmingham hip resurfacing procedure, only recently FDA-approved in the United States and often a better choice than total hip replacement for patients requiring such treatment.

■ TYPICAL TREATMENTS AND COSTS

Cardiovascular:
Coronary Artery Bypass Graft: $8,800
Pacemaker (single-chambered): $6,500
Pacemaker (double-chambered): $9,000

Orthopedic:
Birmingham Hip Resurfacing: $9,900
Joint Replacement:
   Knee: $8,400
   Hip: $9,500
   Ankle: $7,100
   Shoulder: $8,400

Cosmetic:
Breast Augmentation: $3,300-$5,300
Breast Lift/Reduction: $3,300-$5,050
Facelift: $5,700
Liposuction (stomach, hips, and waist): $1,000-$2,650

Dental:
Porcelain Veneer: $420
Crown (all porcelain): $360
Inlays and Onlays: $600-$1,100
Implant (titanium with crown): $1,100

Vision:
Glaucoma: $1,050
LASIK (per eye): $810

Weight Loss:
LAP-BAND System: $6,600
Gastric Bypass: $7,200

■ HEALTH TRAVEL AGENTS

Healthbase Online, Inc.
287 Auburn Street
Newton, MA 02466
Tel: 1 888 691.4584 (US toll-free); 1 617
    418.3436
Fax: 1 800 986.9230 (US toll-free)
Email: info.hb@healthbase.com
Web: www.healthbase.com

Healthbase Online is organized as a one-stop source for all medical tourism needs. It connects patients with internationally accredited hospitals in Thailand, Singapore, India, Belgium, Hungary, Turkey, Mexico, Costa Rica, and Panama. Registered Healthbase members have access to the agency's researching tool, which allows them to explore the various medical procedures available and the hospitals that offer those procedures. Members are guided as they make decisions for themselves using detailed hospital reviews (including accreditation, photos, videos, maps, testimonials and more), physician profiles (qualifications, present and past appointments, and professional experience), and patient testimonials. Members can correspond with partner hospitals and physicians, review personalized estimates from different providers, upload and selectively share their digital medical records, and book their appointments. Other services include medical and dental loan financing and travel insurance. Healthbase charges a flat fee for its services.

IndUSHealth
7413 Six Forks Road, #362
Raleigh, NC 27615
Tel: 1 800 779.1314 (US toll-free)
Fax: 1 888 627.6492 (US toll-free)
Email: info@indushealth.com
Web: www.indushealth.com

For more information on IndUSHealth, see India: Delhi.

Med Journeys
2020 Broadway, Suite 4C
New York, NY 10023
Tel: 1 888 633.5769 (US toll-free); 1 212
    931.0557
Fax: 1 212 656.1134
Email: sonnyk@medjourneys.com
Web: www.medjourneys.com

For more information on Med Journeys, see India: Delhi.

MedRetreat
2042 Laurel Valley Drive
Vernon Hills, IL 60061
Tel: 1 877 876.3373 (US toll-free)
Fax: 1 847 680.0484
Email: customerservice@medretreat.com
Web: www.medretreat.com

For more information on MedRetreat, see Malaysia.

Planet Hospital
23679 Calabasas Road, Suite 150
Calabasas, CA 91302
Tel: 1 800 243.0172 (US toll-free); 1 818
    665.4801
Fax: 1 818 665.4810
Email: rudy@planethospital.com
Web: www.planethospital.com

For more information on Planet Hospital, see Singapore.

The Taj Medical Group, Limited
408 West 57th Street, Suite 9N
New York, NY 10019
Tel: 1 877 799.9797 (US toll-free)
Email: info@tajmedical.com
Web: www.tajmedical.com

For more information on Taj Medical Group,
see India: Delhi.

WorldMed Assist
1230 Mountain Side Court
Concord, CA 94521
Tel: 1 866 999.3848 (US toll-free)
Fax: 1 925 905.5898
Email: whoeber@worldmedassist.com
Web: www.worldmedassist.com

For more information on WorldMed Assist,
see India: Bangalore.

■ HOSPITALS AND CLINICS

Apollo Hospital/Chennai
International Patient Service Center
21, Greams Lane (off Greams Road)
Chennai, Tamil Nadu, INDIA 600 006
Tel: 011 91 44 2829.0200
Fax: 011 91 44 2829.3524
Email: enquiry@apollohospitals.com
Web: www.apollohospitals.com

Apollo Hospital/Chennai, with more than
1,000 beds and an **International Patient
Service Center,** received its JCI accreditation
in February 2006. Seventy percent of Apollo/
Chennai's physicians and surgeons have
trained, studied, or worked in institutions
and hospitals in the US or Western Europe.

Apollo/Chennai is one of the four Apollo
centers of excellence in India. Specialties
include cardiology and cardiothoracic

surgery, cancer care, cosmetic surgery,
nephrology and urology, orthopedics, and
radiology and imaging sciences.

Best-known for its orthopedics and cardiology superspecialties, Apollo/Chennai
has performed thousands of hip resurfacing
surgeries, with a success rate of 98.3 percent. Similarly, the hospital has performed
more than 27,000 heart surgeries, with a
current success rate of 99.6 percent (higher
than most US hospitals' success rates).

For patients interested in alternative
therapies, Apollo/Chennai offers the world's
only comprehensive, hospital-based **Wellness Center,** occupying a full floor of the
hospital. Holistic healing therapies, such as
Ayurvedic medicine, aromatherapy, pranic
healing, yoga, meditation, and music therapy, are offered to international patients as
part of Apollo/Chennai's complimentary
recovery package.

Apollo Dental Centre
21, Greams Road
Opp. M.R.F
Chennai, INDIA 600 006
Tel: 011 91 44 2829.4080
Web: www.apollodentalcentre.com

Apollo actually operates four dental centers
in Chennai, as well as others in Bangalore
and Hyderabad. This one is located adjacent
to the Apollo corporate headquarters and
main Apollo Hospital in Chennai. It offers a
full range of dental care, including crowns
and bridges, inlays and onlays, dentures,
dental implants, root canals, restorative
surgery, cosmetic dentistry, and pediatric
dentistry. Restorations are guaranteed for
two years; advanced crowns and bridges
and injection-molded dentures are guaranteed for five years.

Institute of Cardiovascular Diseases
Madras Medical Mission Hospital
4-A, Dr. J. Jayalalitha Nagar
Mogappair
Chennai, INDIA 600 037
Tel: 011 91 44 2656.1801
Fax: 011 91 44 2656.5510
Email: icvddoctors@mmm.org.in
Web: www.madrasmedicalmission.org

This unit of **Madras Medical Mission Hospital** is one of India's top cardiovascular centers. Its surgeons performed southern India's first heart transplant and India's first bilateral lung transplant, pediatric heart transplant, and simultaneous heart and lung transplant. The parents of ailing children will be happy to learn that the Institute of Cardiovascular Diseases specializes in pediatrics; 25 percent of the institute's patients are kids.

The **Department of Cardiac Surgery** performs approximately 2,000 operations annually, mostly coronary artery bypass procedures, deploying off-pump methodology. Valve replacements are a big specialty, and the institute gives special emphasis to repair techniques that preserve the patient's own valves wherever possible. New and traditional repair techniques, such as chordal shortening, quadrangular resection, and artificial chordae, are used as needed.

The **Paediatric Cardiac Surgical Department** handles the entire spectrum of congenital cardiac anomalies in children from newborns to adolescents. Approximately 8,000 cases of congenital cardiac anomalies have been treated at the institute. The department has performed more than 150 Ross operations in patients as young as three months. Besides operating on the "simpler" anomalies, such as atrial septal defect, ventricular septal defect, and patent ductus arteriosus, the pediatric department handles the more complex anomalies, including hypoplastic left heart syndrome, transposition of great arteries, complete atrioventricular canal defect, and total anomalous pulmonary venous drainage.

Sankara Nethralaya Eye Hospital
"The Temple of the Eye"
18, College Road, Nungambakkam
Chennai, Tamil Nadu, INDIA 600 006
Tel: 011 91 44 2827.1616
Fax: 011 91 44 2825.4180
Email: mrf@snmail.org
Web: www.sankaranethralaya.org

Established in 1978, Sankara Nethralaya Eye Hospital has been recognized by leading Indian media and government sources as one of the country's finest. Daily, the hospital sees 1,200 patients and performs 100 eye operations in 22 operating theaters.

Sankara Nethralaya's ophthalmic subspecialties include cataract and refractive corneal surgery, glaucoma, uveitis, vitreoretinal surgery, pediatric ophthalmology, squint, and neuroophthalmology.

Sankara is particularly proud of its **Ocular Oncology Department,** which diagnoses and treats eye cancer, retinal tumors, and cancers in surrounding structures. Deploying recent innovations, such as transpupillary thermotherapy (TTT), has enabled the clinic to save eyes and lives, according to its founder. The department treats choroidal melanoma and has the expertise and instrumentation to perform complicated surgical procedures, such as total eye-wall resection brachytherapy, which can salvage—instead of removing—affected eyes.

■ RECOVERY ACCOMMODATIONS

Taj Fisherman's Cove
Covelong Beach
Kanchipuram District
Tamil Nadu, INDIA 603 112
Tel: 011 91 44 6741.3333
Fax: 011 91 44 6741.3330
Email: fishcove.chennai@tajhotels.com
Web: www.tajhotels.com

■ HOTELS: DELUXE

Note: Good, safe, reliable, full-service hotels in India aren't cheap, and budget hotels are often lacking in the amenities that help any recovering patient feel more at ease. Deluxe hotels, such as those listed here, are frequently in the $300+ range, and "moderate" hotels are often in the $200–$300 range. A breakfast buffet is usually included. Rates can vary significantly based on season and availability. Hotels in Chennai tend to be slightly less expensive than in other cities in India.

Health travel planners, as well as hospitals' international patient centers, often offer hotel discounts through their partnerships. Check with your agent or clinic before paying full freight.

Taj Connemara
2, Binny Road off Anna Salai
Chennai, INDIA 600 002
Tel: 011 91 44 6600.0000
Fax: 011 91 44 6600.0555
Email: connemara.chennai@tajhotels.com
Web: www.tajhotels.com

The Park Chennai
601, Anna Salai
Chennai, Tamil Nadu, INDIA 600 006
Tel: 011 91 44 4267.6000
Fax: 011 91 44 4214.4100
Email: resv.che@theparkhotels.com
Web: www.theparkhotels.com

■ HOTELS: MODERATE

The Residency Towers
115, Sir Theagaraya Road
T. Nagar
Chennai, INDIA 600 017
Tel: 011 91 44 2815.6363
Fax: 011 91 44 2815.6969
Email: restowers@vsnl.net
Web: www.theresidency.com

Comfort Inn Marina Towers
2A Ponniamman Koiil Street
Egmore
Chennai, INDIA 600 008
Tel: 011 91 44 2858.5454
Fax: 011 91 44 2852.9998
Email: hotelhelp@choicehotels.com
Web: www.choicehotels.com

■ **AT A GLANCE**

Mumbai

Language:	Hindi (English widely spoken in professional and medical circles)
Time Zone:	GMT +5:30
Country Dialing Code:	91
Electricity:	220V, Plug types B & E
Currency:	Rupee
Visa Required?	Yes
Recommended Immunizations:	Hepatitis A; Boosters for Typhoid and Polio; Antimalarial Drugs
Treatment Specialties:	Cardiovascular, Cosmetic, Dental, Fertility/Reproduction, General Surgery, Ophthalmology, Orthopedics, Weight Loss
Leading Hospitals and Clinics:	Asian Heart Institute and Research Center, Jaslok Hospital and Research Centre, Dr. L. H. Hiranandani Hospital, Wockhardt Hospital and Heart Institute, Lilavati Hospital and Research Centre, Rotunda: The Center for Human Reproduction, Shroff Eye Hospital and LASIK Center
JCI-Accredited Hospitals:	Asian Heart Institute and Research Center, Shroff Eye Hospital and LASIK Center, Wockhardt Superspecialty Hospital
Standards and Accreditation:	Ministry of Health and Family Welfare, Medical Council of India, Indian Medical Association, Indian Health Care Federation, British Medical Association (BMA), General Medical Council (GMC), JCI

■ TREATMENT BRIEF

India's most populous city, Mumbai, and its surrounding area are home to 20 million, making it the world's fifth most populated urban center. Formerly Bombay (Portuguese for "good bay"), Mumbai is the economic and entertainment hub of India.

With six large private hospitals and a number of specialty treatment centers serving international patients, Mumbai now counts healthcare as one of its most important economic assets, along with engineering, information technology, and film. ("Bollywood" is king in India, and any hospital visitor with a television will be treated to some lively and colorful cinematic productions.) Mumbai is India's New York, bristling with commercial activity and cultural diversity, extreme in every imaginable way.

Mumbai is headquarters to two large, multispecialty hospitals, the JCI-accredited Wockhardt Hospital and the renowned Jaslok Hospital and Research Centre. Wockhardt's treatment center in Mumbai has established five superspecialty clinics for cardiology, neurology, orthopedics, ophthalmology, and minimally invasive surgery. One of Wockhardt's two superspecialty Heart Institutes is in Mumbai, offering a full range of cardiovascular diagnostics and surgeries.

Jaslok Hospital, one of India's oldest and most venerated, offers 35 specialties, with a fully loaded International Services Department. Mumbai also hosts smaller, prestigious, single-specialty clinics, such as the JCI-accredited Shroff Eye Hospital and LASIK Center, as well as Rotunda: The Center for Human Reproduction.

■ TYPICAL TREATMENTS AND COSTS

Cardiovascular:
Coronary Artery Bypass Graft: $8,800
Pacemaker (single-chambered): $6,500
Pacemaker (double-chambered): $9,000

Orthopedic:
Birmingham Hip Resurfacing: $9,900
Joint Replacement:
   Knee: $8,400
   Hip: $9,500
   Ankle: $7,100
   Shoulder: $8,400

Cosmetic:
Breast Augmentation: $3,300-$5,300
Breast Lift/Reduction: $3,300-$5,050
Facelift: $5,700
Liposuction (stomach, hips, and waist):
   $1,000-$2,650

Dental:
Porcelain Veneer: $420
Crown (all porcelain): $360
Inlays and Onlays: $600-$1,100
Implant (titanium with crown): $1,100

Vision:
Glaucoma: $1,050
LASIK (per eye): $810

Weight Loss:
LAP-BAND System: $6,600
Gastric Bypass: $7,200

■ HEALTH TRAVEL AGENTS

BestMed Journeys
6619 Thirteenth Avenue
Brooklyn, NY 11219
Tel: 1 616 300.8600
Fax: 1 646 300.8601
Email: info@bestmedjourneys.com
Web: www.bestmedjourneys.com

BestMed Journeys entered the medical travel arena in 2007. It serves India, has an in-country office in Chennai, and boasts staff members who speak a variety of Indian dialects as well as English. BestMed offers all the usual services, including passport and visas, airline tickets, ground transportation, food delivery, and laundry services, plus accommodations at one of the agency's fully furnished executive apartments. In Mumbai, BestMed sends health travelers to Dr. L. H. Hiranandani Hospital and Wockhardt Hospital and Heart Institute (see "Hospitals and Clinics," below).

Healthbase Online, Inc.
287 Auburn Street
Newton, MA 02466
Tel: 1 888 691.4584 (US toll-free);
1 617 418.3436
Fax: 1 800 986.9230 (US toll-free)
Email: info.hb@healthbase.com
Web: www.healthbase.com

For more information on Healthbase Online, see India: Chennai.

IndUSHealth
7413 Six Forks Road, #362
Raleigh, NC 27615
Tel: 1 800 779.1314 (US toll-free)
Fax: 1 888 627.6492 (US toll-free)
Email: info@indushealth.com
Web: www.indushealth.com

For more information on IndUSHealth, see India: Delhi.

Medical Tourist Vacations
530 East Patriot Boulevard, #172
Reno, NV 89511
Tel: 1 775 852.5105
Fax: 1 775 852.5105
Email: contact@medicaltouristvacations.com
Web: www.medicaltouristvacations.com

Meditours
1055 Gibson Road
Kelowna, BC, CANADA
Tel: 1 250 765.2842
Email: shaz@meditours.org
Web: www.meditours.org

Established in 2005 and operated by Shaz Pendharkar, this Kelowna, BC-based agency serves US as well as Canadian and world clientele. Meditours specializes in hip and knee surgeries. The agency also works with excellent dentists and plastic surgeons.

Meditours is the exclusive agent for Jaslok Hospital and Research Centre (see "Hospitals and Clinics," below). The agency also serves other established Mumbai-area centers, including the JCI-accredited Shroff Eye Hospital and LASIK Center and Dental Innovations. Ninety-five percent of Meditours patients are American or Canadian. All Meditours-recommended physicians are either US-trained or US board-certified.

In addition, Meditours maintains good relations with Kerala-based hospitals, including the Kerala Institute of Medical Sciences (KIMS) and the Malabar Institute of Medical Sciences. One advantage to treatment in Kerala is its superb resort facilities on the Arabian Sea and scenic rivers. Kerala is also the reputed home of Ayurvedic medicine, and KIMS in Trinvandrum now has a complete floor dedicated to Ayurvedic treatments.

Med Journeys

2020 Broadway, Suite 4C
New York, NY 10023
Tel: 1 888 633.5769 (US toll-free);
   1 212 931.0557
Fax: 1 212 656.1134
Email: sonnyk@medjourneys.com
Web: www.medjourneys.com

For more information on Med Journeys, see India: Delhi.

MedRetreat

2042 Laurel Valley Drive
Vernon Hills, IL 60061
Tel: 1 877 876.3373 (US toll-free)
Fax: 1 847 680.0484
Email: customerservice@medretreat.com
Web: www.medretreat.com

For more information on MedRetreat, see Malaysia.

Planet Hospital

23679 Calabasas Road, Suite 150
Calabasas, CA 91302
Tel: 1 800 243.0172 (US toll-free); 1 818 665.4801
Fax: 1 818 665.4810
Email: rudy@planethospital.com
Web: www.planethospital.com

For more information on Planet Hospital, see Singapore.

Recover Discover Healthcare

G 47, Sector 6, Noida
Uttar Pradesh, INDIA
Tel: 011 91 120 435.9281
Fax: 011 91 120 425.8281
Email: contactus@recoverdiscover.com
Web: www.recoverdiscover.com

For more information on Recover Discover Healthcare, see India: Delhi.

The Taj Medical Group, Limited

408 West 57th Street, Suite 9N
New York, NY 10019
Tel: 1 877 799.9797 (US toll-free)
Email: info@tajmedical.com
Web: www.tajmedical.com

For more information on Taj Medical Group, see India: Delhi.

WorldMed Assist

1230 Mountain Side Court
Concord, CA 94521
Tel: 1 866 999.3848 (US toll-free)
Fax: 1 925 905.5898
Email: whoeber@worldmedassist.com
Web: www.worldmedassist.com

For more information on WorldMed Assist, see India: Bangalore.

■ HOSPITALS AND CLINICS

Asian Heart Institute and Research Center

Bandra Kurla Complex, Bandra (E)
Mumbai, INDIA 400 051
Tel: 011 91 22 6698.6666
Fax: 011 91 22 6698.6506
Email: info@ahirc.com
Web: www.ahirc.com

Asian Heart Institute and Research Center (AHIRC) was established by Contemporary Healthcare Pvt. Ltd. and six of India's top cardiac specialists. A 15-minute drive from Mumbai's domestic and international airports, the hospital forms part of the new Bandra Kurla Complex (BKC), a $250 million business-shopping-healthcare-living complex in northern Mumbai.

In 2005 surgeons at the hospital performed 1,218 coronary surgeries and procedures with a mortality rate of less than 0.5 percent. All coronary procedures at AHIRC deploy the beating-heart technique, which reduces post-operative complications and the length of hospital stays.

In addition to coronary artery surgery, AHIRC specializes in the Maze procedure for atrial fibrillation, valve repair and replacement, and aneurysm surgery of the aorta and other blood vessels. A special pediatric team operates on all types of cardiac conditions in children.

Asian Heart Institute's **International Patients Department** offers airport pickup and dropoff, hotel accommodations and local travel arrangements for companions, consultations with physicians and surgeons, prayer rooms, and Internet facilities.

Jaslok Hospital and Research Centre

15 - Dr. Deshmukh Marg
Pedder Road
Mumbai, INDIA 400 026
Tel: 011 91 6657.3333
Fax: 011 91 2352.0508
Email: info@jaslokhospital.net
Web: www.jaslokhospital.net

Jaslok Hospital and Research Centre is a private multispecialty hospital with 376 beds, 124 full-time resident physicians, and around 100 consulting physicians. Jaslok has its own department of nursing, employing 495 nurses and 60 students.

Jaslok is one of India's top independent private hospitals, with 35 established specialties. Of interest to the international health traveler are radiation oncology, cardiovascular and thoracic surgery, advanced dental surgery, dermatology, ophthalmology, orthopedics, urology, oncosurgery, and nuclear medicine radiation oncology. Jaslok also boasts a **Neuroscience Division,** a **Department of Chest Diseases,** and a **Department of Infertility Management and Assisted Reproduction.**

The hospital's **International Services Department** provides airport pickup, translator, an onsite coordinator for appointments and consultations, locker facilities, and customized cuisine.

Dr. L. H. Hiranandani Hospital

Hill Side Avenue, Hiranandani Gardens
  Powai
Mumbai, INDIA 400 076
Tel: 011 91 22 2576.3300
Fax: 011 91 22 2576.3311
Email: wecare@hiranandanihospital.org
Web: www.hiranandanihospital.org

A newcomer to the Mumbai healthcare scene, the Dr. L. H. Hiranandani Hospital (LHH) opened its doors in early 2004 with 130 beds. More than 30 specialties and subspecialties are offered. LHH's centers of excellence include cardiology (including primary angioplasty), joint replacement and hip resurfacing, human reproduction, bariatric surgery, hair rejuvenation surgery, dental surgery, and ophthalmology.

LHH aggressively promotes its "International Health Checks." Overseas patients can choose silver, gold, or platinum health check packages for liver, diabetic, pulmonary, osteoporosis, renal, thyroid, ophthalmology, and cholesterol tests. Cancer marker tests and mammography are also offered. You can find detailed information about each health check on the LHH Web site under "Overseas Patients."

Lilavati Hospital and Research Centre

A-791, Bandra Reclamation
Bandra (W)
Mumbai, INDIA 400 050
Tel: 011 91 22 2642.1111
Fax: 011 91 22 2640.7655
Email: lilaworld@lilavatihospital.com
Web: www.lilavatihospital.com

Established in 1996, this 329-bed hospital in the heart of Mumbai is known for its cardiovascular and oncology surgeries, orthopedics, and in vitro fertilization (IVF). Lilavati's **LilaWorld Assistant Cell** was established as a special wing of the hospital to accommodate international patients. Amenities include a yoga center, 24-hour pharmacy, temple, and meditation center.

Rotunda: The Center for Human Reproduction

672, Kalpak Gulistan, Perry Cross Road
Opp Brahmakumari Gardens, Bandra (W)
Mumbai, INDIA 400 050
Tel: 011 91 22 655.2000
Fax: 011 91 22 655.3000
Email: rotundachr@gmail.com
Web: www.iwannagetpregnant.com

Fertility consultation and treatment are usually long and emotionally arduous processes. As most couples struggling with these issues know, they are also expensive and not covered by health insurance. Many couples choose to get started abroad, then return to the US to continue treatment and hook up with support groups and ongoing counseling. Founded in 1963, Rotunda is India's most respected fertility treatment facility. In-house pathology, endoscopy, and sonography services allow a couple to undergo all tests under one roof. In addition to the standard fertility services, Rotunda also offers gestational surrogacy services, donor egg in vitro fertilization (IVF), laser-assisted hatching, and a recurrent pregnancy loss clinic. It is India's only lesbian-gay-bisexual-transsexual-friendly center. Rotunda treats about 100 international patients annually.

Shroff Eye Hospital and LASIK Center

222 S. V. Road Bandra (West)
Mumbai, INDIA 400 050
Tel: 011 91 22 6692.1000
Fax: 011 91 22 6694.9880
Email: safalashroff@yahoo.com
Web: www.lasikindia.in

Established in 1919 and family-run since its inception, the Shroff Eye Hospital and LASIK Center is one of only three JCI-accredited

Case Study: Lisa S., San Antonio, Texas

I was diagnosed with complex hyperplasia with atypical cells, which means my uterus is too thick and not viable for carrying a baby. The cost of surrogacy in the US is astronomical, especially if you don't have a volunteer surrogate such as a family member or close friend. So I went to Mumbai, India, where the laws are favorable and the cost is manageable. In Mumbai, I underwent in vitro fertilization using my husband's sperm. My embryos were then implanted in a surrogate mother. We are now expecting twins.

My doctor and his staff were excellent. They accommodated us at every turn, calling us immediately with test results and scheduling appointments that accommodated us and our travel plans. The medical facilities were consistently clean. The staffs were courteous and well organized.

The worst thing was seeing the poverty of India. It was heart wrenching to say the least. We, however, had no problems in India, but we did have some concern about our American doctors resisting cooperation with the Indian team.

We had reverse sticker shock when we saw the prices. We had saved approximately $50,000. Finally, we had found healthcare we could afford! My advice for others who are thinking of going overseas for medical procedures is this: consider using a health travel facilitator. These agents arrange more than travel. In my case, my agent found my doctors, who specialize in IVF and have a surrogacy program. They arranged my medical appointments, got me in direct contact with my doctor when I had medical questions or concerns, and arranged my travel. A facilitator makes planning the trip so much easier, especially if you have not traveled for healthcare before.

vision hospitals in the world. (The other two are in Turkey and Spain.) Drs. Rahul Ashok and Anand Ashok Shroff, along with 23 other physicians and consultants, provide full-service vision diagnosis and treatment, catering to international travelers from 87 countries. Treatments include phacoemulsification cataract surgery, vitreoretinal surgery (for treating advanced diabetic retinopathy, retinal detachment, macular hole, and other retinal diseases), LASIK surgery, glaucoma surgery, squint surgery, keratoplasty and other corneal surgeries, oculoplastic surgery, and other cosmetic treatments.

Shroff Eye Hospital also runs seven superspecialty clinics, including

■ **Diabetic Retinopathy Clinic,** which is dedicated to the identification and long-term care of diabetics at risk for diabetic retinopathy. The clinic is equipped with digital angiography systems, retinal sonography, various lasers, and advanced vitreoretinal surgery equipment to provide treatment to patients with even advanced forms of the disorder.

- **Macular Degeneration Clinic,** for treatment of this disorder common among older people. Digital fluorescein angiography and indocyanine-green angiography are used to diagnose the condition. Treatment is provided in the form of photodynamic therapy.

- **Glaucoma Clinic,** offering a full range of diagnostics, including the Humphrey computerized visual field analyzer, to help prevent further damage to vision.

- **Uveitis Clinic,** including a pathology laboratory that provides the complete range of exams and tests.

- **Cornea Clinic,** providing therapeutic and diagnostic capabilities for corneal disorders, including all aspects of anterior segment imaging, such as corneal topography and pachymetry.

- **Squint/Pediatric Ophthalmology Clinic,** specializing in children with strabismus ("crossed eyes") and amblyopia ("lazy eyes"), and offering prescriptions for glasses and complete eye exams for infants and children. Adults with strabismus who desire strabismus surgery or eye muscle surgery are also seen here.

- The Shroffs are particularly proud of their **LASIK Clinic,** which deploys the latest wavefront-guided LASIK technology. Also known as custom LASIK, the treatment involves new technologies that measure distortions in the eye, providing the physician with the information needed to chart a treatment plan customized to each patient. Shroff was the first eye hospital in India to launch the 500-Hz Concerto Laser; it's one of only six in the world.

Wockhardt Superspecialty Hospital

Mulund Goregaon Link Road
Mumbai, INDIA
Tel: 1 800 730.6373 (US and Canada toll-free); 011 91 22 6799.4444
Email: pthukral@wockhardt.com
Web: www.wockhardt.com

Known throughout Asia and the rest of the world for its specialty centers, Wockhardt is one of India's shining healthcare stars, particularly in the area of heart disease and surgeries. The group, headquartered in Mumbai, first set up a heart hospital in Bangalore in 1990. Wockhardt now operates 15 hospitals across India and plans to expand to 30 hospitals by 2010. Its flagship hospital at Mumbai boasts several centers of excellence, including cardiac care, orthopedics, neurosurgery, and oncology. Wockhardt's Mumbai location also offers its world-renowned **Hip Resurfacing Clinic,** where hundreds of patients from America and Europe have been treated in last few years.

An exclusive partnership with Harvard Medical International (HMI), a division of Boston's Harvard Medical School, gives Wockhardt access to top-flight international medical expertise, along with standards oversight and best practices discipline. Through its HMI partnership, Wockhardt benefits from joint development of new clinical programs, a nursing leadership and development program, continuous improvement programs in care-pathway delivery, and various quality improvement initiatives.

In 2005 Wockhardt Hospital and Heart Institute in Mumbai became the first super-specialty hospital in South Asia to receive JCI accreditation.

Wockhardt Hospital/Mumbai's major specialties include

■ **Advanced Orthopedics and Joint Surgery:** This, one of the largest centers in Asia offering the Birmingham hip resurfacing procedure, attracts hundreds of patients every year from North America and Europe. In addition to hip resurfacing, this center specializes in computer-navigated knee and shoulder joint replacements and in arthroscopic surgery.

■ **Wockhardt Brain and Spine Hospital:** A team of ten specialists, trained mostly in the UK and the US, have created an internationally recognized center for the diagnosis and treatment of brain and spinal conditions. Specialties include stereotactic brain surgery (deploying brain scans, image guidance, and minimally invasive techniques); cerebrovascular surgery (aneurysms); movement disorder surgery (including deep brain stimulation for Parkinson's disease, dystonia, and multiple sclerosis); and various treatments for neuromuscular disorders. The new **Specialty Epilepsy Clinic** deploys up-to-date methods for diagnosing and treating epilepsy and other seizure-related conditions.

■ **Minimal Access Surgeries Centre:** This center offers laparoscopic surgery for appendectomy, gall bladder removal, hernia repair, spleen removal, colorectal polyps and cancers, adrenalectomy, pancreatic tumors, and obesity. It also offers

transurethral resection of prostate (TURP), percutaneous nephrolithotripsy (PCNL), laparoscopic urology, thoracoscopic surgery, and minimal-access cardiac surgeries.

■ **Wockhardt Obesity Surgery Centre:** This center offers a comprehensive range of procedures, including gastric banding, gastric bypass, and sleeve gastrectomy.

■ **Organ Transplants Centre:** The center performs liver and kidney transplants. The hospital adheres strictly to Indian legal norms permitting only live and related donors.

■ **Wockhardt Cancer Hospital:** This hospital offers a complete range of medical and surgical oncology services, and a state-of-the-art center for radiation therapy is scheduled to open soon.

As with many other private Indian hospitals, Wockhardt's outpatient rooms include an attached bathroom, companion sofa-bed, laundry service, color TV with DVD player, and a computer terminal with Internet connection.

■ Wockhardt's **International Patient Service Centre** offers airport pickup and dropoff, travel arrangements, coordination of appointments, arrangements for accommodating companions and family, locker facilities for valuables, and cuisine tailored to suit individual palates.

Wockhardt offers a credit card payment gateway on its Web site, a toll-free phone helpline in the US and the UK, and a 24-hour contact center for international patients.

■ HOTELS: DELUXE

Note: Good, safe, reliable, full-service hotels in India aren't cheap, and budget hotels are often lacking in the amenities that help any recovering patient feel more at ease. Deluxe hotels such as those listed here are frequently in the $300+ range, and "moderate" hotels are often in the $200–$300 range. A breakfast buffet is usually included. Rates can vary significantly based on season and availability.

Health travel planners, as well as hospitals' international patient centers, often offer hotel discounts through their partnerships. Check with your agent or clinic before paying full freight.

Fariyas Hotel
25, off Arthur Bunder Road
Colaba, Mumbai, INDIA 400 005
Tel: 011 91 22 2204.2911
Fax: 011 91 22 2283.4992
Email: info@fariyas.com
Web: www.fariyas.com

Taj President Hotel
90, Cuffe Parade
Mumbai, INDIA 400 005
Tel: 1 866 969.1825 (US toll-free); 011 91 22 6601.1825
Fax: 011 91 22 6665.0303
Email: president.mumbai@tajhotels.com
Web: www.tajhotels.com

Taj Lands End Mumbai Hotel
Bandstand, Bandra (West) Maharashtra
Mumbai, INDIA 400 050
Tel: 1 866 969.1825 (US toll-free); 011 91 22 6668.1234
Fax: 011 91 022 6699.4488
Email: landsend.mumbai@tajhotels.com
Web: www.tajhotels.com

Hotel Leela Kempinski
Sahar
Mumbai, INDIA 400 059
Tel: 011 91 22 6691.1234
Fax: 011 91 22 6691.1455
Email: reservations.mumbai@theleela.com
Web: www.theleela.com/hotel-mumbai.html

■ HOTELS: MODERATE

Sea Princess
969, Juhu Tara Road, Juhu Beach
Maharashtra, Mumbai, INDIA 400 049
Tel: 011 91 22 2661.1111
Fax: 011 91 22 2661.1144
Email: seaprincess@vsnl.com
Web: www.seaprincess.com

Best Western - The Emerald
Juhu Tara Road, Juhu
Mumbai, INDIA 400 049
Tel: 011 91 22 6714.4000
Fax: 011 91 22 6714.4005
Web: www.bestwestern.com

Dream Residency Hotel
Mulund Goregaon Link Road, opposite Wockhardt Hospital
Mulund (West) Mumbai, INDIA 400 080
Tel: 011 91 22 2590.7551

Hotel Executive Enclave
331, Dr. Ambedkar Road
Pali Hill, Bandra (West)
Mumbai, INDIA 400 050
Tel: 011 91 22 6696.9000
Fax: 011 91 22 6696.9001
Email: enclave@vsnl.com
Web: www.executiveenclave.com

DESTINATION: **ISRAEL**

■ **AT A GLANCE**

Jerusalem, Haifa, and Tel Aviv

Language:	Hebrew (English widely spoken)
Time Zone:	GMT +2
Country Dialing Code:	972
Electricity:	230V, Plug type B
Currency:	Shekel
Visa Required?	No
Recommended Immunizations:	Hepatitis A
Treatment Specialties:	Infertility, Cardiology, Orthopedics, General Surgery, Gynecology, Urology
Leading Hospitals and Clinics:	Hadassah University Medical Centers, Assaf Harofeh Medical Center, Chaim Sheba Medical Center, Tel Aviv Sourasky Medical Center, Rabin Medical Center, Herzliya Medical Center
JCI-Accredited Hospitals:	None
Standards and Accreditation:	Academic Council of the Israel Medical Association

■ **TREATMENT BRIEF**

Wars and rumors of wars may make you think twice about Israel as a health travel destination, but that second thought might be worth the effort—and the money. Although many Westerners feel uneasy about the political turmoil of the Middle East, Israel itself is a modern, independent, and advanced nation that has a lot to offer health travelers—and Israel's government is now actively promoting medical tourism. Standards are high, doctors are plentiful and well trained, and the medical technology employed in top hospitals is state-of-the-art.

Israel's 47 general hospitals comprise approximately 13,000 beds. Another 14,000 beds are available for chronic-care patients (including geriatric patients) and some 7,000 for psychiatric patients. Nearly half of those beds are in government-operated facilities. Almost 20 percent are in hospitals run by nonprofit and religious organizations.

Israel has four medical schools, each affiliated with a major university: the Hebrew University Medical School associated with the Hadassah Medical Organization, the Tel Aviv University Medical School, the Technion Medical School in Haifa, and the Ben-Gurion University Medical School in Be'er Sheva. Israel also has two schools of dentistry, one of pharmacology, and 20 nursing schools. Courses for physiotherapists, occupational therapists, nutritionists, x-ray technicians, and laboratory technicians are offered at several institutions.

The top Israeli hospitals are equipped with the same state-of-the-art medical instruments routinely used in diagnosis in the US and Europe. Israel is also known for the design and manufacture of medical equipment. Israel's computer-assisted tomography (CAT) scanners and advanced microcomputer-supported devices are exported widely. The country has pioneered the development and use of laser surgical instruments, computerized monitoring systems, and other life-saving and pain-relieving devices.

No overview of healthcare in Israel would be complete without mention of Israel's in vitro fertilization (IVF) centers, which rank among the world's finest. The IVF unit at Chaim Sheba is the largest in the country. Assuta, IVF Haifa, and Rabin are well known for their excellence. Couples seeking fertility services should also check out Hadassah, Tel Aviv Sourasky, and Herzliya. Prices for fertility services can total a fraction of those found in North America. At one clinic in Israel, for example, the price

of a standard IVF cycle is about $3,000, whereas couples expect to pay $12,000 or more in the US.

For sightseers and history buffs, Israel offers an abundance of both. Jerusalem and its environs abound with religious and historical sites venerated by three of the world's major religions. In Israel's bustling markets, shoppers will find antiques, rugs, jewelry, and more. Israel has 50 national parks, many of which are also historic sites.

Those planning health travel should not overlook the Dead Sea spas and medical centers, which treat a variety of disorders from psoriasis to arthritis pain.

■ TYPICAL TREATMENTS AND COSTS

Cardiovascular:
Coronary Artery Bypass Graft: $25,000
Bypass + Valve Replacement (single): $25,000
Bypass + Valve Replacement (double): $25,000
Pacemaker (single-chambered): $1,000
Pacemaker (double-chambered): $3,000

Orthopedic:
Joint Replacement:
  Knee: $11,000-$18,500
  Hip: $18,000
  Ankle: $18,500
  Shoulder: $18,500

Cosmetic:
Breast Augmentation: $4,000
Breast Lift/Reduction: $8,000
Facelift: $7,800

Liposuction (stomach, hips, and waist):
  $2,500-$7,500
Tummy Tuck: $7,800

Vision:
Glaucoma: $4,500
LASIK (per eye): $1,000

Weight Loss:
LAP-BAND System: $12,500

Fertility/Reproductive Health:
IVF: $3,000-$3,250

Other:
Gall Bladder Removal: $5,000
Prostate Surgery (TURP): $5,000

■ HEALTH TRAVEL AGENTS

IMS Global, Limited
63/12 Hanessim Street, Kfar Ganim
Petach Tikva, ISRAEL 49550
Tel: 1 201 716.2276 (US); 011 972 3908.0570
Fax: 011 972 3909.0764
Email: info@medicaltourismforyou.com
Web: www.medicaltourismforyou.com

Established in 2007, IMS Global arranges
medical travel to 18 medical centers in Israel. IMS has three divisions: one focuses on
fertility, another on children, and the third
on adults. The company provides end-to-
end service and a variety of packages tailored to individual needs. Patients generally
travel from the US, Europe, and the former
Soviet Union. IMS charges no fees for arranging medical travel to Israel unless the
patient wants luxury services.

■ HOSPITALS AND CLINICS

Assaf Harofeh Medical Center
P.O. Beer Yaacov
Zerifin, ISRAEL 70300
Tel: 011 972 8977.9500
Email: assaf@netguide.co.il
Web: http://ahmc.netguide.co.il

Assaf Harofeh Medical Center, one of Israel's
largest, is an 800-bed facility in central
Israel. Located less than ten miles from Tel
Aviv and Ben Gurion Airport, the hospital
cares for a relatively large number of medical travelers, priding itself on offering pleas-
ant and peaceful modern facilities and the
best in Western medicine.

The center provides general medical,
surgical, cardiac, pediatric, neonatal, gynecological, and obstetric services, as well as
24-hour emergency services, intensive care,
and ambulatory psychiatric services. Open-
heart surgery and irradiation therapy are
provided in conjunction with neighboring
hospitals.

The hospital is an academic teaching
facility and part of the Tel Aviv University
Sackler Faculty of Medicine. The first and
largest academic nursing school and Israel's
oldest school of physiotherapy are located
on the hospital grounds.

Assaf Harofeh offers a variety of special
outpatient services for medical travelers.
These include periodic checkups, dialysis
treatments, emergency medical treatment,
and a wide range of diagnostic procedures.

Chaim Sheba Medical Center

Tel Hashomer, ISRAEL 52621
Tel: 011 972 3530.3030
Fax: 011 972 3530.3515
Email: med-tour@sheba.health.gov.il
Web: http://eng.sheba.co.il

With 1,900 beds, Chaim Sheba Medical Center is the largest and most comprehensive tertiary medical center in the Middle East. It is affiliated with the Sackler Faculty of Medicine of Tel Aviv University. Along with a major acute-care hospital and a rehabilitation hospital, Sheba's specialty centers include the **Heart Institute, Cardiac Surgery Department, Orthopedics Department, Eye Institute, Genetics and Fertility Department (IVF), Child Development Department, Burn Unit, Maxillofacial Department, Diagnostic Imaging Institute, Interventional Radiology and Radiosurgery Department, Pediatric Hematooncology Department, Bone Marrow Transplantation Department,** and **Oncology Institute.**

Sheba's efforts to attract medical travelers date back to 1990, when the hospital began to establish official agreements with health ministries in many countries and to treat patients from Russia, the Ukraine, Turkey, Greece, Italy, and Jordan. Sheba's **Department for Medical Tourist Services** is staffed by nurses and an administrative aide who personally assist patients during their medical visits. The staff in this department is fluent in English and all medical reports are provided in English.

For those who wish to remain close to a patient during his or her stay at the hospital, Sheba offers guest accommodations. The Apropo Hotel is located in the **General Hospital**'s shopping mall. **The Rehabilitation Hotel** is located near the **Rehabilitation Center.**

Hadassah University Medical Centers

P.O. Box 12000
Jerusalem, ISRAEL 91120
Tel: 011 972 2677.8555
Fax: 011 972 2677.7500
Email: shivuk@hadassah.org.il
Web: www.hadassah.org.il

The Hadassah University Medical Centers in Jerusalem receive international patients for complicated operations on the knee, hip, eye, brain, and nervous system. The centers boast world-class surgeons and substantial cost savings over medical centers in many other countries. Specialties include oncology, hematology, bone marrow (human cell) transplantation, orthopedic surgery, ophthalmology, cardiac and vascular surgery, and minimally invasive surgeries of all types. Most frequently performed procedures are joint replacements, coronary artery bypasses, heart valve replacements, and colon surgeries.

The Hadassah Web site offers pages in several languages for each medical department, giving Internet users the ability to contact specific treatment centers directly. Hadassah treats about 2,500 international patients annually.

Rabin Medical Center

Jabutinski Street 39
Petah-Tikva, ISRAEL 49100
Tel: 011 972 3937.6666 (Beilinson); 011 972 3937.2222 (Hasharon)
Fax: 011 972 3937.6364
Email: rmc-cs@clalit.org.il
Web: www.clalit.org.il

The Rabin Medical Center (RMC) is located 20 minutes from Tel Aviv. Composed of the Beilinson and Golda-Hasharon campuses, RMC is the largest medical center in Israel. This tertiary-care facility is affiliated with the Tel Aviv University Sackler School of Medicine.

RMC's **Department of Organ Transplantation** performs organ transplants, including kidney, liver, and pancreas. It's the only place in Israel where multiorgan and live-donor liver transplants are performed. The **Department of Cardiothoracic Surgery** is the country's largest, performing over 1,300 procedures annually. One quarter of the operations are performed on children hospitalized in the adjacent **Schneider Children's Medical Center of Israel,** and an additional 300 operations are performed at **Kaplan Hospital** in Rechovot. A heart and lung transplant unit is an integral part of the department.

RMC's **Institute of Oncology** is the largest in Israel, treating patients referred from hospitals throughout the country and abroad. The **Cardiac Catheterization Unit** in the **Department of Cardiology** assists thousands of patients in avoiding surgical procedures with the help of specialists in interventional heart catheterization. The **Pulmonary Institute** treats complex respiratory diseases and critical patients before and after lung transplants. The **Women's Comprehensive Health Center** provides a full range of medical services for women, from puberty through menopause.

RMC provides patients with private accommodations while hospitalized, including single rooms with adjacent bathroom and shower. RMC will help find accommodation for patients' companions in nearby facilities. The center also provides patients with an escort during the entire length of their hospitalization. A medical summary report is provided in English and in other languages as needed at the end of the patient's stay.

Tel Aviv Sourasky Medical Center

6 Weizmann Street
Tel Aviv, ISRAEL 64239
Tel: 011 972 3697.4254
Fax: 011 972 3697.3635
Email: medtour@tasmc.health.gov.il
Web: www.tasmc.org.il

The Tel Aviv Sourasky Medical Center (TASMC) is a full-service healthcare center, with comprehensive medical, surgical, and diagnostic units. It is also the national referral center for both adults and children for various specialties, including oncology, cardiology and cardiothoracic surgery, neurosurgery, orthopedic oncology, orthopedics, surgical oncology, organ transplantation, and microsurgery. TASMC has over 1,100 hospital beds, 60 departments and institutes, and 150 outpatient clinics.

Children are treated at **Dana Children's Hospital,** which offers diagnostic, inpatient, and outpatient care in all pediatric subspecialties, in an atmosphere that maximizes the children's comfort. Women receive specialized care at the **Lis Women's Hospital.** Lis provides cutting-edge services in obstetrics/gynecology, high-risk pregnancy, neonatal intensive care, in vitro fertilization (IVF), and infertility treatments. Furthermore, Lis is considered the country's leading facility for infertility and one of Israel's pioneering hospitals in the field of male infertility.

TASMC's international patients' service staff coordinates consultations, examinations, and treatments, and staff members personally accompany patients and their companions through all stages of medical treatment. International services staff members are fluent in many languages, including English, Russian, French, and Arabic.

Herzliya Medical Center
7 Ramat Yam
Herzliya On-Sea, ISRAEL 46851
Tel: 011 972 9959.2904
Fax: 011 972 9959.2535
Email: inter@hmc-ims.com
Web: www.hmc.co.il

This 93-bed private hospital is located on the Herzliya Promenade, about 15 minutes north of Tel Aviv. It has been in operation since 1982. Its special services include the **Diagnostic Imaging Institute, Gastroenterology Unit, Cardiology Institute, Dialysis Unit, Cytogenetic Institute, Laser Unit, In Vitro Fertilization Unit,** and **Executive Check-Ups.**

Herzliya Medical Center (HMC) was the first private hospital in Israel to perform heart surgery, endoscopic procedures, and neurosurgery. It was also the first in the private sector to offer computed tomography (CT) scanning, catheterization facilities, a cytogenetic laboratory, an intensive care unit, and a psychiatric ward. In 2002 Israel's Ministry of Health ranked HMC in third place in Israel for the number of coronary bypass surgeries performed on adults.

HMC has an **International Department** to assist overseas patients with every aspect of their treatment in Israel. HMC is affiliated with major American and European insurance and assistance companies, in addition to being an international referral center for many embassies and international bodies, including the United Nations. The hospital has agreements and cooperative ventures with several HMOs, supplementary insurance plans, and private medical insurance companies.

Assuta Hospital I.V.F. Center
62 Jabotinski Street
Tel Aviv, ISRAEL
Tel: 011 972 3520.1518
Fax: 011 972 3520.1750
Email: adm@ivfisrael.co.il
Web: www.ivfisrael.co.il

Assuta Hospital I.V.F. Center is one of the largest and most modern in vitro fertilization (IVF) clinics in the Mediterranean region, and it boasts a comparatively high rate of pregnancies. It is located in North Tel Aviv near the seashore, with easy access to Ben Gurion International Airport. Founded in 1987, Assuta offers treatments for both female infertility (mechanical, hormonal, and unexplained) and male infertility, including extraction of sperm from the spermatic duct and testicles, as well as injection of a single sperm into the egg using micromanipulation. The IVF clinic is affiliated with Tel Aviv Assuta Hospital, which has been in operation since 1934.

IVF Haifa
12 Yair Katz Street
Haifa, ISRAEL
Tel: 011 972 4830.9008
Fax: 011 972 4830.0086
Email: ivfisrael@gmail.com
Web: www.ivf.co.il

IVF Haifa started operation in 1996, and it's been helping couples make babies ever since. Located near the Carmel Center in Haifa, the clinic offers the most advanced services in assisted reproductive technologies (ART), including intracytoplasmic sperm insertion (ICSI), microsurgical epididymal sperm aspiration (MESA), testicular sperm aspiration (TESA), and blastocyst culture. Senior physician Dr. Shahar Kol says he is especially proud of the clinic's successful cryobiology laboratory. He and his staff perform over 1,000 oocyte-retrieval procedures a year (and about the same number of thaw cycles).

■ RECOVERY ACCOMMODATIONS

The Ein Kerem Hotel
Hadassah Ein Kerem Medical Center
Jerusalem, ISRAEL
Tel: 011 972 2560.8555
Fax: 011 972 2560.8542
Email: info@einkeremhotel.co.il
Web: www.einkeremhotel.co.il

The Ein Kerem Hotel is situated in the heart of the Hadassah Medical Center, a short walking distance from the hospital wards, outpatient clinics, and various medical facilities. It offers a variety of services geared to assisting outpatients, patients' families and companions, and business travelers.

■ HOTELS: DELUXE

The King David–Jerusalem Hotel
23 King David Street
Jerusalem, ISRAEL 94101
Tel: 1 800 223.7773 (US toll-free); 011 972 2620.8888
Fax: 011 972 2620.8882
Email: kingdavid@danhotels.com
Web: www.danhotels.co.il

Sheraton Tel Aviv
115 Hayarkon Street
Tel Aviv, ISRAEL 63573
Tel: 011 972 3521.1111
Fax: 011 972 3523.3322
Web: www.starwoodhotels.com

Dan Accadia Herzliya Hotel
Ramot-Yam 122 Street
Herzliya Beach, ISRAEL 46851
Tel: 011 972 9959.7070
Fax: 011 972 9959.7090
Email: accadia@danhotels.com
Web: www.danhotels.com

■ HOTELS: MODERATE

Eldan Hotel
24 King David Street
Jerusalem, ISRAEL
Tel: 011 972 2625.2151
Fax: 011 972 2625.2154
Email: jer_hotel@el-dan.com
Web: www.eldanhotel.com

Mount Scopus Hotel
10 Sheikh Jarrah Street
Jerusalem, ISRAEL 91196
Tel: 011 972 2582.8891
Fax: 011 972 2582.8825
Email: mtscopus@netvision.net.il
Web: http://mtscopus.com

Tadmor Hotel
38 Basel Street
Herzliya, ISRAEL
Tel: 011 972 952.5000
Fax: 011 972 957.4560
Web: www.tadmor.co.il

DESTINATION: JORDAN

■ AT A GLANCE

Amman

Language:	Arabic (many medical professionals speak English)
Time Zone:	GMT +2
Country Dialing Code:	962
Electricity:	220V, Plug types B & D
Currency:	Jordanian dinar
Visa Required?	Yes
Recommended Immunizations:	Hepatitis A; Typhoid Booster
Treatment Specialties:	Cardiology, Neurosurgery, In Vitro Fertilization, Minimally Invasive Surgery, Oncology
Leading Hospitals and Clinics:	Jordan Hospital and Medical Center, King Hussein Cancer Center, Al-Essra Hospital, Specialty Hospital
JCI-Accredited Hospitals:	Jordan Hospital and Medical Center, King Hussein Cancer Center
Standards and Accreditation:	JCI; International Society for Quality in Health Care (ISQua); Jordan's Health Care Accreditation and Certification Initiative is a work in progress

■ TREATMENT BRIEF

While Jordan has not yet become a top-ten destination for English-speaking health travelers, it soon will be if its government has its way. In 2004 the Ministry of Health challenged the country's public and private sectors to generate $1 billion annually in medical tourism income by 2010. Official figures show that between 2003 and 2006,

Jordan's health sector generated around $600 million annually in hospital fees from foreign patients alone. More than 100,000 patients entered the country for medical procedures in 2004. While fifty-six private hospitals in Jordan claim to provide services for health travelers, most of their beds are usually filled. Thus, they are expanding to accommodate health travelers.

The Jordanian government sponsors an

office at the airport in Amman to help patients upon arrival, and it seeks to promote medical travel though its embassies abroad. Jordan's health minister predicts that his nation's health travel industry will double in five years. Although Jordan's treatment costs can be as low as one-tenth of those encountered at US medical institutions, the majority of foreign patients still come from other Middle Eastern nations. According to officials, Sudan is the number-one country sending patients to Jordan, followed by Iraq and the Gulf states. Among foreign patients, most come for heart, kidney, neurological, and orthopedic surgeries.

■ TYPICAL TREATMENTS AND COSTS (procedure only)

Cardiovascular:
Coronary Artery Bypass Graft:
$9,500-$15,000
Bypass + Valve Replacement (single):
$12,000 + valve
Bypass + Valve Replacement (double):
$15,000 + valve
Pacemaker (single-chambered): $22,000 +
pacemaker
Pacemaker (double-chambered): $25,000 +
pacemaker

Orthopedic:
Birmingham Hip Resurfacing: $10,000
Joint Replacement:
Knee: $5,000-$8,000 + joint prosthesis
Hip: $5,600-$8,000 + joint prosthesis
Ankle: $10,000 + joint prosthesis
Shoulder: $8,000 + joint prosthesis

Cosmetic:
Breast Augmentation: $2,500-$3,000
Breast Lift/Reduction: $2,700-$3,500
Facelift: $4,000-$4,400
Tummy Tuck: $3,500

Dental:
Porcelain Veneer: $60-$300
Crown (all porcelain): $130-$400
Inlays and Onlays: $30-$250
Implant: $600-$1,000
Extraction (surgical, per tooth): $40-$250

Vision:
Glaucoma: $2,500
LASIK (per eye): $1,000

Weight Loss:
LAP-BAND System: $4,200-$7,200

Other:
Gall Bladder Removal: $900-$2,400
Prostate Surgery (TURP): $1,400-$2,500

■ HOSPITALS AND CLINICS

Jordan Hospital and Medical Center
Queen Nour Street
P.O. Box 520248
Amman, JORDAN 11152
Tel: 011 962 6560.8080
Fax: 011 962 6560.7575
Email: jorhos@jordan-hospital.com
Web: www.jordan-hospital.com

This 300-bed JCI-accredited hospital opened in 1996. In addition to the usual medical and surgical departments, Jordan Hospital and Medical Center provides specialized therapeutic units for emergency medicine, imaging and interventional radiology, nuclear medicine, renal dialysis, lithotripsy, physiotherapy, gastrointestinal and respiratory endoscopy, cardiac catheterization, and intensive care. It offers specialty clinics for diabetes and endocrinology, osteoporosis, in vitro fertilization (IVF), men's diseases, and obesity. The hospital's most often-performed procedures are dialysis, endoscopy, and cardiac catheterization. It served more than 7,000 international patients in 2007. Jordan Hospital is especially proud of its transplantation programs, which include liver, kidney, cornea, and bone marrow. The hospital maintains its own apartments, which are available to recovering patients.

King Hussein Cancer Center

Queen Rania Al Abdullah Street
P.O. Box 1269
Amman, JORDAN 11941
Tel: 011 962 6530.0460
Fax: 011 962 6535.3001
Email: info@khcc.jo
Web: www.khcc.jo

This JCI-accredited facility has earned a reputation as a world-class cancer treatment center for patients from the Middle East. Many of the specialists at King Hussein Cancer Center (KHCC) trained at the best cancer-treatment centers in the world and are recognized experts in their fields. KHCC offers comprehensive cancer management to patients with all types of malignancies, including diagnosis using up-to-date laboratory, pathology, and radiology equipment and treatment protocols that follow the newest and most advanced standards. KHCC offers a full range of cancer-related

services, including screening and community outreach programs.

Al-Essra Hospital

Queen Rania Al-Abdallah Street
Amman, JORDAN 11940
Tel: 011 962 6530.0300
Fax: 011 962 6534.7888
Email: essrahospital@essrahospital.com
Web: www.Essrahospital.com

In the two years following its opening in 2001, Al-Essra Hospital began offering endoscopic surgery, kidney dialysis, cardiovascular surgery, neurosurgery, and pediatric and orthopedic care. While this 60-physician, 160-bed hospital treats more than 20,000 international patients annually (mostly from other Arab countries), fewer than 50 of those patients travel from the US or Canada. Administrators at Al-Essra hope those numbers will change as more Western travelers take advantage of the hospital's facilities, experience, and expertise. The most frequently performed procedures are coronary artery bypass grafts, coronary artery stenting, and laparoscopic fundoplication (a standard surgical method for treating gastroesophageal reflux disease, or GERD). The hospital has a variety of accommodations available for patients and guests, ranging from deluxe suites to basic ward beds.

Specialty Hospital

Jabr Bin Hayan Street
Shmesani
Amman, JORDAN 11193
Tel: 011 962 6500.1111
Fax: 011 962 6569.7425
Email: admin@specialty-hospital.com
Web: www.specialty-hospital.com

Specialty Hospital opened in 1992 with 100 beds; it's now doubled that capacity. While the hospital offers all the usual major departments and units, its best known are cardiovascular surgery, neurosurgery, kidney transplantation, joint replacement, and plastic surgery. Specialty treats more than 4,000 international patients annually, most of them from other countries in the region.

■ HOTELS: DELUXE

Grand Hyatt Amman
Hussein Bin Ali Street, Jabal Amman
P.O. Box 831159
Amman, JORDAN 11183
Tel: 011 962 6465.1234
Fax: 011 962 6465.1634
Email: info.ammgh@hyattintl.com
Web: http://amman.grand.hyatt.com

Kempinski Hotel
Abdul Hamid Shouman Street, Shmeisani
P.O. Box 941045
Amman, JORDAN 11194
Tel: 011 962 6520.0200
Fax: 011 962 6520.0202
Email: reservations.amman@kempinski
 .com
Web: www.kempinski.com

Amman Marriott Hotel
Shmeissani Issam Ajluni Street
P.O. Box 926333
Amman, JORDAN 11190
Tel: 011 962 6560.7607
Fax: 011 962 6567.0100
Web: www.marriott.com/hotels

■ HOTELS: MODERATE

The Regency Palace Hotel
Queen Alya Street / Sports City Road
P.O. Box 927000
Amman, JORDAN 11110
Tel: 011 962 6560.7000
Fax: 011 962 6566.0013
Email: regency@nets.com.jo
Web: www.theregencyhotel.com

Golden Tulip Grand Palace Hotel
Queen Alya Street
P.O. Box 922444
Amman, JORDAN 11192
Tel: 011 962 6569.1131
Fax: 011 962 6563.5143
Email: resv@ammangrandpalace.com
Web: www.goldentulipgrandpalace.com

Rio Jordan Hotel
Queen Rania Al Abdullaj Street
P.O. Box 395, Jubayha
Amman, JORDAN 11941
Tel: 011 962 6532.3291
Fax: 011 962 6534.2262
Email: riohotel@nets.com.jo
Web: http://riojordan-hotel.com

Jerusalem International Hotel
University Road
Amman, JORDAN 11119
Tel: 011 962 6515.1121
Email: alquds@jerusalem.com.jo
Web: www.jerusalem.com.jo

DESTINATION: **MALAYSIA**

■ **AT A GLANCE**

Kuala Lumpur and Penang

Language:	Malay (English widely spoken)
Time Zone:	GMT +8
Country Dialing Code:	60
Electricity:	240V, Plug type D
Currency:	Ringgits
Visa Required?	Not for stays shorter than 90 days; health travelers can arrange for six months
Recommended Immunizations:	Hepatitis A; Boosters for Typhoid and Polio
Treatment Specialties:	Cardiovascular, Cosmetic, Dental, Fertility/Reproductive Health, General Surgery, Ophthalmology, Orthopedics, Stem Cells, Transplant
Leading Hospitals and Clinics:	KPJ Healthcare; Gleneagles Intan Medical Centre, Kuala Lumpur; Prince Court Medical Centre; Gleneagles Medical Centre, Penang; Pantai Medical Centre; Subang Jaya Medical Centre; NCI Cancer Hospital; Institut Jantung Negara (National Heart Institute)
JCI-Accredited Hospitals:	None
Standards and Accreditation:	Association of Private Hospitals of Malaysia (APHM), Malaysian Society for Quality in Health (MSQH); all private medical centers must be approved and licensed by the Malaysia Ministry of Health

■ TREATMENT BRIEF

While most Asia-bound health travelers head to India or Thailand for treatment, Malaysia used to be the international medical community's best-kept secret—but not anymore. In 2005, 230,000 medical travelers sought treatment in Malaysia, and the numbers are growing. Why? Because the country's facilities and expertise are on par with those in India and Thailand, and sometimes the costs are even lower, particularly for the more elaborate cardiovascular and orthopedic procedures. A comparative skip from neighboring Singapore, Malaysia offers excellent facilities and care, with prices 30–50 percent lower.

At least a dozen of Malaysia's 49 private hospitals, including the acclaimed Gleneagles Hospital Group, now serve international patients. Because Malaysia was a long-time British colony until 1957, Western culture is ingrained throughout the country. English is universally and comfortably spoken. Tourist attractions abound, particularly in the squeaky-clean capital of Kuala Lumpur and on the island of Penang, a favorite international beach resort and a medical travel center in its own right.

For those who wish to research Malaysia further, two excellent Web sites provide ample data and easy searching. First check out the Association of Private Hospitals of Malaysia Web site, www.hospitals-malaysia .org. There you'll be able to search by region for all accredited hospitals; within each hospital, drill down to find individual physician's credentials.

At the Malaysia Healthcare Web site, www.malaysiahealthcare.com, you can use the drop-down menus to access the procedure that interests you, and then read about an array of comparative packages offered by the various treatment centers. The site also carries animated tutorials that are easy to understand and impressively presented.

While getting treatment, many international patients take advantage of the exceptional, thorough, and inexpensive physicals offered by most Malaysian private hospitals. A dazzling array of tests and exams, including blood work, bone density scan, chest x-ray, and treadmill can be had for around $500. Malaysian hospitals were the creators of "well-man" and "well-woman" packages: extensive, low-cost physicals and tests promoting preventive care. Packages include pre-employment, executive screening, maternity, and more. Health travelers can also choose from a wide array of diagnostic packages, including heart, stroke, cancer, and bone scan.

■ TYPICAL TREATMENTS AND COSTS

Cardiovascular:
Coronary Artery Bypass Graft:
    $10,600-$13,000
Bypass + Valve Replacement (single):
    $10,600-$16,100
Bypass + Valve Replacement (double):
    $13,600-$18,600
Pacemaker (single-chambered):
    $6,200-$8,000
Pacemaker (double-chambered):
    $7,000-$12,000

Orthopedic:

Birmingham Hip Resurfacing: $14,900

Joint Replacement:

    Knee: $12,700

    Hip: $6,800-$8,150

    Ankle: $12,400

    Shoulder: $11,150

ACL Ligament Reconstruction: $18,600

Other:

Gall Bladder Removal: $3,100-$4,000

Prostate Surgery (TURP): $3,700

■ HEALTH TRAVEL AGENTS

CureOnTour

Bistari, South Block, 39th Floor

Penthouse 3A, Jalan 1/64D off Jalan Putra

Kuala Lumpur, MALAYSIA 50350

Tel: 011 60 3 4043.6090

Fax: 011 60 3 4043.6005

Email: Bernhard@CureOnTour.com

Web: www.CureOnTour.com

This health travel planning company started operations in 2006, providing personalized service to health travelers seeking treatment in the major hospitals of Kuala Lumpur, including Prince Court Medical Centre, Gleneagles Intan Medical Centre, Subang Jaya Medical Centre, Sunway, and Pantai Medical Centre (see "Hospitals and Clinics," below). CureOnTour does not outsource airport pickups; an agency staff member meets arriving clients and assists with every step in the process. The agency arranges flights, accommodations, financing, local transportation, cell phone service, personal nursing (if needed), and special diets. CureOnTour's personal contacts with local hospitals and doctors promise price breaks for the agency's clients.

Malaysia Healthcare

#02-03, 2nd Floor

Crown Regency Serviced Suites

12 Jalan P. Ramlee

Kuala Lumpur, MALAYSIA 50250

Tel: 011 60 327 195.582

Fax: 011 60 321 647.904

Email: info@malaysiahealthcare.com

Web: www.malaysiahealthcare.com

A newcomer to the health travel agent arena, Malaysia Healthcare has formed partnerships with Malaysia's largest hospital networks, such as KPJ Healthcare, Institut Jantung Negara (National Heart Institute), International Specialist Eye Centre, and Twin Towers Medical Centre (see "Hospitals and Clinics," below). Malaysia Healthcare works with eight private, accredited hospitals offering 70 different procedural specialties.

A destination manager is assigned to accompany each patient throughout the visit. The agency offers the usual amenities, including identification and booking of desired medical treatment, all travel booking, pre-treatment medical consultations, and customized holiday planning.

Malaysia Healthcare's impressive Web site (www.malaysiahealthcare.com) allows patients to customize their treatment and holiday arrangements in Malaysia. Besides selecting a hospital in Malaysia, health travelers can review the qualifications of a doctor or a specialist who might perform the required treatment. The portal also allows patients to contact a selected physician directly for consultation on treatment options.

One extra we've not seen elsewhere is this agency's commitment to making the patient's Malaysian physician available by phone or email to the home-country physician. Should pre-operative questions or post-operative complications arise, this is a reassuring service.

MedRetreat
2042 Laurel Valley Drive
Vernon Hills, IL 60061
Tel: 1 877 876.3373 (US toll-free)
Fax: 1 847 680.0484
Email: customerservice@medretreat.com
Web: www.medretreat.com

In operation since 2003, MedRetreat is one of the better-established US-based health travel agencies offering service to Malaysia, Thailand, India, Argentina, Brazil, Costa Rica, El Salvador, South Africa, and Turkey. Members receive personalized service through a boutique-style program designed to meet their specific needs. This proven process includes acquiring hospital information, physicians' credentials, and doctors' consultations; collecting and disseminating medical records; completing price quotations; and arranging procedures, air travel, travel insurance, financing, destination ground transportation, post-operative hotel bookings, passport and visa acquisition, and more. MedRetreat provides 14-hour-per-day access to a US program manager, concierge services in the treatment destination, communications while abroad, and assistance once back home. MedRetreat also offers an unconditional money-back guarantee. Service is free to the healthcare recipient on a first-come, first-served basis. To receive priority service, a Gold Club

Membership is available for $195 (which is deducted from the price of any medical trip booked through MedRetreat).

The Taj Medical Group, Limited
408 West 57th Street, Suite 9N
New York, NY 10019
Tel: 1 877 799.9797 (US toll-free)
Email: info@tajmedical.com
Web: www.tajmedical.com

For more information on Taj Medical Group, see India: Delhi.

■ HOSPITALS AND CLINICS

KPJ Healthcare
No. 1, Jalan Mamanda 9
Taman Dato' Ahmad Razali
Ampang, Selangor, MALAYSIA 68000
Tel: 011 60 3 4270.2500
Fax: 011 60 3 4270.2443
Web: www.kpjhealth.com.my

KPJ Healthcare is not one hospital but a consortium of 17, with healthcare facilities located in most of the major cities and towns in Malaysia. The enterprise totals more than 2,000 beds, 600 physicians and surgeons, and 5,000 staff members. KPJ has developed partnerships and collaborative relationships with hospitals, healthcare companies, and medical training institutes throughout Malaysia and worldwide. More than 15,000 international patients visit a KPJ hospital annually, but as of 2008, only 5 percent of them traveled from the US or Canada. That's likely to change with Malaysia's new initiatives to cut through red tape and promote medical travel.

Case Study: Eileen C., Florida

I limped around for two years on a hip that was bone on bone. I chose to go abroad for surgery because without insurance, I could not afford to have it done in the US. At that point, both of my hips hurt equally, so I planned on having both replaced, as long as I was traveling so far.

The health travel agency I selected suggested I go to Malaysia for surgery, because it was a country that was easy to get around in and was also English speaking. The flight from South Florida to Malaysia was a little uncomfortable. I walked the aisles a lot. Once I arrived in Penang, everyone I met was kind and caring. My hospital room was a suite. My girlfriend traveled to Malaysia and stayed in the hospital with me. My surgeon had a great sense of humor, assuring me that he knew how to replace a hip. After taking new x-rays, he told me I only needed one hip replaced. I greatly appreciated the honesty.

After one week in the hospital with physical therapy, I was released and taken next door to a five-star hotel for two weeks of healing. The doormen at the hotel kept a close eye on me. They pulled out my chairs, helped me up and down stairs, and arranged for rides to go sightseeing. I continued my physical therapy while I was staying in the hotel.

My girlfriend and I saw as much of the island of Penang as we could. We went to the malls, seashore, and night markets. We took a train ride up Penang Hill, overlooking the city of Georgetown.

My medical tourism experience was a good one—with no complications. I was sent home with x-rays and paperwork on everything that was done, in case I needed to see a doctor for any reason. My surgeon kept in touch with me for several months through email, making sure I was keeping up with my exercises. Fortunately, 18 months later, I am still doing well.

The best part of my experience was saving money. I spent a total of $11,000, a savings of about $30,000. Having an agency put the whole package together for me was great. They made it easy and didn't miss a thing. After experiencing medical tourism, I would definitely go abroad for surgery again. It was a journey I will be talking about for years to come.

Gleneagles Intan Medical Centre (Kuala Lumpur)

282 & 286 Jalan Ampang
Kuala Lumpur, MALAYSIA 50450
Tel: 011 60 3 4255.2775
Fax: 011 60 3 4257.9233
Email: inquiry@gleneaglesintan.com.my
Web: www.gimc.com.my

Established in 1996, this 330-bed private hospital is a subsidiary of Parkway Group Healthcare, Asia's largest hospital network, based in Singapore. All of its 103 physicians and surgeons speak English, as does most of the staff. New to the medical travel industry, Gleneagles treated more than 400 US and Canadian patients last year. Treatment specialties include orthopedics, cardiovascular, and general surgery.

The hospital's **International Patients Centre** offers a variety of services, including review of treatment options by specialists and estimated costs at no obligation prior to departure; assistance with visa application (if necessary) and travel arrangements; accommodation bookings and confirmation; airport transfer arrangement; language assistance services; insurance assistance; and post-treatment tour and sightseeing arrangements. Gleneagles's amenities for international patients now include in-room therapeutic spa treatments, such as facials, body massages, and beauty treatments. The goal is to ease the stress of recovery and pamper the recuperating patient.

Prince Court Medical Centre

39, Jalan Kia Pong
Kuala Lumpur, MALAYSIA 50450
Tel: 011 60 3 2160.0000
Fax: 011 60 3 2160.0010
Web: www.princecourt.com

Forbes Magazine has named the Prince Court Medical Centre (PCMC) one of the world's best destinations for medical travel—and with good reason. Affiliated with the Medical University of Vienna, PCMC opened its doors in 2006 with over a million square feet of floor space. Funded by Petronas, a major petroleum company, PCMC offers the atmosphere and service of a five-star hotel.

Its five centers of excellence are the **Heart and Vascular Center; Oncological Center; Mother and Child Center; Center for Cosmetic Surgery, Dermatology and Burn Victims;** and **Center for Urology, Nephrology and Men's Health.** The hospital has more than 300 rooms, all of them either single rooms or private suites.

Gleneagles Medical Centre (Penang)

1, Jalan Pangkor
Penang, MALAYSIA 10050
Tel: 011 60 4 2276.111
Fax: 011 60 4 2262.994
Email: pr@gmc.com.my
Web: www.gleneagles-penang.com

Established in 1973 and now a subsidiary of the giant Parkway Group Healthcare, Gleneagles Medical Centre was the first private hospital in Penang to be awarded three years' full accreditation by the Malaysian Society for Quality in Health (MSQH). The hospital underwent major renovations in the late 1990s, and it is now one of Malaysia's most modern facilities. Specialties include cardiothoracic surgery (adult and pediatric), orthopedic surgery, ophthalmology, oncology, and cardiology. Cataract surgery, heart surgery, and various orthopedic arthroscopies are frequently performed. About 500 patients from the US and Canada sought treatment at this center in 2007.

Institut Jantung Negara (National Heart Institute)

145, Jalan Tun Razak
Kuala Lumpur, MALAYSIA 50400
Tel: 011 60 3 2617.8200
Fax: 011 60 3 2692.5609
Email: info@ijn.com.my
Web: www.ijn.com.my

Institut Jantung Negara (National Heart Institute/IJN) was part of the Kuala Lumpur General Hospital until 1992, when it became a specialist center for cardiovascular and thoracic medicine. Today the hospital has provided cardiac care to over 1 million patients. It's racked up more than 20,000 heart surgeries and 62,000 interventional cardiac procedures. In 2006 surgeons performed the hospital's first video-assisted thoracoscopic ablation fibrillation and its first double-lung transplant. IJN maintains a homograft heart valve bank (homografts are human tissues available for transplantation). The hospital also boasts a comprehensive pulmonary rehabilitation program, conducted through the physiotherapy unit, which helps patients with lung diseases or those who have had lung surgery to improve their breathing and overall health.

IJN often takes referrals of complicated cases from hospitals and doctors throughout Asia and Australia. Health travelers account for about 1,350 outpatient visits and 130 admissions annually. The center supports training, research, and development activities through collaborations with leading international medical establishments, including the UK's Papworth Hospital and Germany's Herz-und.

IJN is located in the heart of Kuala Lumpur's city center, only minutes from train stations and numerous hotels, which range in price from budget to six-star. Hospital service staff can negotiate competitive rates for international patients in nearly all of these hotels.

Pantai Medical Centre

8, Jalan Bukit Pantai
Kuala Lumpur, MALAYSIA 59100
Tel: 011 60 3 2296.0888
Fax: 011 60 3 2282.1557
Email: pmc@pantai.com.my
Web: www.pantai.com.my

Pantai Medical Centre (PMC) is owned by the giant Pantai Group, which has seven hospitals throughout Malaysia. Pantai has forged relationships with a dozen insurance providers worldwide, including Prudential/Cigna and BUPA.

Established in 1974 in the heart of Kuala Lumpur, PMC is Pantai's flagship hospital, with 292 beds and more than 130 specialists. A general hospital, PMC offers nearly every type of diagnostic and treatment, including specialties in urology, cardiology, orthopedics, gastroenterology, endocrinology, and ophthalmology.

The Pantai Executive Screening Program (ESP) is a comprehensive medical examination for early detection of common disorders, such as hypertension, diabetes mellitus, and heart disease. Through these tests, doctors can detect abnormalities in the heart, lungs, liver, kidneys, and urinary tract. PMC's **Haemodialysis Unit** provides inpatient and outpatient treatment for chronic and acute kidney ailments. Pantai's Web site features an impressive roster of specialists, with email addresses for direct contact with physicians and surgeons.

Subang Jaya Medical Centre
Sdn. Bhd., 1, Jalan SS 12/1A
47500 Subang Jaya
Selangor Darul Ehsan, MALAYSIA
Tel: 011 60 3 5639.1466
Fax: 011 60 3 5639.1675
Web: www.sjmc.com.my

Opened in 1995, Subang Jaya Medical Centre (SJMC) is a privately owned and internationally accredited tertiary-care medical center near Kuala Lumpur, a half-hour's drive from Kuala Lumpur International Airport. With the addition of its north wing and **Cancer and Radiosurgery Centre** in 2001, SJMC now has 375 beds and 14 operating theaters, with 89 specialty suites.

SJMC offers the full range of treatments, with subspecialties in cardiovascular and thoracic surgery, oncology and radiosurgery, vascular interventional radiology, blood and marrow transplant, liver transplant surgery, urology, and infertility management.

SJMC's centers of excellence include

■ **Blood Diseases Centre,** which provides a full range of laboratory hematological services for diagnosis of blood disorders; comprehensive treatment for hematological malignancies, such as leukemia, lymphoma, and myeloma; cryopreservation and stem cell storage services for patients undergoing blood/marrow transplants; and blood/marrow transplant using matched unrelated donors for pediatric patients. SJMC is currently the only private hospital in Malaysia to offer blood/marrow transplant services.

■ **Heart Centre,** which is a one-stop treatment center that comprises the **Coronary Care Unit (CCU),** the adjacent **Cardiac Ward,** and the **Cardiovascular Laboratory.** SJMC's Heart Centre is the largest in Malaysia, and more than 2,000 angiograms and angioplasties have been performed since its inception. Noninvasive beating-heart techniques are promoted and practiced by SJMC's Heart Centre specialists.

■ **Vascular Interventional Radiology Centre,** where specialists practice a branch of radiology that combines new catheterization and imaging technologies. Vascular interventional radiology (VIR) offers precise, accurate diagnoses and minimally invasive treatments for blood vessel disorders and diseases of the internal organs. Also known as pinhole surgery, the surgical incision, which is guided by high-resolution imaging equipment, is as small as the tip of a pencil. Procedures performed using VIR generally involve less time, pain, and trauma and lead to shorter hospital stays.

■ **Subang Fertility Centre,** formerly the Pivet Laboratory Malaysia, is a private fertility unit now based at SJMC. Couples who are having difficulty conceiving now have the benefit of the hospital's ancillary support staff and facilities, all under one roof. The center boasts many of Malaysia's firsts, including the first in vitro fertilization (IVF) and first intracytoplasmic sperm injection (ICSI) births in the country. It was also the first center to provide treatment with recombinant drug technology, leading to Malaysia's first IVF and ICSI births resulting from these medications.

■ **Nuclear Medicine and PET/CT Centre,** where radioactive materials are used safely in the diagnosis and treatment of various diseases. The computed tomography (CT) scan is a noninvasive, safe, and relatively painless procedure, usually involving a small injection. Positron emission tomography (PET) is another imaging method used to detect small metabolic changes in diseased tissue. With these techniques, information about various organs can be obtained quickly with little or no pain. SJMC utilizes these sophisticated techniques for bone, lung, renal (kidney), brain, and heart scans in diagnosing cancer, heart disease, neurological conditions, and brain abnormalities.

SJMC's milestones include Malaysia's first related-donor pediatric liver transplant (1995); Malaysia's first liver transplant from a nonblood relative (1995); and first open-heart surgery in a Malaysian private hospital (1985).

NCI Cancer Hospital

PT 13717, Jalan BBN 2/1
71800 Nilai, Negeri Sembilan
Darul Khusus, MALAYSIA
Tel: 011 60 6 850.0999
Fax: 011 60 6 850.0733
Web: www.nci.com.my

Founded in 1999, NCI Cancer Hospital (NCI, formerly known as Nilai Cancer Institute) is a private center in Malaysia specializing in cancer treatment and clinical research. The center is based in Bandar Baru Nilai, about 45 minutes from Kuala Lumpur and just 20 minutes from the Kuala Lumpur International Airport.

NCI provides diagnosis and treatment to cancer patients and conducts clinical research in cooperation with multinational pharmaceutical companies. It was the first facility in Southeast Asia to introduce the Trilogy linear accelerator for precision radiotherapy. The center also employs noninvasive high-intensity ultrasound for cancer treatment.

In 2007 NCI opened a new wing that houses additional treatment facilities and equipment, along with accommodations for patients and their families. NCI's **International Patient Centre** arranges travel, transportation, and lodging, schedules appointments, and assists with visa applications and renewals.

■ HOTELS: DELUXE

Crown Princess
City-Square Centre, Jalan Tun Razak
Kuala Lumpur, MALAYSIA 50400
Tel: 011 60 3 2162.5522
Fax: 011 60 3 2162.4492
Email: crownprincess@crownprincess
.com.my
Web: www.crownprincess.com.my

Hotel Nikko Kuala Lumpur
165, Jalan Ampang
Kuala Lumpur, MALAYSIA 50450
Tel: 011 60 3 2161.1111
Fax: 011 60 3 2161.1122
Email: info@hotelnikko.com.my
Web: www.hotelnikko.com.my

Eastern and Oriental Hotel (Penang)
10 Lebuh Farquhar
Penang, MALAYSIA 10200
Tel: 011 60 4 222.2000
Fax: 011 60 4 261.6333
Email: reservations@e-o-hotel.com
Web: www.e-o-hotel.com

■ HOTELS: MODERATE

Lanson Place Ambassador Row Residences
1, Jalan Ampang Hilir
Kuala Lumpur, MALAYSIA 55000
Tel: 011 60 3 4253.2888
Fax: 011 60 3 4253.1773
Email: enquiry.lpar@lansonplace.com
Web: www.lansonplace.com

SuCasa Service Apartments
222, Jalan Ampang
Kuala Lumpur, MALAYSIA 50450
Tel: 011 60 3 4251.3833
Fax: 011 60 3 4252.1096
Email: ssa@sucasahotel.com
Web: www.sucasahotel.com

G Hotel
168A Persiaran Gurney
Georgetown
Penang, MALAYSIA 11250
Tel: 011 60 4 238.0000
Fax: 011 60 4 238.0088
Email: E.info@ghotel.com.my
Web: www.ghotel.com.my

Sheraton Subang Hotel and Towers
Jalan SS 12/1, 47500
Subang Jaya, Selangor, MALAYSIA
Tel: 011 60 3 5031.6060
Fax: 011 60 3 5031.8686
Email: subang.reservations@sheraton.com
Web: www.sheraton.com/subang

■ **AT A GLANCE**

(1) California and Arizona Borders (2) Texas and New Mexico Borders (3) Coastal

Language:	Spanish (some English)
Time Zone:	GMT -6 & GMT -5
Country Dialing Code:	52
Electricity:	127V, Plug type A
Currency:	Mexican peso
Visa Required?	No
Recommended Immunizations:	Hepatitis A; Typhoid Booster
Treatment Specialties:	Cosmetic, Dental, Ophthalmology
Leading Hospitals and Clinics:	Hospital Angeles, Tijuana; Christus Muguerza Alta Especialidad; Hospital CIMA Hermosillo; Hospital CIMA Santa Engracia
JCI-Accredited Hospitals:	Christus Muguerza Alta Especialidad, Hospital San José Tec de Monterrey
Standards and Accreditation:	Mexican Academy of Dermatology; Mexican Association of Plastic, Reconstructive, and Aesthetic Surgery; American Academy of Cosmetic Dentistry (AACD); American Academy of Implant Dentistry (AAID); JCI

■ **TREATMENT BRIEF**

At first blush, Mexico is a mystery to the aspiring health traveler. Few world-class hospitals exist in Mexico, unlike less-developed India or neighboring Costa Rica. Mexican accreditation standards are weak, and to date Mexico has only two JCI-accredited hospitals, although prospects are improving rapidly for US and Canadian health travelers.

Christus Muguerza Alta Especialidad, which attained JCI accreditation in 2007, is now part of Christus Health in the US, a group serving eight US states, mostly along the US-Mexican border. The merger has made Christus Muguerza the largest health-care provider in Mexico.

Along the US-Mexican border, by the beautiful Mexican coast, or in developed expatriate communities, you'll find dozens of smaller, established clinics that reliably treat tens of thousands of Americans each year. Many of these patients return annually for checkups, dental cleanings, physicals, and a host of other treatments that can be had far less expensively than in Europe and many Asian countries—without the rigors of trans-oceanic travel.

Mexico-bound health travelers usually encounter smaller clinics run by two or three physicians, often second- and even third-generation families. Unassuming yet clean and efficient, they're often as not run by either expatriate US physicians or practitioners trained in the US or Europe.

Quality clinics are located in nearly every major city and resort; yet finding them can be fraught with frustration. Most Web sites throughout Mexico remain in Spanish, and English-speaking physicians are not always available, nor are translation services. The health traveler, in fact, is likely to encounter less English in Mexico than in Malaysia or South Africa, tens of thousands of miles away. English-speaking patients may need to enlist the assistance of health travel agencies to arrange the care they are seeking in Mexico, but be forewarned: many of the health travel agents serving Mexico are partnered with a single clinic or hospital.

Mexico City has 26 million inhabitants and the best and worst of everything, including several world-class hospitals, such as Hospital Angeles. These centers offer state-of-the-art specialties and super-

specialties, including cardiology, oncology, and orthopedics.

Geographical convenience is the big motivation for most Mexico-bound health travelers, and it's no wonder that more than 70 percent of Mexico's US patients reside in California, Texas, or Arizona. Nearby patients from San Diego, Los Angeles, Phoenix, Tucson, and Brownsville simply make the two- to six-hour drive across the border to their clinic of choice, stay a night or two in a hotel, and then drive back. As one veteran multinational patient comments, "A three-hour drive across the border saves me $700 in physicals and dental work every year. That's a no-brainer."

Yet, for folks farther away from the border, and particularly those east of the Mississippi, Mexico may be a less attractive option, unless you have plenty of time to search for a dentist or cosmetic surgeon, or you are traveling to Mexico anyway.

Perhaps more than in any other health travel country, Mexico's leading medical destinations each serve a different type of patient. Thus, we've grouped clinics and accommodations into three destinations:

1) Along the Border: California and Arizona—for patients driving from those and nearby states, as well as for international health travelers. This area includes Tijuana. Nearby San Diego, La Jolla, and Oceanside offer accommodations to suit any budget.

2) Along the Border: Texas and New Mexico—mostly for Texans and New Mexicans. Getting to El Paso International Airport sometimes requires two or more hops, even from larger urban airports, and upscale accommodations are scarce. This area includes Chihuahua and Monterrey.

3) Along the Coast—for those seeking

resorts and recreation to complement their medical treatment. This area includes Cabo San Lucas and Mazatlán. Puerto Vallarta is also a popular destination.

■ TYPICAL TREATMENTS AND COSTS

Cardiovascular:
Coronary Artery Bypass Graft: $27,000
Bypass + Valve Replacement (single): $28,000-$30,000
Bypass + Valve Replacement (double): $35,000
Aortic or Mitral Valve Replacement: $30,000-$35,000

Orthopedic:
Birmingham Hip Resurfacing: $10,200
Joint Replacement:
Knee: $7,000-$14,900
Hip: $8,000-$13,900
Ankle: $10,500
Shoulder: $6,700-$12,000

Cosmetic:
Breast Augmentation: $3,900-$4,200
Breast Lift/Reduction: $4,000
Rhinoplasty (nose): $5,200
Facelift: $5,800-$11,300
Liposuction (stomach, hips, and waist): $2,300-$4,500
Tummy Tuck: $2,200-$8,600

Dental:
Porcelain Veneer: $180-$600
Crown (all porcelain): $339-$650
Inlays and Onlays: $220-$500
Implant: $985-$1,800
Extraction (surgical, per tooth): $120-$350

Vision:
Glaucoma: $1,500-$1,800 (including operating room in some cases)
LASIK (per eye): $650-$1,000 (including operating room in some cases)

Weight Loss:
LAP-BAND System: $7,700-$9,200
Gastric Bypass: $11,000

Other:
Gall Bladder Removal: $3,100-$4,500
Prostate Surgery (TURP): $11,800

■ HEALTH TRAVEL AGENTS

Third-party travel planners for Mexico are scarce, offset by the facts that hospitals and clinics generally offer full services to patients and Mexican phone numbers are readily available to Americans. Similar time zones to the US are also a plus for contacting healthcare providers. We caution you to check out Mexican healthcare referrals carefully.

Healthbase Online, Inc.
287 Auburn Street
Newton, MA 02466
Tel: 1 888 691.4584 (US toll-free);
1 617 418.3436
Fax: 1 800 986.9230 (US toll-free)
Email: info.hb@healthbase.com
Web: www.healthbase.com

For more information on Healthbase Online, see India: Chennai.

Med Journeys
2020 Broadway, Suite 4C
New York, NY 10023
Tel: 1 888 633.5769 (US toll-free);
   1 212 931.0557
Fax: 1 212 656.1134
Email: sonnyk@medjourneys.com
Web: www.medjourneys.com

For more information on Med Journeys,
see India: Delhi.

Planet Hospital
23679 Calabasas Road, Suite 150
Calabasas, CA 91302
Tel: 1 800 243.0172 (US toll-free);
   1 818 665.4801
Fax: 1 818 665.4810
Email: rudy@planethospital.com
Web: www.planethospital.com

For more information on Planet Hospital,
see Singapore.

WorldMed Assist
1230 Mountain Side Court
Concord, CA 94521
Tel: 1 866 999.3848 (US toll-free)
Fax: 1 925 905.5898
Email: whoeber@worldmedassist.com
Web: www.worldmedassist.com

For more information on WorldMed Assist,
see India: Bangalore.

■ HOSPITALS AND CLINICS

CALIFORNIA AND ARIZONA BORDERS

For better or worse, the most accessible
clinics in this region are located in Tijuana,
just over the border from San Diego. With a
nearly insurmountable reputation for illicit
drugs, prostitution, and nonstop revelry,
Tijuana is also the state of Baja's largest city
and a huge cultural and commercial center. Dozens of well-established, reputable
dental and cosmetic surgery clinics exist
alongside the fly-by-nights and hangers-on.
We caution you to choose your healthcare
center carefully. Use a reputable health
travel agency or get a recommendation
from a trusted friend.

Hospital CIMA Hermosillo
Paseo Rio San Miguel #35, Proyecto Rio
   Sonora
Hermosillo, MEXICO
Tel: 1 214 536.3521 (US); 011 52 662
   259.0924
Fax: 011 52 662 259.0999
Email: ogarza@cimahermosillo.com
Web: www.cimahermosillo.com

A subsidiary of the US-owned International
Hospital Corporation, this 52-bed hospital
has been attracting Americans from Arizona and California since it began operation in 1996. Hospital CIMA Hermosillo's
300 physicians offer service in cardiology,
neurosurgery, orthopedics, general surgery,
gynecology, weight-loss surgery, and (a
relatively new area) stem cell transplants.
In 2005 the hospital installed a magnetic
resonance imagery (MRI) Philips 1.5 unit,
allowing its doctors to perform highly
specialized procedures, such as cerebral
angiographies. Other CIMA Hospitals are
located in Monterrey, Chihuahua, and San
José (Costa Rica).

Aesthetic Plastic Surgery Institute (Tijuana)

José Clemente Orozco 2468

Plaza Medical Zona Rio

Tijuana, BC, MEXICO 22320

Tel: 1 866 846.4144 (US toll-free); 011 52 664 634.2310

Email: drsergio@sergiosoberanes.com

Web: www.drsergiosoberanes.com

Aesthetic Plastic Surgery Institute, with two surgeons and a staff of three, treats patients from the US and Canada almost exclusively, many of them referred by the San Diego agency Plastic Surgeons Mexico (www .plasticsurgeons-mexico.com). Head surgeon Sergio Soberanes received his degree at Universidad Autonoma de Baja California's School of Medicine in 1984 and completed his internship at Hospital General de Tijuana. This small clinic is board-certified through the Mexican Association of Plastic, Reconstructive and Aesthetic Surgery, and Dr. Soberanes is a member of the Mexican Council of Aesthetic and Reconstructive Plastic Surgery.

The center's specialties include Botox treatments, brow lifts, eyelid surgery, facelifts, and nose reconstruction. Body contouring procedures include arm, hip, and thigh lifts; breast lifts, augmentation, and reduction; tumescent liposuction; tummy tucks; and vaginal reconstruction and rejuvenation. Weight-loss treatments include LAP-BAND surgery, gastric bypass surgery, and post-bariatric body contouring.

Baja Oral Center (Tijuana)

José Clemente Orozco Street 10122, Suite 408, 4th Floor

Plaza Pacifico Building, Zona Rio

Tijuana, BC, MEXICO

Tel: 1 800 601.3795 (US toll-free); 011 52 664 634.7626

Fax: 011 52 619 270.5368

Email: smile@bajaoralcenter.com

Web: www.bajaoralcenter.com

Six specialists and a staff of 13 run Baja Oral Center, located on three floors of a large office building in the Zona Rio area of Tijuana. Specialties include cosmetic and restorative dentistry, oral and maxillofacial surgery, orthodontics, pediatric dentistry, periodontics, and root canals. The clinic claims to be 100 percent mercury-free.

Baja is equipped with state-of-the-art-treatment rooms, intraoral cameras, and digital x-rays for those who wish to see what the dentist sees. All the dentists speak English.

Clínica Dental Estrella (Tijuana)

Avenida Niños Heroes No. 995, between 3rd & 4th Streets

Zona Centro

Tijuana, BC, MEXICO 22000

Tel: 1 619 308.7989 (US); 011 52 664 688.1651

Fax: 011 52 664 685.0905

Email: info@clinicadentalestrella.com

Web: www.clinicadentalestrella.com

Specializing in implants and prosthodontics (including bridges, crowns, inlays, veneers, and partial and complete dentures), the family-run Clínica Dental Estrella, with four doctors and a staff of ten, claims more than 30 years of combined dentistry experience.

Prosthodontist Jaime Estrella received his three-year specialty in advanced prosthodontic dentistry from California's Loma Linda University, where he also completed a one-year internship in implant surgery.

Implantologist Miguel Estrella received a three-year specialty in advanced implant dentistry from Loma Linda University and training in aesthetic restorations at the Nobel Biocare Training Institute in Yorba Linda, California. He is licensed with the Dental Board of California and is a Member of the American Academy of Implant Dentistry and the American Academy of Osseointegration.

The facility offers an onsite deep-bleaching light system, digital and panoramic x-rays, digital photography, implant tomography, and a sterile surgical suite.

CosMED Plastic Aesthetic Surgical Center (Tijuana)

Calle Mision de San Diego #1527-301
Zona Rio
Tijuana, BC, MEXICO
Tel: 1 877 426.7633 (US toll-free); 011 52 664 634.1903
Web: www.cosmedtj.com

Although smaller than some of its counterparts, CosMED is one of Mexico's most acclaimed cosmetic surgery clinics. Its three surgeons see more than 400 Americans and other international travelers each month for consultation or surgery.

CosMED's surgeons claim more than 30 years of combined practice in cosmetic surgery, and all are board-certified. Specialties include

■ *Facial rejuvenation:* cheek and chin enhancement; collagen injections; ear modification; facial lifts, including eyes, eyebrows, forehead, and neck; lip treatments; and nose reconstruction.

■ *Cosmetic dermatology:* chemical peels, dermabrasion, laser skin resurfacing, and wrinkle and scar improvement.

■ *Body contouring:* Botox injections; breast enlargement, lift, and reduction; buttock implants; liposuction and ultrasonic liposuction; tummy tucks; and spider-vein therapy.

■ *Hair transplants:* minigrafts and micrografts.

CosMED also boasts a full-service spa, housed in the same offices, which offers a 60-minute facial treatment, 35-minute "lunchtime peel," 80-minute four-layer facial, eight-minute deep-cleansing intensifying facial, 35-minute manual lymphatic drainage (recommended before and after facelifts), and skin resurfacing.

CosMED's Web site features an all-video testimonials page. In addition to hearing the expected accolades, prospective patients can view the clinic's impressive surroundings.

Hospital Angeles Tijuana

Avenida Paseo de los Heroes #10999
Zona Rio
Tijuana, CP, MEXICO 22010
Tel-Fax: 011 664 635.1800
Web: www.hospitalangelestijuana.com.mx

Hospital Angeles Tijuana is part of the large Hospital Angeles group. The five-story hospital tower hosts 94 patient rooms and six operating rooms in addition to specialty operating areas.

The hospital has more than 60 specialist physicians, most of whom are US or UK board-certified or have US or UK fellowships.

Specialties include infertility treatments, neurology, orthopedics, and cardiovascular, cosmetic, and general surgery.

Pacific Dental (Tijuana)
Ignacio Comonfort #9317, Suite F
Zona Rio
Tijuana, BC, MEXICO
Tel: 1 877 752.5132 (US toll-free); 011 52 664 634.0835
Email: pacificdental@hotmail.com
Web: www.mexicotijuanadentist.com

Most patients coming to Pacific Dental are Americans seeking the 60 percent dental discount often found in Mexico. The clinic boasts its own crown and bridge laboratory, specializing in porcelain fused to metal and all-ceramic restorations. The latest dental materials are used: Express 2, Finesse, Optec, and Procera. Services include cosmetic and general dentistry, crowns, dentures, implants, porcelain veneers, restorations, root canals, and tooth bonding.

TEXAS AND NEW MEXICO BORDERS:

Somewhat less accessible to the international traveler, several reputable clinics serve Dallas, Houston, San Antonio, El Paso, Albuquerque, Santa Fe, and other nearby US population centers. Health travelers may choose to fly into El Paso or Dallas, and then rent a car and drive across the border.

Rio Dental Clinic (Chihuahua)
Dr. A. Nunez Garcia
3970 Rio Chompoton
Cd. Juarez, Chihuahua, MEXICO
Tel: 1 800 635.7462 (US toll-free)
Fax: 1 915 975.8257
Email: office@riodental.com
Web: www.riodental.com

Owned and run by Americans, Rio Dental Clinic opened its doors in 2005, peopled by a young, talented staff of dentists and specialists. Lead dentist (and co-owner) Jessica Andel has been practicing since her graduation in 2000 from Universidad Autonoma de Ciudad Juarez. Three additional specialists focus on oral surgery, periodontics, and root canal. Rio Dental requires that all dentists and specialists speak English and complete biannual continuing education seminars in Mexico and the US.

Services and specialties include crowns and bridges, dentures and plates, implants, tooth whitening, and routine checkups. Rio Dental provides free transportation to and from most El Paso hotels and from the airport for patients heading directly to their office. Rio Dental treats nearly a thousand across-the-border patients annually.

Imagen Dental
Calzada del Valle
San Pedro Garza Garcia
Nuevo León, Monterrey, MEXICO
Tel: 011 52 81 8185.3503
Fax: 011 52 81 8370.1415
Email: patov@imagendental.com
Web: www.imagendental.com

Despite its name, Imagen Dental does more than dentistry. In business since 1994, Imagen has 19 clinics (18 in Monterrey and one in Nuevo Laredo) and more than 200 physicians and surgeons who provide comprehensive dental, optical (glasses and lenses), and auditory (hearing aid) services. Eye surgeries are performed in the operating rooms of Christus Muguerza Alta Especialidad Hospital (see below). Most of Imagen's dental work is cosmetic and includes implants, veneers, crowns, bridges, gum surgeries, and root canals. One of the Imagen ophthalmologists has performed more than 2,000 eye surgeries.

Imagen uses digital radiology, which emits 80 percent less radiation than normal radiology. The dental clinics employ patient education systems in both English and Spanish and an intraoral camera to show patients pictures and videos of their mouths and teeth. For a patient who needs to return home quickly, Imagen can make Belle Glass Dental Crowns in two hours; these crowns are the same quality as porcelain but are less abrasive against natural teeth. Imagen's audiology laboratory can deliver a hearing aid in two days.

Christus Muguerza Alta Especialidad Hospital

Avenida Hidalgo #2525, Pte. Col. Obispado
Monterrey, Nuevo León, MEXICO 64060
Tel: 011 52 81 8399.3400
Fax: 011 52 81 8174.3484
Email: internationalpatients@
christusmuguerza.com.mx
Web: www.christusmuguerza.com.mx

Christus Muguerza Alta Especialidad was the first hospital in Mexico to achieve JCI accreditation. It is part of the Christus Muguerza Health Group, a nonprofit health system that includes more than 40 hospitals in the US and Mexico. This 200-bed hospital traces its history back to 1934, but it has expanded and gone modern since then, undergoing a major renovation in 2000. Its main areas of expertise include cardiovascular surgery, orthopedics, cardiology, ophthalmology, and general surgery. In 2006 more than 20,000 surgeries were performed at Alta Especialidad, including endoscopic, vascular, and ophthalmic procedures. Most

frequently performed procedures include cataract removal, knee arthroscopy, gall bladder removal, and angiography.

Hospital CIMA Santa Engracia

Avenida Frida Kahlo 180
Valle Oriente Garza Garcia
Monterrey, Nuevo León, MEXICO 66260
Tel: 011 52 81 8368.7777
Fax: 011 52 81 8368.7746
Email: mtarabay@santaengracia.com
Web: www.santaengracia.com

Seventy beds and 200 physicians support Hospital CIMA Santa Engracia's specialties in orthopedics, urology, obstetrics and gynecology, pediatrics, and otolaryngology (ear, nose, and throat). Its most frequently performed procedures are weight-loss and orthopedic surgeries. English-speaking patients need to be careful here; the main language is Spanish and fewer than half the physicians speak English. Monterrey is, however, a short 90-minute flight from Dallas, and CIMA is US-managed. More than 300 international patients seek treatment here annually. Ground transportation is provided as part of the costs, and CIMA's **International Patients Services** will arrange hotel accommodations within minutes of the hospital. Weight-loss surgery packages include hotel stay.

COASTAL

We've focused on the most popular resorts, most accessible by air (one stop or less from most major US airports, with ample accommodations for every lifestyle). Health travelers heading for these destinations have usually budgeted additional time to allow for recovery as well as a week or more of sightseeing or relaxing.

Mexican Dental Vacation (Mazatlán)

Olas Altas #1
Centro Historico
Mazatlán, Sinaloa, MEXICO 82000
Tel: 011 52 669 981.8236
Fax: 011 52 669 981.8236
Email: mdvmaz@yahoo.com
Web: www.mexicandentalvacation.com

Mexican Dental Vacation (MDV) was founded by Canadian businessman Nick Konev to provide first-class dental care at huge savings. Dr. Stephen Mackey, DDS, is now working with MDV after more than 30 years of experience in the Seattle area. MDV specializes in implants, and the office performs seven to ten implants each week. Other specialties include bridges, root canals, bone graft and sinus lift surgeries, and cosmetic work, such as bleaching and crowns. Prices at MDV are comparable to those at other dental offices in Mazatlán. MDV offers the newest state-of-the-art equipment, an autoclave to steam-sterilize all equipment (which not every office in Mexico has), and a competent, English-speaking staff.

A word of caution: as in the US, there are often delays in dental work, so plan a few extra days in Mazatlán, just in case. In addition, some treatments, such as implants, are a two-step process with several months of healing between procedures, meaning two visits to the land of the sun. MDV can arrange timeshares at four-star resorts for health travelers in Mazatlán for around $400 per week.

Miguelangelo Plastic Surgery Clinic (Cabo San Lucas)

Transpeninsular Highway Km 6.7
Cabo San Lucas, BC Sur, MEXICO 23454
Tel: 1 800 386.2226 (US toll-free); 011 52 624 104.3583
Fax: 011 52 624 104.3587
Web: http://miguelangeloclinic.com

One of Mexico's top cosmetic surgery clinics, the one-doctor Miguelangelo Plastic Surgery Clinic is renowned mostly for its founder, owner, and head surgeon, Miguelangelo Gonzalez. The clinic has a staff of ten. Up to 90 percent of its patients come from the US or Canada.

Angel's Touch Dental Clinic (Cabo San Lucas)

Plazas Doradas Building Local #10 & #11
Carretera Transpeninsular
Cabo San Lucas, BC Sur, MEXICO
Tel: 1 866 331.3996 (US toll-free); 011 52 624 142.6192
Fax: 011 52 624 142.2459
Email: info@angelsdental.com
Web: www.angelsdental.com

Owner and head dentist Rosy Peña opened her clinic in 1981 in the central plaza of San José del Cabo. Angel's Touch now has a staff of six, including a general dentist, dental surgeon, endodontist, orthodontist, periodontist, and odontopediatrist. The clinic sees more than 120 US patients each month.

Services include amalgam/mercury filling removal (price includes tooth-color-matching resin replacement fillings), bridges, crowns (porcelain over metal or 100 percent porcelain), dentures, extractions, fillings, implants (traditional or one-day for laterals only), partials (traditional and ValPlast or Teflon), periodontal work (including gum reduction, osseous treatment, and deep periodontal cleaning), and root canals.

■ RECOVERY ACCOMMODATIONS

Christus Muguerza Alta Especialidad reports special relationships with two hotels that it often recommends to its international patients:

Hotel Chipinque
Meseta de Chipinque #1000
San Pedro, Garza Garcia
Monterrey, Nuevo León, MEXICO
Tel: 011 81 8173.1777
Fax: 011 81 8350.0841
Email: ventas@hotelchipinque.com
Web: www.hotelchipinque.com/
indexenglish.htm

Located near the summit of the Sierra Madre Oriental at 5,000 feet and just 15 minutes from the heart of San Pedro Garza Garcia, Nuevo León, Hotel Chipinque lies in a serene natural setting that promotes a relaxing recovery.

Hotel Hacienda Cola de Caballo
Carretera a Cola de Caballo Km 6
El Cercado, Santiago, Nuevo León, MEXICO 67320
Tel: 011 81 8285.0260
Fax: 011 81 8285.0660
Email: hotel@coladecaballo.com
Web: www.coladecaballo.com/Ingles/
homeingles.htm

Hotel Hacienda Cola de Caballo is located near a natural waterfall called Cola de Caballo (which means "horse's tail") in the middle of the Sierra Madres, 30 minutes from Monterrey on the National Highway.

■ HOTELS: DELUXE

Although the deluxe hotels listed are at the higher end of accommodations given, featured amenities vary by location.

CALIFORNIA AND ARIZONA BORDERS:

Grand Hotel Tijuana
Boulevard Agua Caliente 4500
Col. Aviacion, CP
Tijuana, BC, MEXICO 22420
Tel: 1 866 472.6385 (US toll-free)
Fax: 011 52 624 681.7016
Email: reservations@grandhoteltij.com.mx
Web: www.grandhoteltij.com.mx

Hotel Real Del Rio
Avenida José Maria Velazco #1409-A
Zona Rio
Tijuana, BC, MEXICO 22320
Tel: 1 877 517.6479 (US toll-free); 011 52 664
634.3100
Email: hospedaje@realdelrio.com
Web: www.realdelrio.com

Hotel Del Coronado
1500 Orange Avenue
Coronado, CA 92118
Tel: 1 800 468.3533 (US toll-free); 011 52 619
435.6611
Email: delinquiries@hoteldel.com
Web: www.hoteldel.com

Hotel Fiesta Americana Hermosillo
Boulevard Eusebio Kino 369
Col. Lomas Pitic
Hermosillo, Sonora, MEXICO 83010
Tel: 011 52 662 259.6000
Fax: 011 52 662 259.6061
Web: www.fiestamericana.com

TEXAS AND NEW MEXICO BORDERS:

Camino Real
101 South El Paso Street
El Paso, TX 79901
Tel: 1 800 901.2300 (US toll-free); 1 915
534.3000
Fax: 1 915 534.3024
Email: elpaso@caminoreal.com.mx
Web: www.caminoreal.com.mx

Pueblo Bonito Mazatlán
Avenida Camaron Sabalo 2121
Mazatlán, MEXICO 82110
Tel: 011 52 669 989.8900; 011 52 669
989.0525
Fax: 011 52 669 914.1723; 011 52 669
988.0718
Email: iquintero@pueblobonito.com.mx
Web: www.pueblobonito-mazatlan.com

Fiesta Inn Ciudad Juarez
Paseo Triunfo de la Republica 3451
Colonia Circuito Pronaf
Ciudad Juarez, Chihuahua, MEXICO 32315

Tel: 011 52 656 686.0700
Fax: 011 52 656 686.0701
Web: www.fiestainn.com

Hotel Quinta Real Monterrey
Diego Rivera #500 Fraccionamiento Valle
Oriente
San Pedro Garza Garcia, Nuevo León,
MEXICO 66260
Tel: 1 866 621.9288 (US and Canada toll-
free); 011 52 81 8368.1000
Fax: 011 52 81 8368.1070
Email: reservaciones@quintareal.com
Web: www.quintareal.com

Presidente Intercontinental Monterrey
José Vasconcelos 300
Oriente, San Pedro Garza Garcia
Monterrey, NLE, MEXICO 66260
Tel: 011 52 81 8368.6000
Fax: 011 52 81 8368.6040
Web: www.ichotelsgroup.com

Sheraton Ambassador
Avenida Hidalgo 310 Oriente
Monterrey, Nuevo León, MEXICO 64000
Tel: 011 52 81 8380.7000
Fax: 011 52 81 8345.1984
Email: Monterrey.Sheraton@Sheraton.com
Web: www.starwoodhotels.com

Colonial Hotel
Avenida Abraham Lincoln 1355
Ciudad Juarez, MEXICO 32310
Tel: 1 800 782.6926 (US toll-free); 011 52 656
613.5050
Email: reservacionescjs@hotelescolonial
.com
Web: www.hotelescolonial.com

COASTAL

One and Only Palmilla
Km 7.5 Carretera Transpeninsular
San José del Cabo
BCP, MEXICO 23400
Tel: 1 866 829.2777 (US toll-free); 011 52 624
146.7000
Fax: 011 52 624 146.7001
Email: reservations@oneandonlyresorts
.com
Web: www.oneandonlyresorts.com

**Sheraton Hacienda del Mar Resort and
Spa Los Cabos**
Corredor Turistico Km 10, Lote D
Cabo San Lucas, Baja California Sur, MEXICO
23410
Tel: 011 52 624 145.8000
Fax: 011 52 624 145.8002
Email: information@sheratonhacienda
delmar.com
Web: www.sheraton.com/HaciendaDelMar

Hotel El Tapatio and Resort
Boulevard Aeropuerto #4275, Tiaquepaque
Guadalajara, Jalisco, CP, MEXICO 45588
Tel: 1 800 327.1847 (US toll-free); 011 52 33
3837.2929
Fax: 011 52 33 3635.6664
Web: www.hotel-tapatio.com

Hotel Villa Ganz
Lopez Cotilla #1739, Col. Lafayette 44140
Guadalajara, Jalisco, MEXICO
Tel: 1 800 813.2333 (US toll-free); 011 52 33
3120.1416
Email: info@villaganz.com
Web: www.villaganz.com

■ HOTELS: MODERATE

CALIFORNIA AND ARIZONA BORDERS:

Hotel Colonial Hermosillo
Vado del Rio #9, Villa DE
Hermosillo, MEXICO 83280
Tel: 011 52 662 259.0000
Fax: 011 52 662 250.0773
Web: www.hotelscolonial.com

Grand Tijuana Hotel
Boulevard Agua Caliente #4500,
  Col. Aviación
CP 22420
Tijuana, BC, MEXICO
Tel: 1 866 495.1879 (US toll-free); 011 664
681.7000
Fax: 011 664 681.7016
Email: ventasmx@grandhoteltij.com.mx
Web: www.grandhoteltij.com.mx

Best Western Americana Inn
815 West San Ysidro Boulevard
San Diego, CA 92173
Tel: 1 800 WESTERN (US toll-free); 1 619
428.5521
Fax: 1 619 428.0693
Web: http://book.bestwestern.com

TEXAS AND NEW MEXICO BORDERS:

Courtyard by Marriott San Jeronimo
Avenida San Jerónimo 1012, Col. San
  Jerónimo
Monterrey, Nuevo León, MEXICO 64640
Tel: 1 800 561.4761 (US toll-free); 011 52 81
8389.7900
Fax: 011 52 81 8389.7910
Web: www.marriott.com

Hampton Inn Monterrey–Gallerias Obispado Hotel
Avenida Gonzalitos No. 415 Sur Obispado
Monterrey, Nuevo León, MEXICO 64060
Tel: 011 52 81 8625.2450
Fax: 011 52 81 8625.2451
Web: www.hamptoninn.com

Novotel Monterrey Valle
Avenida Lazaro Cardenas 3000
Esq. Dr. Alt, Valley Oriente
San Pedro Garza Garcia, Nuevo León,
    MEXICO 66269
Tel: 011 52 81 8133.8133
Fax: 011 52 81 8133.8134
Email: H3551@accor.com
Web: www.novotel.com

COASTAL

Costa de Oro Beach Hotel
Avenida Camaron Sabalo 710
Mazatlán, MEXICO 82110
Tel: 011 52 669 913.5344
Fax: 011 52 669 914.4209
Web: www.costaoro.com

Best Western Posada Freeman
79 Olas Altas Beach
Mazatlán, MEXICO 82000
Tel: 011 52 669 985.6060
Fax: 011 52 669 985.6064
Web: http://book.bestwestern.com

El Encanto Inn
Calle Morelos #133
San José del Cabo, BCS, MEXICO
Tel: 011 52 624 142.0388
Fax: 011 52 624 142.4620
Email: info@elencantoinn.com
Web: www.elencantoinn.com

Tropicana Inn
Boulevard Mijares #30 Colonia Centro
San José del Cabo, BCS, MEXICO 23400
Tel: 011 52 624 142.1580
Email: gtehotel@tropicanainn.com.mx
Web: www.tropicanacabo.com/hotel/

DESTINATION: **NEW ZEALAND**

■ AT A GLANCE

Auckland

Language:	English
Time Zone:	GMT +12
Country Dialing Code:	64
Electricity:	230V, Plug type C
Currency:	New Zealand dollar
Visa Required?	Not for stays shorter than 90 days
Recommended Immunizations:	None
Treatment Specialties:	Cardiology, Orthopedics, General Surgery, Gynecology, Urology
Leading Hospitals and Clinics:	Mercy Hospital, Ascot Hospital
JCI-Accredited Hospitals:	None
Standards and Accreditation:	New Zealand Council of Healthcare Standards, International Society for Quality in Health Care (ISQua)

■ TREATMENT BRIEF

While health travel is a new concept for New Zealand, the government has begun promoting health services for international patients in recent years. In 2007, 500–750 medical travelers sought care there. While most traveled from neighboring Pacific islands, the number of patients from the US, Canada, and the UK is increasing. The main attractions are affordability and quality care in an English-speaking country. Tourism services are well established in New Zealand, and healthcare standards are of the high caliber applied in Australia and a number of other Commonwealth countries. Although costs are not substantially lower than in the US (when travel and accommodations are taken into account), some health travelers choose New Zealand for its cultural familiarity, temperate climate, and eye-popping scenery.

■ TYPICAL TREATMENTS AND COSTS (including airfare, lodging, and insurance)

Cardiovascular:

Coronary Artery Bypass Graft: $37,000
Bypass + Valve Replacement (single): $40,000
Bypass + Valve Replacement (double): $40,000
Pacemaker (single-chambered): $20,000
Pacemaker (double-chambered): $20.000

Orthopedic:

Birmingham Hip Resurfacing: $20,000
Joint Replacement:
  Knee: $22,000
  Hip: $25,000
  Ankle: $22,000
  Shoulder: $20,000

Other:

Gall Bladder Removal: $12,000
Prostate Surgery (TURP): $11,000

■ HEALTH TRAVEL AGENTS

Medtral Limited
Mercy Specialist Center
100 Mountain Road
P.O. Box 99-894
Epson, Auckland, NEW ZEALAND
Tel: 1 866 206.3582 (US toll-free); 011 64 9 623.6588
Fax: 1 866 761.4627 (US toll-free); 011 64 9 623.6587
Email: edward.watson@medtral.com
Web: www.medtral.com

This new agency, established in 2007, arranges private surgical and recuperative care for medical travelers from throughout the world. Medtral New Zealand offers numerous packages priced competitively with other health travel destinations. Many Medtral-affiliated doctors were trained in the US, Canada, or the UK. Medtral arranges flights and accommodations, airport transportation, appointment and procedure schedules, and in-country support. The agency also collaborates with doctors in the patient's home country to ensure information transfer and appropriate post-procedure follow-up.

■ HOSPITALS AND CLINICS

Mercy Hospital
98 Mountain Road
Epsom, Auckland, NEW ZEALAND
Tel-Fax: 011 64 9 623.5747
Email: andrew.wong@mercyascot.com
Web: www.mercyascot.co.nz

and

Ascot Hospital
30 Greenlane Road
Remuera, Auckland, NEW ZEALAND
Tel: 011 64 9 520.9530
Fax: 011 64 9 623.5745
Email: andrew.wong@mercyascot.com
Web: www.mercyascot.co.nz

MercyAscot is a New Zealand-owned private hospital and clinics facility formed from the integration of two private surgical hospitals, Mercy Hospital and Ascot Hospital. Mercy is the teaching hospital of the University of Auckland, founded in 1900. Ascot is the newer facility, established in 1999. Mercy and Ascot boast standards comparable to those of Australian hospitals. They are best known for services in cardiology, orthopedics, general surgery, gynecology, and urology. The most often-performed procedures are arthroscopies, discectomies, and total hip joint replacements. Two hundred physicians regularly serve at Mercy and Ascot. Travel packages for these hospitals are arranged through Medtral (see "Health Travel Agents," above).

■ HOTELS: DELUXE

The Westin Auckland, Lighter Quay
21 Viaduct Harbour Avenue
Lighter Quay, Auckland NEW ZEALAND 1010
Tel: 011 64 9 909.9000
Fax: 011 64 9 909.9001
Email: westin.auckland@westin.com
Web: www.starwoodhotels.com

The Langham, Auckland
83 Symonds Street, P.O. Box 2771
Auckland 1, NEW ZEALAND
Tel: 011 64 9 379.5132
Fax: 011 64 9 377.9367
Email: akl.pabx@langhamhotels.com
Web: http://auckland.langhamhotels.co.nz

■ HOTELS: MODERATE

Novotel Ellerslie
72-112 Greenlane Road East
Ellerslie, Auckland, NEW ZEALAND 1050
Tel: 011 64 9 529.9090
Fax: 011 64 9 529.9092
Email: h3060-re01@accor.com
Web: www.novotel.com

Oaks Smartstay Apartments on Hobson
188 Hobson Street
Auckland, NEW ZEALAND 1036
Tel: 011 64 9 337.5800
Fax: 011 64 9 337.5900
Email: oaksonhobson@theoaksgroup.co.nz
Web: www.theoaksgroup.com.au

DESTINATION: PANAMA

■ AT A GLANCE

Panama City

Language:	Spanish (English widely spoken)
Time Zone:	GMT -5
Country Dialing Code:	507
Electricity:	120V, Plug type A
Currency:	US dollar or Panamanian balboa
Visa Required?	Purchase on arrival for 90 days
Recommended Immunizations:	Yellow Fever; Hepatitis A; Typhoid Booster
Treatment Specialties:	Cosmetic Surgery, In Vitro Fertilization, Orthopedics, Dental, LASIK Eye Surgery
Leading Hospitals and Clinics:	Clinica Hospital San Fernando, Centro Médico Paitilla, Hospital Nacional, Hospital Punta Pacífica
JCI-Accredited Hospitals:	None
Standards and Accreditation:	American Hospital Association, Latin American Hospital Federation, Panamanian Private Hospital Association

■ TREATMENT BRIEF

If health travel makes sense to you, but a 20+-hour flight to the other side of the world doesn't, then a Western Hemisphere nation, such as Panama, may be a good choice. While its healthcare offerings aren't on the same scale as in its Eastern counterparts, the same attributes that attract tourists to Panama attract health travelers as well: the climate is Caribbean (usually without the hurricanes!), the scenery outside the cities is appealing, and the cultural diversity of this crossroads nation is enlightening. Panama's strategic geographic position makes it a trade center, and the Canal makes it a hub of commerce in the Americas. Daily direct flights from Miami, Los Angeles, Houston, and New York get you there in four hours or less. That's one reason why Panama's tourist industry is growing by nearly 20 percent annually. Baby boomers are another, as they're retiring to Panama in droves, and there's no shortage of retirement and resort communities to attract them.

While Panama is a relative newcomer to global healthcare, the country adopted US healthcare standards de facto during its long affiliation with the US. Panamanian agents and hospitals are competing in the global healthcare market with highly credentialed doctors, new facilities, and the latest in high-tech equipment. Many physicians and surgeons are US-trained and board-certified. Treatment specialties include dental implants, plastic surgery, assisted reproduction, cardiology, cosmetic dentistry, and orthopedics.

Besides location and high-quality healthcare, Panama offers other advantages to health travelers: the US dollar is an official currency, and most doctors speak fluent English. Best of all are the prices: they can be half what you'd expect in the US or Europe.

■ TYPICAL TREATMENTS AND COSTS (not including doctors' fees)

Cardiovascular:
Coronary Artery Bypass Graft:
 $9,500-$15,000
Bypass + Valve Replacement (single):
 $12,000-$15,000
Bypass + Valve Replacement (double):
 $15,000-$18,000
Pacemaker (single-chambered):
 $2,000-$4,400
Pacemaker (double-chambered):
 $3,000-$5,700

Orthopedic:
Joint Replacement:
 Knee: $5,900-$8,000
 Hip: $4,000-$7,000
 Ankle: $1,900
 Shoulder: $6,000

Cosmetic:
Breast Augmentation: $1,500-$2,000
Breast Lift/Reduction: $1,500-$3,000
Facelift: $2,000-$3,000
Liposuction (stomach, hips, and waist):
 $1,600-$4,000
Tummy Tuck: $1,500

Dental:
Porcelain Veneer: $500
Crown (all porcelain): $500
Inlays and Onlays: $350
Implant: $1,000
Root Canal: $200-$400
Extraction (surgical, per tooth): $175

Vision:
Glaucoma (per eye): $2,500
LASIK (both eyes): $2,500

Weight Loss:
LAP-BAND System: $2,300-$7,000

Other:
Gall Bladder Removal: $1,200
Prostate Surgery (TURP): $3,200
Gynecologic Laparoscopy: $1,850
Hysterectomy:
 Abdominal: $1,800
 Vaginal: $1,400

■ HEALTH TRAVEL AGENTS

Healthbase Online, Inc.
287 Auburn Street
Newton, MA 02466
Tel: 1 888 691.4584 (US toll-free);
1 617 418.3436
Fax: 1 800 986.9230 (US toll-free)
Email: info.hb@healthbase.com
Web: www.healthbase.com

For more information on Healthbase
Online, see India: Chennai.

Pana-Health
Royal Center Building, Tower A
Marbella
Panama City, PANAMA
Tel: 1 888 825.7567 (US toll-free); 011 507
223.6766
Email: nford@pana-health.com
Web: www.pana-health.com

Pana-Health is a group of healthcare specialists who have joined together to serve
international patients and promote health
travel to Panama. Pana-Health's standard
package includes the transfer of confidential medical information and arrangements for appointments, patient-doctor
telephone consultations, hotel accommodations, and in-country transportation.
Pana-Health organizes all aspects of care,
including pre-treatment lab work, x-rays,
hospital pre-admission, hospital discharge,
and post-treatment follow-up care. Pana-
Health usually refers patients to either
Centro Médico Paitilla or Clinica Hospital
San Fernando.

Planet Hospital
23679 Calabasas Road, Suite 150
Calabasas, CA 91302
Tel: 1 800 243.0172 (US toll-free); 1 818
665.4801
Fax: 1 818 665.4810
Email: rudy@planethospital.com
Web: www.planethospital.com

For more information on Planet Hospital,
see Singapore.

■ HOSPITALS AND CLINICS

Clinica Hospital San Fernando
Via España Final
P.O. Box 0834-00363
Panama City, PANAMA
Tel: 011 507 305.6399
Fax: 011 507 305.7000
Email: elewis@hospitalsanfernando.com;
tmendez@hospitalsanfernando.com
Web: www.hospitalsanfernando.com

In operation since 1949, the 159-bed Clinica
Hospital San Fernando provides medical
services in radiology and diagnostic imaging, gynecology and obstetrics, respiratory
medicine and allergies, oncology, cardiology, nuclear medicine, and urology. Specialties include orthopedics, general surgery,
cardiovascular surgery, ambulatory surgery,
and LASIK vision correction. The most frequently performed procedures are knee
and hip replacements, laparoscopic gall
bladder removal, and LAP-BAND or gastric
bypass surgery.

San Fernando boasts affiliations with
Tulane University, Children's Hospital–
Miami, Baptist Medical Center–Miami,

Christus Health, and Christus Muguerza. The number of international patients receiving care at San Fernando now exceeds 5,000 annually. Most doctors speak English, as do staff members of the **International Affairs Office,** whose services include 24/7 fully bilingual assistance, preferred providers' appointments, preferred appointments for any medical test, a fully bilingual pharmacy that dispenses FDA-approved medications, hotel and air reservations, verification of benefits from US-based insurance companies, and coordination with a local tour company for sightseeing.

Centro Médico Paitilla

Avenida Balboa y Calle 53
Panama City, PANAMA 0816-03075
Tel: 011 507 265.8891
Fax: 011 507 265.8862
Email: aclientes@cmpaitilla.com
Web: www.centromedicopaitilla.com

This 166-bed private hospital has been in operation since 1975. Today Centro Médico Paitilla (CMP) employs more than 250 physicians and surgeons, many of them trained and board-certified in the US. The hospital has an "academic agreement" with the Cleveland Clinic and is certified as a training facility by the American Heart Association. During the time when US military bases were operational in Panama, CMP was one of two hospitals authorized to provide medical services to US military personnel and their families. Treatment specialties include oncology, cardiology, vascular surgery, orthopedics, and neurology. Procedures most frequently performed are open-heart surgery, orthopedic prosthesis implants, and cardiac catheterization with stenting. CMP

offers numerous special services within its departments of medicine, pediatrics, surgery, psychiatry, obstetrics and gynecology, odontology, imaging and radiology, and complementary medicine.

Hospital Nacional

Avenida Cuba & 38th–39th Streets
Panama City, PANAMA
Tel: 011 507 207.8100
Fax: 011 507 207.8337
Email: mercadeo@hospitalnacional.com
Web: www.hospitalnacional.com

Although the 80-bed private Hospital Nacional traces its history back to a small clinic that opened in the 1970s, the new facility is modern. Services include medical imaging (x-ray, magnetic resonance imaging [MRI], ultrasound, nuclear medicine, and fluoroscopy), angiography, mammography, bone densitometry, endoscopy, physical therapy, hyperbaric oxygen therapy, cardiologic testing (including Holter monitor, electrocardiography [EKG], echocardiography, and stress tests), and hemodialysis.

Hospital Nacional maintains agreements for care of active and retired US Army patients. These patients are within the programs Tricare Standard, Tricare Prime (Latin America), and Tricare for Life. Hospital Nacional's **International Insurance Department** handles the insurance policies of foreign companies as a special service for medical travelers. Covered patients can receive care without prepayment because the department bills insurance companies directly.

Hospital Punta Pacifica
Punta Pacifica Avenue, Paitilla
Panama City, PANAMA 0831-01593
Tel: 011 507 204.8000
Fax: 011 507 204.8010
Email: info@hpp.com.pa
Web: www.hospitalpuntapacifica.com

This 101-bed hospital opened in 2006, offering 52 private rooms. More than 350 physicians and surgeons are accredited to practice in this Johns Hopkins–affiliated hospital. All speak English, and Punta Pacifica offers supplementary English language education for all staff. Departments include urology, cardiology, orthopedics, physiotherapy and rehabilitation, gastroenterology, endoscopy, pediatrics, neurology, dermatology, gynecology and obstetrics, nephrology, endocrinology, oncology, and chemotherapy. Specialties include general and laparoscopic surgery, orthopedics, cardiovascular procedures (including minimally invasive techniques), neurosurgery, colonoscopy, endoscopy, angiography, and plastic surgery. Rates are estimated to be 30 percent less than for comparable treatments in the US. Punta Pacifica attracts 200 patients from the US and Canada annually.

■ RECOVERY ACCOMMODATIONS

In 2008 there were no recovery lodges in Panama, but that may change soon, as construction plans are in the works.

Case Study: Sandra E., Arizona

I had wanted to get my breasts redone for some time. I already had breast implants, but they had became saggy and misshapen after I had a child in 2000. I saw a plastic surgeon here in Arizona. He told me that I needed a breast lift and new implants. The cost would be $10,000.

I saw an article in the October 2007 issue of *Good Housekeeping* about medical tourism and about the agents who arrange medical travel. I chose one of them, and the agency booked me with a Harvard-trained surgeon in Panama. I had no problems with the trip. It was no different from flying to New York, except I had to go through customs.

In Panama, I got a high-quality surgeon whom I could never have afforded here. He and his team took wonderful care of me before, during, and after the surgery. I saved $4,000 by having my surgery in Panama.

My husband needs about $12,000 worth of dental work (US prices). Once I pay off my surgery on my Visa card, I will accompany him to Panama to get the work done. The dentists there are US-trained and certified. The work will cost us less than half, including flight and hotel!

■ HOTELS: DELUXE

Marriott Hotel
Calle 52 y Ricardo Arias
Area Bancaria
Panama City, PANAMA
Tel: 011 507 210.9100
Fax: 011 507 210.9110
Web: www.marriott.com

InterContinental Miramar Panama
Miramar Plaza, Avenida Balboa
Panama City, PANAMA
Tel: 011 507 206.8888
Fax: 011 507 223.4891
Email: panama@interconti.com
Web: www.miramarpanama.com

Radisson Decapolis Hotel
Avenida Balboa-Multicentro
Panama City, PANAMA 0833-0293
Tel: 1 888 201.1718 (US toll-free); 011 507 215.5000
Fax: 011 507 215.5715
Email: hotel.information@decapolishotel .com
Web: www.radisson.com/panamacitypan

■ HOTELS: MODERATE

Courtyard Marriott Real Hotel
Via Israel Multiplaza Pacific Mall
Panama City, PANAMA
Tel: 011 507 301.0101
Web: www.marriott.com/courtyard

Plaza Paitilla Inn
P.O. Box 0816-03579, Zona 5
Panama City, PANAMA
Tel: 011 507 208.0600
Fax: 011 507 208.0619
Email: reservaciones@plazapaitillainn.com
Web: www.plazapaitillainn.com

Four Points by Sheraton Panama
Street 53, Marbela & Avenue 5A-B South
Panama City, PANAMA 832-0239
Tel: 011 507 265.3636
Fax: 011 507 265.3550
Web: www.starwoodhotels.com

El Dorado Country Inn and Suites Hotel
El Dorado Shopping District
Brostella Avenue & El Dorado Boulevard
Panama City, PANAMA
Tel: 011 507 300.3700
Fax: 011 507 236.9320
Email: Sales@PanamaCanalCountry.com
Web: www.panamacanalcountry.com/ eldorado

DESTINATION: **PHILIPPINES**

■ AT A GLANCE

Manila and Quezon City

Language:	90 different languages and dialects (English is used in schools and most people speak it)
Time Zone:	GMT +8
Country Dialing Code:	63
Electricity:	110V & 220V, Plug types A & B
Currency:	Philippine peso
Visa Required?	On arrival for 21 days; can be extended
Recommended Immunizations:	Typhoid; Hepatitis A; Antimalarial Drugs
Treatment Specialties:	Cardiology, Cardiovascular Surgery, Oncology, Orthopedics, Cosmetic Surgery
Leading Hospitals and Clinics:	St. Luke's Medical Center, The Medical City, Asian Hospital and Medical Center
JCI-Accredited Hospitals:	St. Luke's Medical Center, The Medical City
Standards and Accreditation:	Philippine Department of Health, JCI

■ TREATMENT BRIEF

Medical travel is getting a lot of attention in the Philippines these days. In 2004 the Philippine Medical Tourism Program was launched as a public- and private-sector initiative. In 2006 the Philippines held its first-ever convention on medical tourism, with the theme of "Only in the Philippines: Tender Loving (Health) Care." In 2007 the *International Medical Travel Journal* reported that the Philippines were experiencing a new wave of medical travelers. The nation's former health secretary, Alfredo Bengzon, estimated that 5 percent of admissions at The Medical City in Pasig City were visitors from other countries, and he put the total number of medical travelers at nearly 100,000 annually. The big areas of demand are bariatric surgery, cosmetic surgery, ophthalmology, and dental work.

Despite all the press, however, the infrastructure of the Philippines does not yet appear ready for the discerning medical traveler. Those who seek medical care in the Philippines need to steel their nerves for Web sites that don't work, emails that bounce back, and patient inquiries that go unanswered. Although two hospitals have recently become JCI-accredited, customer service is generally poor throughout the nation's network of hospitals. Or, as one medical travel consultant put it, "Why journey to Asia's sixth leading destination when there are five others to choose from?"

There are other drawbacks. Manila is an even longer flight from the US than to most other Asian cities, often involving three or more hops. Once you're there, prepare for culture shock. The capital city, Manila, a huge urban archipelago, is chaotic and loud; the crime rate is high.

The picture is not entirely bleak, however. For those willing to do their homework, there's significant money to be saved. Knee replacement surgery in the Philippines might set you back $6,000, for example, compared to $40,000 or more in the US. And the best hospitals in the Philippines boast facilities and Western-trained physicians comparable to those at desirable medical destinations in other Asian nations. Nurses in the Philippines have earned an international reputation for excellence. So with the Philippines' growing commitment to medical travel, that nation's ability to deliver may better match its promises in the years to come.

■ TYPICAL TREATMENTS AND COSTS

Cardiovascular:
Coronary Artery Bypass Graft:
$19,000-$25,000

Orthopedic:
Joint Replacement:
Hip: $8,300-$12,200
Knee: $9,300-$10,800

Cosmetic:
Breast Augmentation: $5,250
Breast Lift/Reduction: $5,400
Tummy Tuck: $5,350

■ HEALTH TRAVEL AGENTS

Planet Hospital
23679 Calabasas Road, Suite 150
Calabasas, CA 91302
Tel: 1 800 243.0172 (US toll-free);
1 818 665.4801
Fax: 1 818 665.4810
Email: rudy@planethospital.com
Web: www.planethospital.com

For more information on Planet Hospital, see Singapore.

■ HOSPITALS AND CLINICS

St. Luke's Medical Center
279 E. Rodriguez Sr. Boulevard
Quezon City, PHILIPPINES 1102
Tel: 011 632 723.1206
Fax: 011 632 726.3911
Email: info@stluke.com.ph
Web: www.stluke.com.ph

While St. Luke's Medical Center (SLMC) has been around since 1903, there's nothing old-fashioned about this huge operation. The 650-bed hospital has nine institutes, 13 departments, and 19 centers, most equipped with the best of modern technology and staffed by internationally trained specialists. More than 1,700 physicians and surgeons are affiliated with SLMC; they see patients in more than 450 private clinics. SLMC received JCI accreditation in 2003.

SLMC offers all the usual specialties, including cardiovascular medicine, neurology and neurosurgery, cancer, ophthalmology, and treatments for digestive and liver diseases. SLMC's **International Patient Care Center** recommends medical specialists and makes appointments. It handles hospital admissions and discharges, travel planning, and airport transfers, plus translator, secretarial, and concierge services.

The Medical City
Ortigas Avenue
Pasig City
Metro Manila, PHILIPPINES
Tel: 011 63 2 635.6789
Email: mail@medicalcity.com.ph
Web: www.medicalcity.com.ph

The Medical City (TMC) is a 500-bed, private, JCI-accredited, tertiary-care hospital that's been operating since the 1970s. TMC's 350 physicians offer the full range of diagnostic and therapeutic services, utilizing state-of-the-art technology, such as computed tomography (CT), magnetic resonance imaging (MRI), and cardiac catheterization. Clinical departments and specialty units include surgery, anesthesiology, pediatrics, obstetric-gynecology, ophthalmology, otolaryngology, psychiatry, and rehabilitation medicine, as well as diagnostic and intervention units for diagnostic radiology, radiotherapy, nuclear medicine, stroke care, and intensive care.

Asian Hospital and Medical Center
2205 Civic Drive
Filinvest Corporate City, Alabang
Muntinlups City, PHILIPPINES 1780
Tel: 011 63 2 771.9000
Fax: 011 63 2 876.5761
Email: his@asianhospital.com
Web: www.asianhospital.com

Asian Hospital and Medical Center (AHMC) is the first major private hospital with tertiary-care facilities in the southern Luzon corridor of metropolitan Manila. Owned by Thailand's well-known Bumrungrad International, AHMC opened its doors in 2002. Its units include bone marrow transplant, cardiac catheterization, cardiovascular rehab, women's health, clinical nutrition, dermatology, gastrointestinal endoscopy, extracorporeal shockwave lithotripsy, eye laser and diagnosis, hemodialysis, outpatient chemotherapy, pharmacy, physical rehab, and interventional and vascular radiology.

AHMC's **International Center** arranges accommodations, transportation, and concierge services, including porters, postal deliveries, and business services. The most popular services for international patients include comprehensive executive health screening, cosmetic surgery, advanced laparoscopic and bariatric surgery, joint replacement surgery, and cardiovascular surgery.

Philippine Heart Center
East Avenue
Quezon City, PHILIPPINES 1100
Tel: 011 63 2 925.2401
Email: info@phc.gov.ph
Web: www.phc.gov.ph

Nearly a million children and adults afflicted with heart disease and related ailments have been treated at the Philippine Heart Center since it opened its doors on Valentine's Day in 1975. The center is organized to diagnose, treat, and rehabilitate patients of every age with every kind of cardiovascular disorder. Diagnostic support services include a hemodynamics cardiovascular laboratory, computed tomography (CT), electrophysiology, nuclear medicine, hemodialysis, and radiology. The **Noninvasive Cardiac Laboratory** provides complete cardiac diagnosis through inter-related noninvasive methods and procedures, such as 2D echocardiogram with color Doppler and stress (treadmill) testing. The **Diagnostic Radiology Laboratory** provides radiological services to patients, including fluoroscopic contrast examinations, tomogram of specific organs or structures, portable radiography and fluoroscopy, and diagnostic (noncardiac) ultrasound. The **Pulmonary Medicine Laboratory** diagnoses, evaluates, and manages patients with problems in the respiratory system.

The center's three main units are the **Department of Cardiovascular Surgery and Anesthesia, Department of Cardiovascular Medicine,** and **Department of Allied Medical and Surgical Specialties.** The hospital has six operating suites with

facilities and support staff for five simultaneous open-heart procedures plus one additional simultaneous closed-heart, thoracic, vascular, or general surgical procedure.

■ HOTELS: DELUXE

Makati Shangri-La Hotel
Ayala Avenue at Makati Avenue
Makati City, Manila, PHILIPPINES 1200
Tel: 011 63 2 813.8888
Fax: 011 63 2 813.5499
Email: slm@shangri-la.com
Web: www.shangri-la.com

Edsa Shangri-La Hotel
Ortigas Centre
Mandaluyong City, PHILIPPINES 1650
Tel: 011 63 2 633.8888
Fax: 011 63 2 631.1067
Email: esl@shangri-la.com
Web: www.shangri-la.com

Discovery Suites
25 ADB Avenue, Ortigas Center
Pasig City, PHILIPPINES
Tel: 011 63 2 683.8222
Fax: 011 63 2 683.8111
Web: www.discoverysuites.com

■ HOTELS: MODERATE

Holiday Inn Galleria Manila
One Asia Development Bank Avenue
Pasig, Manila, PHILIPPINES 1655
Tel: 1 800 315.2621 (US toll-free); 011 63 2
   633.7111
Fax: 011 63 2 633.2824
Web: www.ichotelsgroup.com

The Richmonde Hotel
21 San Miguel Avenue, Ortigas Center
Pasig City, Metro Manila, PHILIPPINES 1600
Tel: 011 63 2 638.7777
Fax: 011 63 2 638.8567
Web: www.richmondehotel.com

DESTINATION: SINGAPORE

■ AT A GLANCE

Singapore City

Language:	English (primary language), Mandarin, Malay, Tamil
Time Zone:	GMT +8
Country Dialing Code:	65
Electricity:	230V, Plug type G
Currency:	Singapore dollar (SGD)
Visa Required?	Not for stays shorter than 90 days
Recommended Immunizations:	Hepatitis A; Boosters for Typhoid and Polio
Treatment Specialties:	Cardiovascular, Gastroenterology, General Surgery, Hepatology, Neurology, Oncology, Ophthalmology, Orthopedics, Stem Cell Therapy
Leading Hospitals and Clinics:	National Healthcare Group, Parkway Group Healthcare, Raffles Medical Group, Singapore Health Services (SingHealth)
JCI-Accredited Hospitals:	Alexandra Hospital, Changi General Hospital, East Shore Hospital, Gleneagles Hospital and Medical Centre, Institute of Mental Health/ Woodbridge Hospital, Johns Hopkins Singapore International Medical Centre, KK Women's and Children's Hospital, Mount Elizabeth Hospital, National Heart Centre, National Skin Centre, National University Hospital, Singapore General Hospital, Tan Tock Seng Hospital
Standards and Accreditation:	Specialists Accreditation Board, Singapore Ministry of Health, JCI

■ TREATMENT BRIEF

Like Malaysia, Singapore is less familiar to US patients as a health travel destination than Thailand and India. However, Singapore has been an international healthcare destination since the 1980s, and more than 400,000 international patients visited Singapore in 2006.

The country boasts 13 JCI-accredited hospitals and centers and the most JCI-accredited facilities in Asia. Singapore is also home to Asia's second largest hospital network, Parkway Group Healthcare, with 1,500 beds, 1,400 specialists, and three JCI-accredited treatment centers.

In 2000 the World Health Organization ranked Singapore's healthcare system number one in Asia and sixth in the world. Singapore has one of the lowest infant (1.9/1,000 births) and maternal (0.0 to 1.0/1,000 live or stillbirths) mortality rates in the world. Life expectancy averages 79.3 years; males live an average of 77.4 years and females, 81.3 years.

The Health Manpower Development Program, sponsored by the Ministry of Health, sends Singapore doctors to the best medical centers around the world, and they return to serve, bringing with them a quality of services to match international standards.

Having invested a great deal of time, money, and energy in the quality of its healthcare professionals, facilities, and infrastructure through the past decades of economic plenty, Singapore finds itself in the curious position of having insufficient sick people to sustain the quality of healthcare services it has developed. Singapore's medical system must serve a larger population than its 4.5 million people—hence, the large "insourcing" of patients.

SingaporeMedicine Initiative: In 2003 the government of Singapore launched the SingaporeMedicine Initiative to develop and maintain Singapore as a medical travel destination and to consolidate its considerable medical offerings. The Singapore government supports the healthcare industry for both local and international patients. Research partnerships with US universities, such as Johns Hopkins and Duke Medical Center, along with formal relationships with GlaxoSmithKline and Novartis, underscore Singapore's sustained commitment to cutting-edge healthcare. Singapore as a medical destination is uniquely supported by a multifaceted medical hub, with research and development (bench, translational, and clinical), medical conferences and training, pharmaceutical and medical device manufacturing, and headquartering of multinational healthcare corporations.

Healthcare Specialties: Singapore boasts a wider range of healthcare services than most other countries. Highlights include the Biopolis Biotechnology Research Center, SingHealth's National Cancer Centre Singapore, and National Neuroscience Institute.

The new hub of Singapore's health sciences effort is the $300 million Biopolis, a seven-building, 2-million-square-foot biotechnology research center that opened in late 2003. Among other projects, Biopolis houses a stem cell bank to parlay some of the world's most liberal laws on the use of human embryonic cells into research and experimentation. Researchers hope that stem cells, the all-purpose building blocks that turn into specific tissues (such as bone, muscle, or nerves), can be cultivated and used to treat congenital defects, injuries, and a host of other maladies. Dozens of US and European scientists have been lured to Biopolis, which has, in turn, yielded partnerships with prominent universities, research centers, and pharmaceutical and healthcare companies.

The National Cancer Centre is one of Asia's leading hospitals for oncology diagnosis and treatment. This multidisciplinary research and treatment complex offers specialties in bone, breast, brain, cervical, colon, liver, lymph, lung, ovarian, and prostate cancers. The National Neuroscience Institute, the leading regional specialist center for treatment, education, and research in the neurosciences, has the world's first integrated neuroscience center, the BrainSuite. It has an operating theater equipped for high-precision radiosurgery and advanced image-guidance navigation.

Health travelers enjoy the widespread use of English as the preferred business language. Because Singapore is one of Asia's wealthiest nations and has Southeast Asia's highest standard of living, medical travelers are spared the glaring cultural and economic contrasts often seen in India, Central America, and South America. Most of Singapore is squeaky clean, with some city streets so filled with US retail storefronts that they feel eerily like home.

While most treatments are far less costly than in the US, Singapore remains one of Asia's more expensive medical stops, catering largely to patrons from adjacent countries, the Middle East, Europe, and Africa,

who are seeking higher quality care and are willing to pay for it. The slightly higher prices are offset by shorter stays, better outcomes, and quicker returns to active life.

Those seeking scenic side trips or exotic vacations should know that Singapore is entirely urban and suburban, offering few opportunities for rural or beach excursions. However, Malaysia and Thailand, both excellent medical destinations in their own right, are relatively short hops by air from Singapore and offer additional vacation options.

■ TYPICAL TREATMENTS AND COSTS

Cardiovascular:
Coronary Artery Bypass Graft:
$12,050-$20,500
Bypass + Valve Replacement:
Single Valve: $21,000-$23,500
Double Valve: $22,500-$25,000
Pacemaker (single-chambered): $550
Pacemaker (double-chambered): $750
Angiography: $2,500-$3,750
Angioplasty: $9,950-$16,400

Orthopedic:
Birmingham Hip Resurfacing: $12,000
Carpal Tunnel: $850-$1,250
Joint Replacement:
Knee: $8,350-$10,900
Hip: $12,000
Ankle: $4,500-$6,000
Shoulder: $5,500-$6,800

Cosmetic:

Botox: $300-$1,000

Breast Augmentation: $5,000-$10,000

Breast Lift/Reduction: $5,000-$10,000

Breast Reconstruction: $3,500-$5,000

Facelift: $5,000-$10,000

Liposuction (stomach, hips, and waist):
$3,000-$10,000

Tummy Tuck: $4,000-$8,000

Dental:

Porcelain Veneer: $250-$300

Crown (all porcelain): $275-$325

Inlays and Onlays: $425

Implant: $2,500-$3,200

Extraction (surgical, per tooth): $50-$125

Vision:

Cataract (per eye): $1,850-$4,000

Glaucoma (per eye): $500-$4,150

LASIK (per eye): $925-$1,800

Weight Loss:

LAP-BAND System: $8,800

Gastric Bypass: $13,000-$40,000

Other:

Gall Bladder Removal: $1,950-$3,850

Hernia Repair (one): $1,950-$3,350

Prostate Surgery (TURP): $3,550-$6,950

■ HEALTH TRAVEL AGENTS

ChoiceMed Health

9 Tan Quee Lan Street, #02-02 TQL Suites

SINGAPORE 188098

Tel: 011 65 6884.9375

Fax: 011 65 6884.9376

Email: inquiries@choicemed.com

Web: www.choicemed.com

This newcomer in the health travel arena started up in 2007, hoping to establish a track record for service in five coordinated areas: hassle-free trip planning, attentive and caring doctors, premium hospital service, excellent airlines and luxury hotels, and a dedicated, round-the-clock concierge service. ChoiceMed offers a standard package that includes all consultations and procedural costs, medications, room charge, rehab, x-rays, flights and hotel (for two), concierge service, local transport, and a leased mobile phone. The agency sends clients to the JCI-accredited National University Hospital, KK Women's and Children's Hospital, and Changi General Hospital.

Companion Global Healthcare, Inc.

c/o Blue Cross Blue Shield of South Carolina

I-20 at Alpine Road, AF-324

Columbia, SC 29219

Tel: 1 803 264.3256

Fax: 1 803 264.7063

Email: David.Boucher@BCBSSC.com

Web: www.CompanionGlobalHealthcare
.com

For more information on Companion Global Healthcare, see Thailand.

Healthbase Online, Inc.

287 Auburn Street

Newton, MA 02466

Tel: 1 888 691.4584 (US toll-free); 1 617
418.3436

Fax: 1 800 986.9230 (US toll-free)

Email: info.hb@healthbase.com

Web: www.healthbase.com

For more information on Healthbase Online, see India: Chennai.

International Medical Resources, LLC
9492 Good Lion Road
Columbia, MD 21045
Tel: 1 410 992.3436
Fax: 1 410 992.3437
Email: info@medinfoonline.com
Web: www.medinfoonline.com

For more information on International Medical Resources, see Thailand.

Planet Hospital
23679 Calabasas Road, Suite 150
Calabasas, CA 91302
Tel: 1 800 243.0172 (US toll-free); 1 818
665.4801
Fax: 1 818 665.4810
Email: rudy@planethospital.com
Web: www.planethospital.com

Rudy Rupak founded Planet Hospital in 2002, after being impressed with the quality of care his fiancée received when she fell ill in Thailand. This agency has since sent more than 1,200 patients abroad for medical care. Planet Hospital currently serves 12 countries, including Belgium, Costa Rica, India, Mexico, Singapore, Thailand, the Philippines, Panama, El Salvador, Cyprus, and Malta. The company has concierges in every city it serves, and company representatives personally inspect every hospital and doctor it recommends.

Planet Hospital currently serves several self-insured employers who have contracted with the agency to help their employees save money. Specialties include cardiovascular services, orthopedics, cosmetic surgery, dental care, fertility/ reproduction (including surrogacy), and oncology. Planet Hospital is the only medical travel company that has been a member of the Better Business Bureau since 2002 with an AA rating.

The company's Web site offers a comprehensive list of major hospitals in its service area, along with a sampling of its top recommended physicians and their credentials. A robust testimonials page features real clients with real names. At this writing, Planet Hospital is sending five patients per day abroad for treatment from its offices in California, Saudi Arabia, the UK, Canada, and France.

The Taj Medical Group, Limited
408 West 57th Street, Suite 9N
New York, NY 10019
Tel: 1 877 799.9797 (US toll-free)
Email: info@tajmedical.com
Web: www.tajmedical.com

For more information on Taj Medical Group, see India: Delhi.

■ HOSPITALS AND CLINICS

Essentially all four healthcare provider groups in Singapore are private limited companies. National Healthcare Group and Singapore Health Services (also known as SingHealth) are public-sector services, owned by the government. Private providers include Parkway Group Healthcare and many other medical centers, such as the Johns Hopkins Singapore International Medical Centre.

Sorting through these four healthcare groups and their 24 hospitals and clinics can be daunting! The following lists the hospitals most frequently used by international patients.

National Healthcare Group

Institute of Mental Health/Woodbridge
  Hospital*
Johns Hopkins Singapore International
  Medical Centre*
National University Hospital*
Tan Tock Seng Hospital*
Alexandra Hospital*
National Skin Center*

Parkway Group Healthcare

Gleneagles Hospital*
Mount Elizabeth Hospital*
East Shore Hospital*

Singapore Health Services (SingHealth)

Hospitals
  Changi General Hospital*
  KK Women's and Children's Hospital*
  Singapore General Hospital*
National Centres
  Cancer
  Dental
  Heart*
  Eye
  Neuroscience Institute

Other Medical Groups and Centers

AsiaMedic
eMenders Medical Specialist Group
Mount Alvernia Hospital
Pacific Healthcare
Raffles Hospital
Thomson Medical Centre
Surgeons International

*JCI-accredited

■ NATIONAL HEALTHCARE GROUP

National Healthcare Group (NHG) is a major
public healthcare provider in Singapore,
recognized at home and abroad for the
quality of its medical expertise and facilities. National University Hospital (see
below) was Singapore's first public-sector
institution to achieve JCI accreditation.

The institutions in the NHG provide
a full range of healthcare services, from
health screening to tertiary specialist services to medical research. Health travelers
use the group's one-stop **International Patient Liaison Centre** (IPLC) that facilitates
access to all NHG services. The IPLC acts as a
liaison between NHG and referral resources,
patients and families, and payers outside of
Singapore.

As a major healthcare provider in Singapore, NHG offers an integrated network of
nine primary healthcare polyclinics, three
acute-care hospitals, one psychiatric hospital, one national center, three specialty
institutes, and five business divisions.

National University Hospital
5 Lower Kent Ridge Road
SINGAPORE 119074
Tel: 011 65 6779.2777
Fax: 011 65 6777.8065
Email: iplc@nhg.com.sg
Web: www.nuh.com.sg

National University Hospital (NUH) is an
acute-care tertiary hospital. It was also the
first hospital in Singapore to be accredited
by JCI. NUH offers a full range of services
and facilities, including specialist clinics and
centers, clinical support services (such as

dietetics and diagnostic imaging), dental services, nursing care, and support groups for liver transplant and breast cancer patients. Its departments include cardiology, cardiothoracic and vascular surgery, gastroenterology and hematology, hepatology, oncology, hand and reconstructive microsurgery, neonatology, obstetrics and gynecology, ophthalmology, orthopedic surgery, head and neck surgery, pathology, pediatric surgery, urology, oral and maxillofacial surgery, and restorative dentistry. The hospital's clinicians also serve on the Faculty of Medicine at the National University of Singapore.

Tan Tock Seng Hospital
11 Jalan Tan Tock Seng
SINGAPORE 308433
Tel: 011 65 6779.2777
Fax: 011 65 6777.8065
Email: iplc@nhg.com.sg
Web: www.ttsh.com.sg

Established in 1844, Tan Tock Seng Hospital (TTSH) is Singapore's second largest acute-care hospital, with 1,400 beds. With strengths in geriatric medicine, infectious disease management, rehabilitation medicine, respiratory medicine, rheumatology, allergy, and immunology, TTSH is also a major referral center for diagnostic radiology, emergency medicine, ophthalmology, gastroenterology, otolaryngology, and orthopedic surgery. The hospital includes two major specialty centers: one in rehabilitation medicine and communicable diseases, and the other in research on treatments for emerging diseases.

Johns Hopkins Singapore International Medical Centre
11 Jalan Tan Tock Seng
SINGAPORE 308433
Tel: 011 65 6880.2236
Fax: 011 65 6880.2223
Email: iploffice@imc.jhmi.edu
Web: www.imc.jhmi.edu

Johns Hopkins Singapore (JHS) was established by the US university of the same name in 1998 as its base of medical operations in Southeast Asia. Physicians from Johns Hopkins in Baltimore collaborate with Singapore medical institutions and physicians, providing inpatient care to manage and treat disease; outpatient care to screen for, diagnose, monitor, and treat early-stage and advanced cancers; second opinions on complex medical conditions; and consultations with referring physicians.

Research and educational activities are carried out by the **Division of Biomedical Sciences,** an academic division of the medical school, with a focus on cellular and immunotherapies and a specific interest in stem cell, virology, and cancer research.

In 2005 the medical center relocated to its current premises in Tan Tock Seng Hospital, which expanded its facilities considerably. The increased space has enabled JHS to increase the number of beds available for chemotherapy patients and other inpatients.

Alexandra Hospital
International Patient Services
Level 3 Administrative Block
378 Alexandra Road
SINGAPORE 159964
Tel: 011 65 6476.8828
Fax: 011 65 6379.3880
Email: ips@alexhosp.com.sg
Web: www.alexhosp.com.sg

Formerly the British Military Hospital, Alexandra Hospital received a complete makeover in 2000 under NHG's auspices. Besides offering patient-centered service and promoting medical excellence through its research infrastructure, the hospital prides itself on its tranquil and healing environment. Because research shows that greenery speeds recovery, the hospital offers its patients a therapeutic garden that includes a 100-species butterfly trail, an ecological garden, a fragrant garden, and a medicinal garden with 100 types of healing plants.

One innovation at Alexandra is a platform that allows post-surgery patients to update nurses by sending pictures of their wounds via multimedia message service or email. The hospital ranks highest in the Singapore Ministry of Health's patient satisfaction survey.

Specialties include cardiology, dentistry, diabetes diagnosis and treatment, endocrinology, gastroenterology, general surgery, neurology, ophthalmology, orthopedics, and neck and head surgery. Alexandra was the first hospital in Southeast Asia to perform a limb reattachment.

■ PARKWAY GROUP HEALTHCARE

Parkway Group Healthcare (http://singapore.parkwayhealth.com) is a wholly owned subsidiary of Parkway Holdings Limited. Another of Asia's massive private healthcare organizations, Parkway has an extensive network of hospitals and integrated healthcare facilities throughout Singapore. Its **International Patient Assistance Centre** (www.ipac.sg) is a one-stop service for international patients visiting its affiliated hospitals.

Gleneagles Hospital and Medical Centre
6A Napier Road
SINGAPORE 258500
Tel: 011 65 6735.5000
Fax: 011 65 6732.6733
Email: ipac@parkway.sg
Website: www.gleneagles.com.sg

Established in 1957 and purchased by Parkway Group Healthcare in 1987, the JCI-accredited Gleneagles Hospital and Medical Centre is a 380-bed, private, tertiary, acute-care hospital. It has established partnerships with Johns Hopkins Hospital (US) and Thames Valley Hospital (UK). With a total of 280 specialists, the hospital is a leading center for the care and treatment of cardiac patients. It is also a regional referral center with proven technology, being the first hospital in Southeast Asia to use a robotic surgiscope for neurosurgery, spinal surgery, and ear, nose, and throat surgeries.

Parkway set up the **Asian Centre for Liver Diseases and Transplantation** (ACLDT) at Gleneagles in 1994. ACLDT is the first private center in Asia dedicated to the treatment of all types of liver diseases, including liver cancer, hepatitis, alcoholic cirrhosis, and pediatric liver diseases. Gleneagles was the first hospital in Southeast Asia to perform a living-donor liver transplant.

Other specialties include cancer treatment, cardiology, cardiothoracic and vascular surgery, gastroenterology and hepatology, hematology, lithotripsy, neuroscience, oral and maxillofacial surgery, neonatology, obstetrics and gynecology, ophthalmology, orthopedics, pediatrics, sports and exercise medicine, and urology.

Mount Elizabeth Hospital
3 Mount Elizabeth
SINGAPORE 228510
Tel: 011 65 6735.5000
Fax: 011 65 6732.6733
Email: ipac@parkway.sg
Website: www.mountelizabeth.com.sg

Mount Elizabeth Hospital (MEH) is a 505-bed, private, tertiary, acute-care hospital. It has performed the largest number of cardiac surgeries and neurosurgeries in the private sector in the region.

The **Mount Elizabeth Oncology Centre** (MEOC) provides comprehensive facilities for treating a wide range of cancers. MEOC was the first center in Asia to provide TomoTherapy, one of the latest radiation treatments for cancer. Other technologies used by MEOC in treating cancer tumors include intensity-modulated radiation therapy, which is beneficial in cases where a tumor occurs very close to a critical organ; external radiation therapy; radiosurgery or stereotactic radiotherapy, used to treat tumors in the head and upper neck; and brachytherapy for cancers of the cervix,

lung, esophagus, bile ducts, nose, and throat.

MEH's **Hematology and Stem Cell Transplant Centre** (HSCTC) is the first facility in Southeast Asia to offer stem cell transplant therapy. The center specializes in treating blood disorders, such as leukemia, thalassemia, and sickle cell anemia, and advanced cancers, such as those of the kidney, pancreas, and ovary.

**Specialist Dental Group
(Henry Lee Dental Surgery)**
3 Mount Elizabeth Medical Centre, #08-10
   & #08-08
Mount Elizabeth Medical Centre
SINGAPORE 228510
Tel: 011 65 6734.9393
Fax: 011 65 6733.6032
Email: info@specialistdentalgroup.com
Web: www.specialistdentalgroup.com

Specialist Dental Group started treating international patients in 1979. Patients come from Australia, the US, the UK, Russia, Mongolia, Fiji, the Maldives, Bangladesh, Indonesia, and Malaysia. Services include dental implants, whitening, crowns, veneers, dentures, root canals, gum treatments, wisdom tooth extraction, orthodontics, and treatment of jaw disorders.

Specialist also features the "Teeth-in-an-Hour" system. Conventional implant treatment requires an intermediate stage of temporary implants that must stay in place for several weeks. With Teeth-in-an-Hour by Nobelbiocare, however, implants and replacement teeth can be placed at the same time. The process is completed in about an hour, and the patient leaves with his or her final teeth at the end of the appointment.

Recently the practice has doubled its

office space and doubled the number of dental specialists working there. The clinic's location at the Mount Elizabeth Medical Centre, next to the hospital, has resulted in a dental team experienced in the treatment of medically compromised patients, including people with heart problems, diabetes, cancer, or immunosuppression.

The clinic's internationally trained team includes dental specialists certified by American and Canadian Boards of Prosthodontists. Online appointment booking is available.

■ SINGAPORE HEALTH SERVICES (SINGHEALTH)

Singapore Health Services (SingHealth) is Singapore's largest group of healthcare institutions, with three hospitals, five national specialty centers, and a network of primary healthcare clinics.

■ HOSPITALS

Changi General Hospital
2 Simei Street 3
SINGAPORE 529889
Tel: 011 65 8125.8293
Fax: 011 65 6782.1353
Email: international@cgh.com.sg
Web: www.cgh.com.sg

Changi General Hospital (CGH) is located only ten minutes from Singapore International Airport. It offers a comprehensive range of medical, surgical, and paramedical services and a medical center for international travelers. CGH is an emerging expert in various specialties, such as gastroenterology, dermatology, obstructive sleep apnea, sports medicine, prostate management, male impotence, urinary incontinence, cartilage transplant, arthroscopy, one-stop breast care, and multiphasic health screening. The hospital is also well equipped with modern technology, such as magnetic resonance imaging (MRI), Spirul computed tomography (CT), and cardiac catheterization.

KK Women's and Children's Hospital
100 Bukit Timah Road
SINGAPORE 229899
Tel: 011 65 6394.8888
Fax: 011 65 6292.5145
Email: international@kkh.com.sg
Web: www.kkh.com.sg

KK Women's and Children's Hospital (KKH) is the largest facility in Singapore providing specialized care for women, babies, and children. KKH is a major tertiary referral center for high-risk obstetrics, gynecological oncology, urogynecology, neonatology, pediatrics, pediatric bone-marrow transplants, and pediatric open-heart surgeries. It is also a teaching hospital affiliated with the National University of Singapore.

The **KK Women's Hospital** contains a breast center and other subspecialty units, such as minimally invasive surgery; plastic, reconstructive, and aesthetic surgery; and sports medicine. The **KK Breast Centre** is a one-stop center for breast health.

The **KK Minimally Invasive Surgery Centre** (KKMIS) is a specialized gynecological center with expertise in endoscopic surgery. A highly qualified team of laparoscopic surgeons performs minimally invasive surgery for uterine fibroids, ovarian cysts, endometriosis, sterilization, reversal of sterilization, and tubal surgery.

The **KK Children's Hospital** offers a wide range of pediatric medical and surgical services. The **Cleft and Craniofacial Centre** is the only dedicated, comprehensive craniofacial service in Singapore. KKH's **Children's Cancer Centre** is one of the largest pediatric children's cancer centers in Southeast Asia.

Singapore General Hospital
Outram Road
SINGAPORE 169608
Tel: 011 65 6326.5656
Fax: 011 65 6326.5900
Email: ims@sgh.com.sg
Web: www.sgh.com.sg

Established in 1821, Singapore General Hospital (SGH) is Singapore's oldest and largest acute-care tertiary hospital. It is dedicated to research and providing multidisciplinary medical care. Backed by state-of-the-art facilities, it offers team-based, high-quality patient care and has 29 clinical specialties.

Its four specialty centers are the **National Cancer Centre, National Dental Centre, National Heart Centre,** and the **Singapore National Eye Centre.** SGH is also the national referral center for plastic surgery and burns, renal medicine, nuclear medicine, pathology, and hematology.

Specialties include colorectal surgery, dermatology, diagnostic radiology, endocrinology, gastroenterology, geriatric medicine, hematology, hand surgery, internal medicine, neonatal and developmental medicine, neurology, neurosurgery, nuclear medicine and positron emission tomography (PET), obstetrics and gynecology, orthopedic surgery, pathology, rehabilitative

medicine, renal medicine, respiratory and critical care medicine, rheumatology and immunology, urology, plastic surgery, reconstructive surgery, aesthetic surgery, and surgery of the ear, nose, and throat.

■ NATIONAL CENTERS

National Cancer Centre Singapore
11 Hospital Drive
SINGAPORE 169610
Tel: 011 65 6236.9433
Fax: 011 65 6536.0611
Email: foreign_patient@nccs.com.sg
Web: www.nccs.com.sg

The National Cancer Centre Singapore (NCCS) is a national and regional center dedicated to the prevention and treatment of cancers, including thoracic, hepatobiliary (liver and bile ducts), pancreatic, head, and neck cancers. It sees over 50 percent of the cancer patients in Singapore.

As a one-stop specialist center housing Singapore's largest pool of oncologists, NCCS uses advanced equipment and employs the latest therapies, including minitransplants and targeted therapies that maximize outcomes and minimize undesirable side effects.

Physically and operationally designed to provide integrated, holistic, patient-centered clinical services, the center promotes cross-consultation among oncologists of different specialties. Patients can therefore be assessed by more than one specialist during the same visit. NCCS also conducts clinical and basic research and develops public cancer education programs directed toward prevention and treatment.

National Dental Centre
4, Second Hospital Avenue
SINGAPORE 168938
Tel: 011 65 6324.2215
Fax: 011 65 6324.8810
Email: appointment@ndc.com.sg
Web: www.ndc.com.sg

The National Dental Centre (NDC) is Singapore's referral center for patients needing specialized oral healthcare services. NDC attends to more than 160,000 patients yearly, supported by fully trained support staff, 92 fully equipped dental treatment rooms, and a day-surgery center with six operating theatres. Interdepartmental teams offer an integrated environment for managing the full spectrum of oral healthcare services.

National Heart Centre
Mistri Wing
17 Third Hospital Avenue
SINGAPORE 168752
Tel: 011 65 6326.5656
Fax: 011 65 6326.5900
Email: ims@singhealth.com.sg
Web: www.nhc.com.sg

The National Heart Centre (NHC) is the national referral center for cardiovascular diseases in Singapore. It provides comprehensive preventive, diagnostic, therapeutic, and rehabilitative cardiac services to local and overseas patients. NHC's multidisciplinary team of professionals carries out approximately 75,000 cardiac investigative procedures and over 6,000 heart operations annually. To date, NHC has performed 24 heart transplants, and the survival rate of its heart transplant patients compares favorably with international standards established in other institutions. NHC's lung

transplantation program was started in 1999; it offers hope for some patients who have final-stage lung disease.

Singapore National Eye Centre
11 Third Hospital Avenue
SINGAPORE 168751
Tel: 011 65 6100.9393
Fax: 011 65 6222.9393
Email: ips@snec.com.sg
Web: www.snec.com.sg

The Singapore National Eye Centre (SNEC) has a staff of 450 medical, paramedical, and administrative personnel. SNEC is actively involved in clinical trials and research into the causes and treatments of major eye conditions, such as myopia and glaucoma. It is the only center outside of the US that teaches the use of the automated lamellar keratoplasty instrument in performing endothelial keratoplasty, a corneal transplant procedure that does not require the removal of the entire cornea. Other SNEC specialties include cataract and comprehensive ophthalmology, cornea and external eye disease, glaucoma, neuroophthalmology, ocular inflammation and immunology, oculoplastic and aesthetic eye surgery, pediatric ophthalmology and strabismus correction, refractive surgery, and vitreoretinal surgery.

National Neuroscience Institute
11 Jalan Tan Tock Seng
SINGAPORE 308433
Tel: 011 65 9637.9718
Fax: 011 65 6357.7103
Email: nni_secretariat@nni.com.sg
Web: www.nni.com.sg

The National Neuroscience Institute (NNI) is the international specialist center for the management and care of neurological diseases. It provides treatment for a broad range of illnesses that affect the brain, spine, nerves, and muscle. The team of NNI clinicians attends to the largest number of outpatient cases and inpatient admissions for neurological diseases in Singapore. Its medical care is complemented by state-of-the-art medical equipment and imaging technology. It is the only institute in Singapore with a dedicated neuroradiology department.

NNI is one of the few centers in Asia capable of participating in international clinical trials for new medications, particularly for stroke treatment. In the area of technology, NNI is the first in Southeast Asia to launch the 3 TESLA magnetic resonance imagery (MRI) scanner, a highly accurate instrument that provides better neuro-imaging for patients with stroke, epilepsy, and other neurological diseases.

National Skin Centre
1 Mandalay Road
SINGAPORE 308205
Tel: 011 65 6253.4455
Fax: 011 65 6253.3225
Email: nurseadvice@nsc.gov.sg
Web: www.nsc.gov.sg

The National Skin Centre is an outpatient dermatological center that provides specialized dermatological services and conducts research in dermatology. It is the national and regional referral center for treatment of complex skin diseases; it is also a training center for local and international skin specialists and paramedical personnel. The center offers clinics for contact dermatitis, occupational dermatoses, cutaneous infection, dermatological and laser surgery, drug eruption, hair and nail disorders, immunodermatology, lymphoma, pediatric dermatology, phototherapy, and the treatment of wounds and ulcers.

■ RAFFLES MEDICAL GROUP

Raffles Hospital
585 North Bridge Road
SINGAPORE 188770
Tel: 011 65 6311.1666
Fax: 011 65 6311.2333
Email: enquiries@raffleshospital.com
Web: www.raffleshospital.com

Raffles Medical Group (RMG) is one of the largest private healthcare providers in Singapore. RMG consists of an extensive network of 60 Raffles Medical Clinics islandwide and a flagship hospital, Raffles Hospital. RMG's holistic approach to healthcare led to the inception of **Raffles Health,** a preventive care unit that offers a full range of nutraceuticals, supplements, vitamins, and medical diagnostic equipment.

Raffles Hospital is a full-service private hospital that offers a full complement of specialist services combined with some of the most advanced medical technology. The hospital also offers several outpatient specialty clinics, including **Raffles Aesthetics Centre, Raffles Cancer Centre, Raffles Children's Centre, Raffles DentiCare, Raffles Heart Centre, Raffles Surgery Centre,** and **Raffles Women's Centre.** As an alternative or complement to Western medicine, **Raffles Chinese Medicine** offers services in herbal medicine, acupuncture, and acupressure.

■ HOTELS: DELUXE

Four Seasons Hotel Singapore
190 Orchard Boulevard
SINGAPORE 248646
Tel: 011 65 6734.1110
Fax: 011 65 6733.0682
Email: businesscentre.sin@fourseasons
.com
Web: www.fourseasons.com/singapore

Furama Riverfront Singapore
405 Havelock Road
SINGAPORE 169633
Tel: 011 65 6333.8898
Fax: 011 65 6733.1588
Email: riverfront@furama.com
Web: www.riverfront.furama.com

Grand Hyatt Singapore
10 Scotts Road
SINGAPORE 228211
Tel: 011 65 6738.1234
Fax: 011 65 6732.1696
Email: sales.sg@hyattintl.com
Web: www.singapore.grand.hyatt.com

Intercontinental Singapore
80 Middle Road
SINGAPORE 188966
Tel: 011 65 6338.7600
Fax: 011 65 6338.7366
Email: singapore@interconti.com
Web: www.singapore.intercontinental.com

■ HOTELS: MODERATE

Golden Landmark Hotel
390 Victoria Street
SINGAPORE 188061
Tel: 011 65 6297.2828
Fax: 011 65 6298.2038
Email: info@goldenlandmark.com.sg
Web: www.goldenlandmark.com.sg

New Orchid Hotel
347 Balestier Road
SINGAPORE 329777
Tel: 011 65 6253.2112
Fax: 011 65 6255.6033
Email: neworchidhotel@hotmail.com
Web: www.avipclub.com/sg/neworchid

Park View Hotel
81 Beach Road
SINGAPORE 189692
Tel: 011 65 6338.8558
Fax: 011 65 6334.8558
Email: parkview@parkview.com.sg
Web: www.parkview.com.sg

Allson Hotel Singapore
101 Victoria Street
SINGAPORE 188018
Tel: 011 65 6336.0811
Fax: 011 65 6339.7019
Email: allson.res@pacific.net.sg
Web: www.allsonhotelsingapore.com

DESTINATION:
SOUTH AFRICA (CAPE TOWN AND JOHANNESBURG)

■ AT A GLANCE

Cape Town and Johannesburg

Language:	Afrikaans and 12 other languages (English widely spoken)
Time Zone:	GMT +2
Country Dialing Code:	27
Electricity:	230V, Plug types M & C
Currency:	Rand
Visa Required?	No
Recommended Immunizations:	Hepatitis A; Boosters for Typhoid and Polio
Treatment Specialties:	Addiction Recovery, Cardiovascular, Cosmetic, Dental, Ophthalmology, Orthopedics
Leading Hospitals and Clinics:	Bay View Private Hospital, Cape Town Medi-Clinic, Carter Gordon Clinic, Christiaan Barnard Memorial Hospital, Kingsbury Hospital, Netcare Olivedale Hospital, Pretoria Eye Institute, The Rosebank Clinic
JCI-Accredited Hospitals:	None
Standards and Accreditations:	South African Medical Association, Health Professions Council of South Africa, The Council for Health Service Accreditation of Southern Africa (a member of the International Society for Quality in Health Care [ISQua]), Association of Plastic and Reconstructive Surgeons of South Africa, International Society of Aesthetic Plastic Surgery

■ TREATMENT BRIEF

Since Dr. Christiaan Barnard performed the world's first heart transplant operation in 1967, South Africa and medicine have been synonymous. Capitalizing on its superb medical reputation as one way of overcoming the stigma of apartheid, South Africa has emerged as a world-class destination for health travelers.

Because of South Africa's long travel times and relatively high treatment costs, most health travelers choose this country for its privacy, unique sightseeing opportunities, or both. For those who do not wish friends and family to know about their cosmetic and other elective procedures, what better excuse for a month's absence than an African safari? Or for patients with a more charitable bent, South Africa and its neighboring nations offer vast opportunities for a few weeks' volunteer work. Either option is a convenient way to pass a month or two and then return home rested and healed.

Those sensitive to cultural and language differences may prefer South Africa over some South American, Asian, or European countries because they're more likely to be greeted in English. Cape Town and Johannesburg—South Africa's two main medical cities—are distinctly Anglo-centric within a melting pot of cultures and social classes.

Long known as a center of high-quality cosmetic surgeries coupled with first-rate surgeons, South Africa has nearly as long a history of excellent dental care, particularly restorative and cosmetic. More recently, orthopedic surgery—primarily hip and knee work—is attracting European health travelers who are willing to pay higher treatment costs to avoid the cultural rigors of India or Brazil.

South Africa also boasts an enviable stable of well-established health travel agents whose services can be a godsend to any prospective international patient. The newly formed Medical Tourism Association of South Africa helps to maintain quality standards and service and to foster excellent relationships among patients, treatment centers, in-country third-party facilities, and international partners.

A word of caution: if you're thinking "exotic far-flung vacation" when you think South Africa, you're on the right track. You need to remember, however, that most cosmetic surgery protocols specifically caution against exposure to the sun after treatment. Since there's no shortage of sun in that part of the world, plan to take your safari, bush trip, or beach getaway prior to your procedure.

■ TYPICAL TREATMENTS AND COSTS

Cardiovascular:
Bypass + Valve Replacement (single): $40,250

Cosmetic:
Breast Augmentation: $4,300-$5,200
Breast Lift/Reduction: $6,300-$6,900
Facelift: $6,500-$7,200
Liposuction (stomach, hips, and waist): $4,500-$5,750
Tummy Tuck: $4,800-$5,750

Dental:
Crown: $860–$920
Implant: $1,900–$2,400
Extraction (surgical, per tooth): $320–$360

Vision:
LASIK (per eye): $2,530–$2,875

■ HEALTH TRAVEL AGENTS

MedRetreat
2042 Laurel Valley Drive
Vernon Hills, IL 60061
Tel: 1 877 876.3373 (US toll-free)
Fax: 1 847 680.0484
Email: customerservice@medretreat.com
Web: www.medretreat.com

For more information on MedRetreat, see
Malaysia.

Surgeon and Safari
158 Mount Street, Bryanston, Sandton
Johannesburg, Gauteng, SOUTH AFRICA
Tel: 011 27 82 395.3356
Email: lorraine@surgeon-and-safari.co.za
Web: www.surgeon-and-safari.co.za

This is perhaps the best known of all cosmetic surgery travel agencies. Its founder, Lorraine Melvill, opened Surgeon and Safari to UK clients in 2000. Now more than one-third of its patients are from the US. Sometimes jokingly referred to as the "beauty and the beast" agency, Surgeon and Safari provides A-to-Z services, including help with medical evaluation and consultations, appointments with surgeons, airport transport, and medical transfers. A Surgeon and Safari representative personally accompanies each patient to all medical appoint-

ments and stays with him or her on the day of surgery.

The agency most often refers patients to The Rosebank Clinic (see "Hospitals and Clinics," below) and Castenhof Hospital in Johannesburg.

Those planning surgery in Johannesburg may want to look into Surgeon and Safari's recovery lodgings. Available only to the agency's patients, the private houses provide most hotel amenities, plus round-the-clock recuperation assistance for guests. Prices at Surgeon and Safari's recovery retreat are about half those of a five-star Johannesburg hotel. In addition to cosmetic and plastic surgery procedures, Surgeon and Safari has recently begun offering dental care, ophthalmology, and orthopedics.

Surgical Attractions
45 Bristol Road
Parkwood, Johannesburg
Gauteng, SOUTH AFRICA
Tel: 011 27 11 880.5122
Fax: 011 27 11 788.9043
Email: info@surgicalattractions.com
Web: www.surgicalattractions.com

Ingrid Lomas established Surgical Attractions in 2002. Since then she has served more than 5,500 international patients. Her main office is in Johannesburg, although her agency arranges medical treatment in both Cape Town and Johannesburg, often sending patients to The Rosebank Clinic or Christiaan Barnard Memorial Hospital (see "Hospitals and Clinics," below). Surgical Attractions arranges telephone consultations between patients and physicians and facilitates continuing email communication. The agency offers a full range of additional services, including pre-operative and post-operative care, recuperation accommodation, a companion care service, rejuvenation holiday tours, and transportation to and from airports and medical facilities. For those who wish additional travel services, Surgical Attractions can arrange in-country travel and assist with international travel and other nonmedical travel details.

If you want to avoid hotels, Surgical Attractions also maintains partnerships in Cape Town and Johannesburg with various guest care lodges, which are the private homes of nurses who care for recovering patients. These accommodations provide medical assistance 24/7, companionship for patients traveling alone, and three home-cooked meals a day.

■ HOSPITALS AND CLINICS

While no South African hospitals currently carry JCI accreditation, several are in progress toward that goal. The country has long enjoyed a reliable medical infrastructure in compliance with the accreditation standards of international associations and a host of in-country accreditation agencies. The standards apply to general practice as well as to cosmetic and dental surgery.

Regarding cosmetic surgery in South Africa, few dedicated clinics exist. Plastic surgery (including cosmetic and reconstructive) is more likely to be performed by a well-regarded specialist in an excellent private hospital. Patients interested in traveling to South Africa for cosmetic surgery should consult a health travel agent who specializes in that arena.

Bay View Private Hospital
Corner Alhof & Ryk Tulbach Streets
Mossel Bay, SOUTH AFRICA 6500
Tel: 011 27 44 691.3718
Fax: 011 27 44 691.3717
Email: bayview@pixie.co.za
Web: www.bayviewprivatehospital.com

One of South Africa's finest hospitals occupies one of the world's most beautiful settings for a treatment center. Set along the Garden Route, a three-hour eastward coastal drive (or 40-minute flight) from Cape Town, Bay View Private Hospital overlooks the Indian Ocean, where porpoises can be seen frolicking outside patients' rooms.

Established in 1995, Bay View now has 106 beds. The hospital prides itself on the high-profile care administered in the center's geographical remoteness. Twenty-three physicians and surgeons and a staff of 300 have seen thousands of international patients over the past decade. Bay View performs more than 200 cardiac surgeries and 1,800 orthopedic surgeries annually.

The hospital is best known for its **Cardiac Cath Lab,** founded in 1999 by Christiaan Barnard. At Bay View the full gamut of heart diagnostics and surgeries is performed at less than half the cost of comparable treatments in the US.

In addition to the full range of orthopedic surgeries, Bay View's **Orthopedics Clinic** also offers the Birmingham hip resurfacing procedure. This popular alternative to traditional hip replacement, only recently authorized in the US, costs about $10,000 at Bay View. Patients specifically seeking this procedure may consider South Africa a more convenient destination than India or Southeast Asia.

Other specialties include urology, gastroenterology, general and endoscopic surgery, neurology and neurosurgery, and ophthalmology.

While the hospital's international clientele hails mostly from the UK and Germany, Bay View's **International Services Director** can help US patients with bookings, hotels, and transportation. Bay View pays for the 40-minute flight from Cape Town to the clinic.

Cape Town Medi-Clinic

P.O. Box 12199, Mill Street 8010
21 Hof Street, Oranjezicht 8001
Cape Town, SOUTH AFRICA
Tel: 011 27 21 464.5500
Email: hospmngrcapet@mediclinic.co.za
Web: www.capetownmc.co.za

Located in the quiet Cape Town suburb of Oranjezicht, the 150-bed Cape Town Medi-Clinic is one of 40 private hospitals that form the Medi-Clinic Group, one of the largest private hospital groups in Africa.

Five operating theaters carry out general and superspecialties, including cardiothoracic surgery, clinical sexology, dentistry, dermatology, general surgery, neurology and neurosurgery, orthopedics, pediatric surgery, plastic and reconstructive surgery, spinal surgery, and urology.

Carter Gordon Clinic

13 Anthony Street
Plettenberg Bay
Western Cape, SOUTH AFRICA 6600
Tel: 011 27 44 533.3041
Fax: 011 27 44 533.1298
Email: info@my-rehab.co.za
Web: www.my-rehab.co.za

Many individuals grappling with addiction and emotional dependency require extended clinical, supervised help. Some are advised to undergo the more rigorous programs (à la Hazelton or Betty Ford) in a professional setting far away from home, family, friends, and work.

Opened in 2006 by two addiction and recovery specialists, the 15-bed Carter Gordon Clinic is patterned after the "Minnesota Model," combining a longer-term stay with the Alcoholics Anonymous 12-step program. All types of substance addiction and addictive behaviors are addressed, including alcoholism and addictions to narcotics, sex, and gambling. Rigorous group and individual counseling make up a good part of the day, with morning walks on the beach and evening tours at game parks and nearby marvels.

More than half of Carter Gordon's clients arrive from the UK, Holland, and Germany. The clinic is experiencing such growth in demand from overseas that a new facility is being constructed that will accommodate 30 patients with a mix of single and shared suite-style bedrooms, several counseling rooms for group and one-on-one sessions, and expanded recreational facilities.

The clinic is a five-hour drive east from Cape Town to reposed Plettenberg Bay, the jewel of South Africa's famed Garden Route. Clients can arrange to be met by a driver at Cape Town International Airport.

Carter Gordon's typical recovery programs last six weeks, and take patients through the first five steps of the AA 12-step program. For patients needing a clinically monitored regimen, the $10,500 fee (inclusive of lodging, meals, and activities) is a bargain compared to similar programs in the US. The clinic is currently seeking accreditation through the Department of Social Development as well as the Board of Health Care Funders.

Christiaan Barnard Memorial Hospital

181 Longmarket Street
Cape Town, SOUTH AFRICA 8001
Tel: 011 27 21 480.6111
Fax: 011 27 21 424.0826
Email: info@netcare.co.za
Web: www.netcare.co.za (then search for Barnard)

Named after South Africa's famed heart transplant pioneer, Christiaan Barnard Memorial Hospital is most noted for cardiac and kidney transplant surgeries, although it provides a variety of medical services with top-flight surgeons specializing in cardiac surgery, urology, orthopedics, and dental care. The hospital treats many heads of states, partly because of its reputation for confidentiality. This hospital is part of the giant Netcare Group network, which provides more than a quarter of the healthcare available in South Africa.

Kingsbury Hospital

Wilderness Road
Claremont, SOUTH AFRICA 7700
Tel: 011 27 21 670.4000
Fax: 011 27 21 683.5138
Email: Frances.Johnston@lifehealthcare
.co.za
Web: www.lifehealthcare.co.za

Located near Cape Town, Kingsbury Hospital is part of the Life Healthcare network, which manages 62 facilities throughout South Africa. The hospital's 134 beds and seven operating theaters support the usual gamut of medical disciplines, including

treatment of breast diseases, colorectal surgery, dentistry, dermatology, gastroenterology, general surgery, neurology and neurosurgery, ophthalmology, orthopedics, plastic and reconstructive surgery, urology, and vascular surgery.

Kingsbury boasts two superspecialties, which are

■ *Repair of abdominal aortic aneurysm:* Most often diagnosed in men over the age of 60, an abdominal aortic aneurysm is a dilation of the body's largest artery, which lies in the abdominal cavity. If an undetected aneurysm enlarges, its sudden rupture is usually fatal. Kingsbury has invested in sophisticated ultrasound detection and diagnosis, as well as in a revolutionary technique for treatment that involves inserting stent grafts through the groin into the affected artery—without having to open up the abdomen.

■ *Obesity surgery:* Recognizing the epidemic rise of obesity worldwide (and its associated maladies of heart attack, stroke, high blood pressure, cancer, depression, arthritis, and sleep disorders), Kingsbury's **Chrysalis Clinic** takes a holistic approach to obesity and weight loss. A team of specialists carefully examines a patient's history and health status and then works with the patient to consider all options. Nonsurgical options are considered first, involving a combination of dietetic treatment, exercise, pharmacological treatment, and psychotherapy. Patients are assessed by an endocrinologist/physician, a dietician, a surgeon, a biokineticist, and a psychiatrist or psychologist from the Chrysalis Clinic team. A program is then developed around the findings, which may include surgical interventions.

Netcare Olivedale Hospital

Pres Fouche / Windsor Way

Olivedale

Johannesburg, SOUTH AFRICA

Tel: 011 27 11 777.2000

Fax: 011 27 11 462.8382

Email: elainer@olivedale.netcare.co.za

Web: www.olivedaleclinic.co.za

Netcare Olivedale Hospital is owned and managed by the Netcare Group. Since 1996, Netcare has grown to include 44 hospitals in South Africa, totaling more than 7,600 beds and 3,300 associated medical practitioners. Olivedale's 263 beds and 11 operating theaters make it one of the largest in the network. The hospital's specialties include cardiology and cardiothoracic surgeries, diabetes diagnosis and treatment, general surgery, neurology, nuclear medicine, oncology, ophthalmology, orthopedics, and urology.

Pretoria Eye Institute

630 Schoeman Street

Arcadia

Pretoria, SOUTH AFRICA

Tel: 011 27 12 343.5873

Fax: 011 27 12 344.4541

Email: info@eyeinstitute.co.za

Web: www.eyeinstitute.co.za

Pretoria Eye Institute (PEI) was Africa's first private eye hospital. Its 40-bed facility treats 6,000 patients per month, and more than 7,200 surgeries are performed annually in six operating theaters. PEI's 20-chair day facility is manned by a separate ophthalmic staff.

Surgeries performed by 18 ophthalmologists are offered for cataract retinal detachment, diabetic retinopathy, glaucoma, refractive/LASIK procedures, lens implantation, and macular degeneration. The institute is situated close to several embassies in Pretoria, and some of the savvier diplomatic travelers schedule eye exams, LASIK treatments, and other procedures while there. PEI also serves a large crowd of patients from the UK, who come to take advantage of the considerable cost savings.

The Rosebank Hospital

14 Sturdee Avenue

Johannesburg, SOUTH AFRICA 2196

Tel: 011 27 11 328.0500

Fax: 011 27 11 328.0510

Email: info@netcare.co.za

Web: www.netcare.co.za (then search for Rosebank)

The Rosebank Hospital has earned an international reputation for excellence in plastic and reconstructive surgery. The hospital also has a close association with the **Centre for Sports Medicine and Orthopaedics,** which places it in a unique position to meet the medical needs of both professional and leisure sportsmen and sportswomen.

Located in the northern suburbs of Johannesburg, Rosebank is a part of the Netcare Group, South Africa's largest hospital and doctors' network. This 132-bed private hospital offers 24-hour care. Patients generally spend one or two nights in the clinic after surgery, and private rooms are available. Each self-contained ward has an in-suite bathroom, radio, satellite television, and telephone.

■ RECOVERY ACCOMMODATIONS

At this writing, independent recovery re-treats have not appeared on the scene in South Africa, except for those managed by Surgeon and Safari. Because of the large number of medical travelers visiting South Africa, most deluxe hotels are responsive to the care and dietary needs of traveling pa-tients. If you need specialized medical care, ask your health travel agent to recommend suitable accommodations.

■ HOTELS: DELUXE

Mount Nelson Hotel
76 Orange Street
Cape Town, SOUTH AFRICA 8001
Tel: 011 27 21 483.1000
Fax: 011 27 21 483.1001
Email: reservations@mountnelson.co.za
Web: www.mountnelson.co.za

The Table Bay Hotel
Victoria and Alfred Waterfront, Quay 6
Cape Town, SOUTH AFRICA 8001
Tel: 011 27 21 701.1202
Fax: 011 27 21 406.5686
Email: tablebay@accommodationsouth
africa.co.za
Web: http://tablebay.accommodation
southafrica.co.za

The Westcliff Hotel
67 Jan Smuts Avenue
Westcliff
Johannesburg, SOUTH AFRICA
Tel: 011 27 11 481.6000
Fax: 011 27 11 646.3500

Email: reservations@westcliff.co.za
Web: www.westcliff.co.za

Hyatt Regency Johannesburg
Park Hyatt Johannesburg
191 Oxford Road
Rosebank
Johannesburg, SOUTH AFRICA 2132
Tel: 011 27 11 280.1234
Fax: 011 27 11 280.1238
Email: Reservations.JOHPH@hyattintl.com
Web: http://johannesburg.regency.hyatt
.com

■ HOTELS: MODERATE

Highlands Country House Hotel
36 Tennant Road
Kenilworth
Cape Town, SOUTH AFRICA 7708
Tel: 011 27 21 797.8810
Fax: 011 27 21 761.0017
Email: info@highlands.co.za
Web: www.highlands.co.za

Hilton Sandton Johannesburg
138 Rivonia Road
Sandton, SOUTH AFRICA 2146
Tel: 1 800 664.6835 (US toll-free); 011 27 11
322.1888
Fax: 011 27 11 322.1818
Email: reservations.sandton@hilton.com
Web: www.hilton.com

Melrose Place
12a North Street / 30 Victoria Avenue
Melrose, Johannesburg, SOUTH AFRICA
Tel: 011 27 11 442.5231
Fax: 011 27 11 880.2371
Web: www.melroseplace.co.za

DESTINATION: **SOUTH KOREA**

■ AT A GLANCE

Seoul

Language:	Korean (English spoken by many health professionals)
Time Zone:	GMT +9
Country Dialing Code:	82
Electricity:	110V & 220V, Plug types A & B
Currency:	Won
Visa Required?	Not for stays shorter than 30 days; longer stays may require a visa
Recommended Immunizations:	Hepatitis A; Typhoid Booster
Treatment Specialties:	Oncology, Cardiology, Ophthalmology, Orthopedics, Dental
Leading Hospitals and Clinics:	Severance Hospital, Yonsei University Health System; Cheongshim International Medical Center; Wooridul Spine Hospital; Jaseng Hospital of Oriental Medicine
JCI-Accredited Hospitals:	Severance Hospital, Yonsei University Health System
Standards and Accreditation:	Korean Ministry of Health and Welfare, JCI

■ TREATMENT BRIEF

Like many Asian nations, South Korea has developed economically and culturally far more quickly than the average American may realize. After many years of postwar governmental strife, Korea launched one of the planet's fastest growing economies—now the third largest economy in Asia (behind Japan and China) and the eleventh largest in the world.

Korea is also one of the world's most technologically and scientifically advanced countries; it's the only one in the world with nationwide 100 Mbit/s broadband Internet access and full HDTV broadcasting. Ninety percent of all Korean homes are connected to high-speed broadband Internet. A bullet-train network zips travelers around the country at speeds exceeding 220 kilometers (130 miles) an hour. Hyundai and Samsung are located here, a reminder of Korea's formidable ability to compete in major industry sectors.

Healthcare is no exception, and Korea's star as a health travel destination is rapidly rising. While language and cultural barriers persist, Korea boasts a network of 20 modern international hospitals, including Severance Hospital, the world's largest JCI-accredited hospital, with more than 2,000 beds.

The Korean penchant for technology is revealed in its hospitals, where most are fully digitized and electronic health records are the rule. Visitors can even watch their granny's colonoscopy on a television monitor in the hospital lobby (optional!).

Korea's foray into medical tourism began with service to Japanese patients, and despite a sometimes uneasy political relationship between the two countries, patients flock from Japan to take advantage of the huge cost savings and excellent care Korea has to offer. The Korean government has initiated a set of measures to promote medical tourism by aiding hospitals in their marketing and by easing regulations. The government is also pushing to simplify the process of issuing visas for overseas patients, especially those from Asian nations.

In addition to the usual range of general surgeries, Korea's hospitals and clinics are known for cosmetic surgeries and treatments for spinal disorders and cancer. In the center of the country, Daegu hosts the most famous herbal medicine market in South Korea, dating from 1658. On the southern coast, Busan is one of Asia's seashore hotspots, where medical travelers flock to Hanyang University Medical Center for its low-cost comprehensive health screenings.

Medical travelers who react adversely to the heat and humidity of Southeast Asia will find Korea's northern mountainous climate more to their liking. And Korea Airlines offers nonstops from at least a dozen US and Canadian cities; its northern geography shortens flights to a long, but manageable, 11–14 hours.

■ TYPICAL TREATMENTS AND COSTS

Cardiovascular:
Coronary Artery Bypass Graft: $40,400

Orthopedic:
Joint Replacement:
  Knee (one): $19,060
  Knee (two): $29,720
  Hip: $21,930
  Ankle: $18,430
  Disc: $18,500

■ HEALTH TRAVEL AGENTS

The Taj Medical Group, Limited
408 West 57th Street, Suite 9N
New York, NY 10019
Tel: 1 877 799.9797 (US toll-free)
Email: info@tajmedical.com
Web: www.tajmedical.com

For more information on Taj Medical Group, see India: Delhi.

■ HOSPITALS AND CLINICS

Severance Hospital, Yonsei University Health System
250 Seongsanno (134 Sinchon-Dong)
Seodaemun-Gu
Seoul, SOUTH KOREA 120-752
Tel: 011 82 2 2228.1485
Fax: 011 82 2 2363.0396
Email: dylandavis@yuhs.ac
Web: www.yuhs.or.kr/en

Yonsei University Health System (YUHS) was established in 1885 as Korea's first institution practicing and teaching western medicine. YUHS consists of two graduate schools, three colleges, and five hospitals, which together see more than 2.7 million outpatients and nearly 1 million inpatients yearly. With more than 3,000 beds, the latest state-of-the-art equipment, an advanced information technology infrastructure, and a world-class medical team, YUHS is working to become a hub for medical services in East Asia.

Today its flagship hospital, Severance, is the world's largest JCI-accredited hospital. It boasts 975 physicians and surgeons and 3,800 staff. Severance is best known for its services in oncology, cardiology, ophthalmology, orthopedics, and dentistry. It has six specialty centers: **Cancer, Children's, Rehabilitation, Cardiovascular, Dental,** and **Eye, Ear, Nose, and Throat.** It is the referral center for US military personnel in Korea and the on-call hospital for US presidential visits. Severance offers comprehensive VIP Health Screenings and the services of an **International Healthcare Center.** Physicians and surgeons speak English. In 2006 approximately 2,300 inpatients from the US and Canada received medical services at Severance.

Cheongshim International Medical Center
460, Songsan-Ri, Sorak-Myeon
Gapyeong-Gun
Gyeonggi-Do, SOUTH KOREA 477-855
Tel: 1 82 31 589.4641
Fax: 1 82 31 589.4476
Email: master@cheongshim.com
Web: http://eng.csmc.or.kr

This small hospital opened its doors in 2003. Thirteen physicians and surgeons tend to patients in 250 beds. Cheongshim International Medical Center specializes in health screenings, women's services, and rehabilitation. The center provides customer-specific cultural and administrative services for all nationalities and promises a total-care service with high-quality treatment, minimal medical fees, and administrative help in applying for medical insurance coverage. The **International Medical Clinic** for foreign patients has single-bed and double-bed rooms. The hospital is proud of its beautiful mountain setting. Cheongshim runs tourism programs by boat and ferry service and coordinates treatment with tourism through nearby golf, spa, marine sports, and hiking facilities. About 10 percent of its 24,000 patients annually come from outside the country.

Wooridul Spine Hospital
47-4 Chungdam-Dong
Gangnam-Gu
Seoul, SOUTH KOREA 135-100
Tel: 011 82 2513.8157
Fax: 011 82 2513.8386
Email: wipc@wooridul.com.kr
Web: www.wooridul.com

Founded in 1982, Wooridul Spine Hospital (WSH) now has branch hospitals in Seoul, Gimpo Airport, Busan, and Daegu, under direct management of WSH. New WSH hospitals in Jeju Island, China, and Malaysia are expected in the near future. The four centers operating now employ more than 120 doctors who specialize in spinal procedures. The most often performed are microscopic surgery and fusion, endoscopic surgery, and anterior surgery and fusion.

WSH has earned a reputation as a pioneer of minimally invasive spinal surgery. The hospital prides itself on treating people in their seventies and eighties who have other physical ailments, such as diabetes mellitus or hypertension. WSH physicians also provide training to doctors from Europe and the Americas. About 330 doctors in orthopedics and neurosurgery have learned new techniques of spinal treatment from WSH since 1993.

WSH has been developing new nonsurgical techniques for the treatment of spinal disorders. A new pain-management system called computer-guided spinal microtherapy combines computed tomography (CT) scanning with a 3D camera. The system allows doctors to visualize a pressed nerve and administer an injection or stimulate the affected nerve.

In 2005 WSH opened the **Wooridul International Patients Center** (WIPC) to facilitate the access of international patients and provide better medical care. The WIPC is located at Chungdam-dong WSH in Seoul, providing various consultations and business services to international patients. English, Japanese, Chinese, French, and Spanish interpreters are available.

Jaseng Hospital of Oriental Medicine
635 Shinsa-Dong
Gangnam-Gu
Seoul, SOUTH KOREA
Tel: 011 82 2 3218.2167
Email: enjaseng@jaseng.co.kr
Web: www.jaseng.net

For those seeking nonsurgical treatments for spinal disorders, complaints of the bones and joints, or abnormalities of the throat, mouth, and jaw, Jaseng Hospital of Oriental Medicine may well be the answer. The **Jaseng Spine Center, Jaseng Bone and Joint Center,** and **Jaseng Throat, Mouth, and Jaw Center** offer a wealth of treatment options, and patients undergo thorough clinical examination, radiological testing, and evaluation by an appropriate specialist. Here 25 doctors provide a personalized mix of treatments, which may include acupuncture, spinal manipulation, and herbal medication. Motion Style Treatment (MST) requires patients with musculoskeletal dysfunctions to move around while acupuncture needles are in place. This technique is said to regulate the function of blood vessels and stimulate *chi* (energy flow within the body). Precisely measured and positioned doses of bee venom may be used to alleviate inflammation and reduce back pain. Herbal acupuncture uses injections of medicinal herbal extract into acupuncture points to treat pain in the lower back, leg, and joints, as well as some chronic diseases.

CHUNA is a unique manipulation practiced at Jaseng to realign displaced bones and joints. Other treatments at Jaseng include physical therapy, compression therapy, aquapressure, air pressure therapy, electric stimulation, hot-pack massage, microcurrent, and ultrasonic current. Jaseng's **Wellness Center** promotes optimal health through prevention and treatment of obesity, allergies, chronic fatigue, and more. More than 500 patients from the US and Canada seek treatment at Jaseng annually.

Park Hyatt Seoul
995-14 Daechi 3-Dong
Gangnam-Gu
Seoul, SOUTH KOREA 135-502
Tel: 011 82 2 2016.1234
Fax: 011 82 2 2016.1200
Email: seoul.park@hyattintl.com
Web: http://seoul.park.hyatt.com

■ HOTELS: DELUXE

Grand InterContinental Seoul
159-8, Samseong-Dong
Gangnam-Gu
Seoul, SOUTH KOREA 135-732
Tel: 1 800 496.7621 (US toll-free); 011 82 2555.5656
Fax: 011 82 2559.7990
Web: www.ichotelsgroup.com

Lotte Hotel
1, Sogong-Dong
Jung-Gu
Seoul, SOUTH KOREA 100-721
Tel: 1 201 944.1117 (NY office); 011 82 2 771.1000
Fax: 1 201 994.1146 (NY office); 011 82 2 752.3758
Email: nylotte@hotmail.com
Web: www.lottehotel.co.kr

Grand Hilton Seoul
201-1 Hongeun-Dong
Seodaemun-Ku
Seoul, SOUTH KOREA 120-710
Tel: 011 82 2 3216.5656
Fax: 011 82 2 3216.7799
Email: grandseoul@hilton.com
Web: www1.hilton.com

■ HOTELS: MODERATE

Hotel Seokyo
354-5 Seogyo-Dong
Mapo-Gu
Seoul, SOUTH KOREA
Tel: 011 82 2330.7770
Fax: 011 82 2333.3388
Email: webmaster@hotelseokyo.co.kr
Web: www.hotelseokyo.co.kr

Imperial Palace Hotel
248-7 Nonhyun-Dong
Kangnam-Gu
Seoul, SOUTH KOREA
Tel: 011 82 2 3440.8000
Fax: 011 82 2 3440.8200
Web: www.imperialpalace.co.kr

Yonsei University Guest House
Shinchon-Dong 134
Seodaemun-Gu
Seoul, SOUTH KOREA
Tel: 011 82 2361.3291 (Yonsei University)
Email: ysid@bubble.yonsei.ac.kr
Web: www.yonsei.ac.kr/eng (Yonsei University)

DESTINATION: **TAIWAN**

■ AT A GLANCE

Taipei, Taoyuan City, and Tainan City

Language:	Mandarin Chinese, Taiwanese, Hakka (English spoken by many health professionals)
Time Zone:	GMT +8
Country Dialing Code:	886
Electricity:	110V, Plug type A
Currency:	Taiwan dollar
Visa Required?	30 days given on arrival; medical travelers can apply for six months
Recommended Immunizations:	Hepatitis A
Treatment Specialties:	Cardiology, Orthopedics, Weight Loss, Fertility, Health Screenings, Ophthalmology
Leading Hospitals and Clinics:	Min-Sheng General Hospital, Taipei Medical University–Municipal Wan Fang Hospital, E-Da Hospital, Chang Bing Show Chwan Memorial Hospital, Chang Gung Memorial Hospital, National Taiwan University Hospital, National Cheng Kung University Hospital
JCI-Accredited Hospitals:	Min-Sheng General Hospital, Taipei Medical University–Municipal Wan Fang Hospital, Koo Foundation Sun Yat-Sen Cancer Center
Standards and Accreditation:	Taiwan Joint Commission on Hospital Accreditation, Taiwan Hospital Association, Public Hospital Association, Taiwan College of Healthcare Executives, JCI

■ TREATMENT BRIEF

One of the original Four Asia Tigers, Taiwan has grown by leaps and bounds over the past 50 years to become a fully modernized, industrialized nation and a top player in the global economy. While cultural barriers still exist, American visitors will be comforted by the Taiwanese love of basketball and baseball, the proliferation of 24-hour convenience stores, the enthusiastic cheerleading performances, and the ubiquitous billiards and karaoke. Western art forms thrive in Taiwan. (Taiwanese film director Ang Lee produced the Oscar winners *Crouching Tiger, Hidden Dragon* and *Brokeback Mountain*.)

Although suffering from pollution and traffic snarls, Taiwan's principal cities are modern, friendly, and safe, with a brand-new, high-speed bullet-train system connecting the island's major industrial and population centers. Situated off the coast of mainland China between South Korea and Hong Kong, Taiwan enjoys a more temperate climate than India, Malaysia, or Singapore—a real plus for many Western medical travelers. Taiwan's beautiful and wild mountainous region on the east side of the island provides an array of luxury recovery accommodations, vacation attractions, and sightseeing opportunities.

Taiwan applies some of the world's highest healthcare standards, with dozens of new hospitals and clinics, mostly located in Taipei, its capital. Two are JCI-accredited: Min-Sheng General Hospital and Taipei Medical University–Municipal Wan Fang Hospital. While medical travelers from nearby Japan are a major market, recent centralized efforts are underway to westernize Taiwan's health centers and promote medical tourism from the US, UK, and other English-speaking nations.

While US healthcare languishes in an expensive, often counterproductive "heal the sick" mindset, Taiwan's focus is clearly preventive. Comprehensive healthcare screenings abound, and Taiwan's close cultural ties to China have produced a wealth of alternative and complementary therapies and procedures. Customer service is excellent, at times over-the-top; one example is Chang Bing Show Chwan Health Care Center Park, which boasts a modern art gallery, a children's museum, and a 200-seat movie theater for patients. Taiwan's specialties include cardiology, orthopedics, weight-loss surgery, and fertility treatments. Costs are generally on par with Thailand and Singapore—with savings of 30–60 percent over comparable care in the US.

■ TYPICAL TREATMENTS AND COSTS

Note: Some lower prices are for the procedure only; higher prices may include anesthesia, medications, hospital stay, lab work, and nursing expenses. Make sure you find out exactly what you are paying for and what extra costs you may incur.

Cardiovascular:
Coronary Artery Bypass Graft:
  $25,000-$30,300
Bypass + Valve Replacement (single): $12,400
Bypass + Valve Replacement (double): $14,520
Pacemaker (single-chambered):
  $4,600-$20,000
Pacemaker (double-chambered):
  $6,150-$18,000

Orthopedic:
Birmingham Hip Resurfacing: $6,000
Joint Replacement:
  Knee: $2,200-$10,610
  Hip: $2,200-$8,790
  Ankle: $1,000-$8,000
  Shoulder: $1,000-$6,060

Cosmetic:
Breast Augmentation: $4,600-$11,000
Breast Lift/Reduction: $4,700-$11,000
Facelift: $2,000-$15,200
Liposuction (stomach, hips, and waist):
  $1,850-$13,400
Tummy Tuck: $3,700-$11,000

Dental:
Porcelain Veneer: $315-$615
Crown (all porcelain): $615-$1,070
Inlays and Onlays: $455-$615
Implant: $3,750-$5,000
Extraction (surgical, per tooth): $15-$300

Vision:
Glaucoma: $615
LASIK (per eye): $612-$1,580

Weight Loss:
LAP-BAND System: $10,000

Other:
Gall Bladder Removal: $1,700-$4,500
Prostate Surgery (TURP): $1,500-$4,000

■ HOSPITALS AND CLINICS

Min-Sheng General Hospital
21F, #168 Jin-Kuo Road
Taoyuan City
Taoyuan County, TAIWAN 330
Tel: 011 886 3317.9599
Fax: 011 886 3316.4300
Email: liao33@gmail.com
Web: www.e-ms.com.tw

Established in 2001, Min-Sheng General Hospital has more than 600 beds and 120 physicians and surgeons. Min-Sheng staff members pride themselves on seamless care and one-on-one services to patients. Its **International Department** boasts "selective, low-risk, highly competitive health services and packages"—some of them set up to work with US health insurance plans. Such packages include coronary artery bypass graft, percutaneous transluminal coronary angioplasty (PTCA), cardiac catheterization, total knee and total hip replacement, LASIK eye surgery, hernia repair, weight-loss surgery, colporrhaphy (surgical repair of a defect in the vaginal wall), vaginal hysterectomy, liposuction, tummy tuck, breast augmentation or reduction, and laminectomy (a spinal surgery for relieving back pain).

While Min-Sheng has been serving its local patients for more than 30 years, its international services have expanded since its JCI accreditation in 2006. Min-Sheng's specialty centers focus on minimally invasive surgery, nephrology, emergency and acute care, digital imaging and digitally guided surgery, oncology, cardiology, gynecology, fertility treatment, plastic and cosmetic surgery, three-dimensional stereotactical

scanning, sleep medicine, LASIK eye surgery, and VIP Health Screenings.

For health travelers, Min-Sheng arranges airport pickup (average 20 minutes
from airport to hospital), taxi service, hotel
accommodations (including wheelchair-
accessible rooms and special diets), a
24-hour immediate phone connection to
hospital staff, and an embassy connection
for emergencies. Guidebooks and tours are
also available.

**Taipei Medical University–Municipal Wan
Fang Hospital**
No. 111 Hsing-Long Road, Section 3
Taipei, TAIWAN 116
Tel: 011 886 2 2930.7930
Fax: 011 886 2 2933.5221
Email: grace@wanfang.gov.tw
Web: www.wanfang.gov.tw

Taipei Medical University–Municipal Wan
Fang Hospital is a regional teaching hospital with 750 beds, employing 66 physicians
and 215 surgeons. Less than 20 percent of
them speak English. Doctors in training at
Taipei Medical University do their intern-
ships at Wan Fang. Located on a 22-acre
campus near a major freeway in Taipei,
Wan Fang has been operating since 1997 as
Taiwan's first publicly owned but privately
operated hospital. Wan Fang received its JCI
accreditation in 2006.

Wan Fang is best known for neurosurgery, cardiology, orthopedics, infertility
treatments, and laser cosmetic surgery
(nearly 5,000 annually). Wan Fang's **Laser
Cosmetic Center** offers a wide range of
dermatological treatments, ranging from
Botox injections to microinvasive surgery
for osmidrosis (secretion of foul-smelling
sweat). Wan Fang's most frequent cardio-

vascular surgeries include cardiac catheterization and stenting (about 800 cases per
year); other frequently performed procedures are open reduction and fixation of
fractures of the extremities (more than 700
cases annually). Some 8,000 international
patients seek treatment at Wan Fang each
year, most of them from nearby Asian countries, including Japan, China, Korea, and
Myanmar.

Bair's Eye Clinic
No. 192-4 Beitun Road
Beitun District
Taichung City, TAIWAN 406
Tel: 011 886 4 2234.6699
Email: mail@eyelasik.com.tw
Web: www.eyelasik.com.tw

Bair's Eye Clinic in Taichung City performs
LASIK surgery on 20–30 foreigners each
month. Specialists at Bair formulate a
treatment plan custom-designed for each
patient. Laser in situ keratomileusis (LASIK)
is currently the most common type of laser
vision-correction procedure. It corrects
nearsightedness, farsightedness, and
astigmatism.

The clinic offers custom wave-front
LASIK procedures (also known as custom
ablation). For patients with thin corneas
or large pupils, Bair offers photorefrac-
tive keratectomy (PRK). Laser epithelial
keratomileusis (LASEK) is an effective procedure for patients who have thin or flat
corneas. For nearsighted or farsighted patients, an implant called a phakic intraocular lens (IOL) is inserted under the surface of
the eye to serve as an internal contact lens.
In a procedure utilizing intrastromal corneal
ring segments (ICRS), two slim half-rings
are inserted around the edges of the cor-

nea to adjust the vision of myopic patients by flattening the curvature of the cornea. Potential candidates for treatment at Bair's must meet certain requirements for general and eye health. Visit the Web site to check the criteria.

E-Da Hospital

No. 1 Jiau-Shu Tsuen Road
Yan-Chao Shiang
Kaohsiung County, TAIWAN 824
Tel: 011 886 7 615.0011
Fax: 011 886 7 615.5352
Email: ed103221@edah.org.tw
Web: www.edah.org.tw

E-Da Hospital opened its doors in 2004. Two hundred physicians and surgeons at this regional teaching hospital treat patients in a 1,170-bed facility that boasts impressive modern architecture and luxurious interior décor, complete with pianists performing in the lobby, light and water shows, art exhibits, and numerous cultural activities.

E-Da's doctors specialize in minimally invasive surgeries, esophageal and voice reconstruction, total joint replacement, brachial plexus injury, hyperhidrosis (excessive sweating), Gamma Knife radiosurgery, prostate laser surgery, sleep assessments, and cardiac catheterization. E-Da employs technologically advanced equipment, including Gamma Knife, 64-slice computed tomography (CT), and magnetic resonance imaging (MRI).

Chin-Kun Huang International Endoscopic Obesity Center is part of E-Da Hospital. Surgeons there perform mostly gastric bypass operations, with smaller numbers of LAP-BAND and sleeve gastrectomies. The cost of gastric bypass is about $16,000 including all travel costs, compared

to about $30,000 in the US, according to E-Da representatives. The center is a member of the Asia Pacific Bariatric Surgery Society and the International Federation for the Surgery of Obesity.

E-Da's **International Service Center** team offers advice on physicians and procedures, assistance with visa applications, and arrangements for local accommodations. Case managers offer email and teleconferencing communication with physicians, as well as assistance with local and international travel. An Internet platform is provided for Web-conferencing once patients return home.

Chang Bing Show Chwan Health Care Center Park

No. 6 Lugong Road
Lukang Zhen
Changhua County, TAIWAN 505
Tel: 011 886 921 888.611
Fax: 011 886 2 2351.7988
Email: brady@24drs.com; tobrady@gmail
   .com
Web: www.cbshow.org.tw/en

Chang Bing Show Chwan Health Care Center Park is a new concept in healthcare design: a "health park" that integrates treatment facilities, an art gallery, a movie theater, and a museum along with restaurants, retail stores, recreational facilities, and convenient transportation into what its planners call "a unique and holistic healthcare experience." Show Chwan staffers work to integrate a patient-centered philosophy with the latest medical technology, including positron emission tomography (PET) and computed tomography (CT) scanning, robotic arm (minimally invasive) surgery, Gamma Knife radiosurgery, and more.

The hospital opened in 2006, with 1,000 beds and nearly 400 physicians and surgeons. It's affiliated with Johns Hopkins University Welch Center, Tokyo Women's Hospital, Vancouver General in Canada, and Garfield Medical Center in Los Angeles. Its treatment specialties include orthopedics, cardiovascular surgery, gastroenterology, neurology and neurosurgery, and various cosmetic procedures.

Chang Gung Memorial Hospital
No. 5 Fusing Street
Gueishan Township
Taoyuan County, TAIWAN 333
Tel: 011 886 3 319.6200
Fax: 011 886 3 319.8001
Email: isc@cgmh.org.tw
Web: www.cgmh.org.tw

Chang Gung Memorial Hospital (CGMH) is part of a larger healthcare system that includes Chang Gung University, Chang Gung Institute of Nursing, Acute Hospital, Chronic Hospital, and the Chang Gung Nursing Home and Aging Village. Administrators say that among the people of Taiwan, one in every seven chooses to visit Chang Gung Memorial Hospital for medical care.

Chang Gung was founded in 1976 by the chairman of Formosa Plastics Corporation, a global petrochemical company. It is a nonprofit hospital that stresses medical research and education as well as clinical services. Its 800 physicians and surgeons serve patients occupying almost 4,000 beds. Overall, nearly 9,000 people work in the Chang Gung system.

The hospital's specialty centers include the **Cancer Center, Cosmetic Center, Genomic Medicine Research Laboratory, Perinatal Medicine Unit, Liver Research**

Unit, Liver Transplant Center, and **Reproductive Center.** Most frequently performed procedures include repair of cleft lip and palate, facial bone reshaping, joint replacements, and living-donor liver transplants. Some 500 international patients seek treatment at Chang Gung annually. Recovery lodging is available in the **Chang Gung Health and Culture Village.**

National Taiwan University Hospital
No. 7 Chung-Shan South Road
Taipei, TAIWAN 100
Tel: 011 886 2 231.23456
Fax: 011 886 2 239.10708
Email: Jin670@ntuh.gov.tw
Web: http://ntuh.mc.ntu.edu.tw

Established in 1895, National Taiwan University Hospital (NTUH) is an affiliated teaching hospital of the National Taiwan University College of Medicine. NTUH provides comprehensive ranges of specialty and subspecialty services. The main hospital and two branch hospitals house more than 2,500 beds. More than 1,000 physicians, surgeons, attending doctors, and residents serve patients at NTUH. Most of the physicians and many of the staff members speak English.

Treatment specialties include cardiovascular disease, infertility, orthopedic procedures for joint disease and joint replacement, liver disease, and oncology. Frequently performed procedures include cardiac diagnosis and treatment, breast cancer surgery, and joint replacements of the knee, hip, and ankle. In 2003 NTUH received worldwide recognition for its management of Severe Acute Respiratory Syndrome (SARS) epidemics in Taiwan.

That same year, the hospital reported the world's first successful use of autologous stem cell transplantation to treat nasopharyngeal cancer. NTUH also boasts the world's largest clinical trials of HPV-008 vaccines for cervical cancer, the first successful positive cross-match living-donor kidney transplant in Asia, and the world's first successful endoscopic potassium-titanyl-phosphate KTP laser surgery for recurrent nasopharyngeal cancer. It's also a pioneer in testing interferon therapy for the treatment of chronic hepatitis.

More than 13,000 international patients received treatment at NTUH in 2006, approximately 2,400 of them from the US and Canada.

National Cheng Kung University Hospital
No. 138 Sheng Li Road
Tainan City, TAIWAN 70403
Tel: 011 886 6 235.3535
Fax: 011 886 6 236.9602
Email: thp@mail.hosp.ncku.edu.tw
Web: www.hosp.ncku.edu.tw

Located in the northern district of Tainan City, National Cheng Kung University Hospital opened in 1988. The hospital has more than 20 departments and specialty centers, including internal medicine, surgery, urology, otolaryngology, psychiatry, neurology, anesthesiology, family medicine, orthopedics, ophthalmology, physical rehabilitation, obstetrics and gynecology, pediatrics, dermatology, pathology, dentistry, emergency medicine, diagnostic radiology, radiation oncology, genetics, and nuclear medicine. It is best known for its cardiovascular medicine, orthopedic and plastic surgery, transplantations, and emergency/critical-care services. The hospital's most frequently performed procedures are joint replacements and cardiac catheterizations.

■ HOTELS: DELUXE OR MODERATE

Note: Taiwan's hotels are divided into three classes: international tourist class, tourist class, and ordinary. Legally licensed hotels post their certifications, and most health travelers should make sure that their accommodations have earned the highest rating—as have the ones listed here—and are also recommended by one or more of our featured hospitals. Even for some of Taiwan's best hotels, prices are moderate by US standards.

TAIPEI

Fullon Hotel Sanyin
No. 63 Dasyue Road
Sansia Township
Taipei County, TAIWAN 237
Tel: 011 886 2 867 21.234
Fax: 011 886 2 867 20.036
Email: rsvn_sy@fullon-hotels.com.tw
Web: www.fullon-hotels.com.tw

Shangri-La's Far Eastern Plaza Hotel
No. 201 Tun Hwa South Road, Section 2
Taipei, TAIWAN 106
Tel: 011 886 2 2378.8888
Fax: 011 886 2 2377.7777
Email: tpe@shangri-la.com
Web: www.shangri-la.com

The Grand Hotel
No. 1, Chung Shan N. Road, Section 4
Taipei, TAIWAN 104
Tel: 011 886 2 2886.8888
Fax: 011 886 2 2885.2885
Web: www.grand-hotel.org

Sheraton Taipei Hotel
No. 12 Chung Hsiao East Road, Section 1
Taipei, TAIWAN 100
Tel: 011 886 2 2321.5511
Fax: 011 886 2 2394.4240
Email: sheraton@sheraton-taipei.com
Web: www.sheraton-taipei.com

Grand Formosa Regent Taipei
41 Chung Shan N. Road, Section 2
Taipei, TAIWAN 104
Tel: 011 886 2 2523.8000
Fax: 011 886 2 2523.2828
Email: customerservice@grandformosa
    .com.tw
Web: www.grandformosa.com.tw

Caesar Park Hotel Taipei
No. 38 Chung Hsiao West Road, Section 1
Taipei, TAIWAN
Tel: 011 886 2 2311.5151
Fax: 011 886 2 2331.9944
Web: www.caesarpark.com.tw

Grand Hyatt Taipei
No. 2 Song Shou Road
Taipei, TAIWAN 11051
Tel: 011 886 2 2720.1234
Fax: 011 886 2 2720.1111
Email: grandhyatttaipei@hyattintl.com
Web: http://taipei.grand.hyatt.com

TAIPEI (REGIONAL)

Monarch Plaza Hotel
No. 300 Chuang Ching Road, Section 1
Tao Yuan, TAIWAN 330
Tel: 011 886 3 316.9900
Fax: 011 886 3 316.5047
Email: eo1@monarch-hotels.com
Web: www.monarch-hotels.com.tw

Ta Shee Resort Hotel
166 Jih-Shin Road, Yung-Fu, Ta-Shee
Tao Yuan, TAIWAN
Tel: 011 886 3 387.6688
Fax: 011 886 3 387.5288
Web: www.tasheeresort.com.tw

TAINAN

Tayih Landis Tainan
No. 660 Shi Men Road, Section 1
Tainan, TAIWAN 700
Tel: 011 886 6 213.5555
Fax: 011 886 6 213.5599
Email: pr@tayihlandis.com.tw
Web: www.tayihlandis.com.tw

Evergreen Plaza Hotel
No. 1 Lane 366, Section 3
Jhonghua E. Road
Tainan, TAIWAN
Tel: 011 886 6 289.9988
Fax: 011 886 6 289.6699
Web: www.orientaltravel.com

Hotel Tainan
1 Cheng Gong Road
Tainan, TAIWAN
Tel: 011 886 6 228.9101
Fax: 011 886 6 226.8502
Email: Ghotel-tainan@hotel-tainan.com.tw
Web: www.hotel-tainan.com.tw

KAOHSIUNG

The Ambassador Hotel Kaohsiung
202 Misheng 2nd Road
Kaohsiung, TAIWAN
Tel: 011 886 7 211.5211
Fax: 011 886 7 281.1115
Web: www.ambhotel.com.tw

The Splendor, Kaohsiung

No. 1 Tzu-Chiang 3rd Road
Kaohsiung City, TAIWAN 802
Tel: 011 886 566.8000
Fax: 011 885 566.8080
Web: www.thesplendor-khh.com

Hotel Kingdom

42 Wufu 4th Road
Kaohsiung, TAIWAN
Tel: 011 886 7 551.8211
Fax: 011 886 7 521.0403
Email: service@hotelkingdom.com.tw
Web: www.hotelkingdom.com.tw

■ **AT A GLANCE**

Bangkok and Phuket

Language:	Thai (English widely spoken in business and medical circles)
Time Zone:	GMT +7
Country Dialing Code:	66
Electricity:	220V, Plug types A, B, & C
Currency:	Thai baht
Visa Required?	Yes
Recommended Immunizations:	Hepatitis A; Boosters for Typhoid and Polio
Treatment Specialties:	Cardiovascular, Cosmetic, Dental, Gender Reassignment, Neurology, Oncology, Ophthalmology, Orthopedics, Weight Loss
Leading Hospitals and Clinics:	Bangkok Hospital Group Medical Center, Bumrungrad International Hospital, Samitivej Sukhumvit Hospital, Bangkok Dental Group, Bangkok International Dental Center, Bangkok Hospital Phuket, Phuket International Hospital
JCI-Accredited Hospitals:	Bangkok Hospital Group Medical Center, Bumrungrad International Hospital, Samitivej Sukhumvit Hospital
Standards and Accreditation:	Institute of Hospital Quality Improvement and Accreditation, Society of Plastic and Reconstructive Surgeons of Thailand, Thai Association of Orthodontists, JCI

■ TREATMENT BRIEF

Although it now shares the spotlight with India, Singapore, and Malaysia, the Kingdom of Thailand is the rightful wellspring of contemporary medical travel. Eleven years ago, with the crash of the Thai bhat, business and governmental leaders capitalized on Thailand's excellent medical infrastructure to attract international patients from nearby countries with less robust healthcare choices. Patients from Japan, Vietnam, Korea, and China were rapidly followed by European clients. Now thousands of Americans and Canadians head to Bangkok or Phuket, mostly to save on elective surgeries with lower costs that more than compensate for the uncomfortably long flight.

Thailand's huge medical calling card is Bangkok's venerated, JCI-accredited Bumrungrad International Hospital, covering a million-square-foot complex in downtown Bangkok. More than 900 full-time and consulting physicians representing every imaginable specialty and subspecialty practice there.

Bumrungrad has set the pace for both the quality and quantity of contemporary international healthcare throughout Asia and the world. Bumrungrad's large presence is not without its competition, and the equally impressive Dusit Medical Group owns and operates a network of 17 hospitals throughout Thailand, including Bangkok International Hospital, Bangkok Hospital Phuket, Bangkok General Hospital, and Samitivej Sukhumvit Hospital.

Although not Thailand's native tongue, English is widely spoken in Thai cities and resort centers, and English is taught as a second language in Thai schools. While extremes of wealth and poverty can be readily witnessed, health travelers may feel more comfortable in Thai culture than in India or Africa.

Sex and the City … Thai-Style

No discussion of healthcare in Thailand would be complete without at least a mention of sex-change treatments or gender reassignment surgery. Difficult to obtain in the US without a good deal of red tape, sex reassignment treatment options are probably more available in Bangkok than anywhere else on the planet.

Women can choose from a smorgasbord ranging from vaginoplasty (a rejuvenative tightening of the vagina) to full female-to-male gender reassignment; men are offered single or full orchiectomy (testicle removal), penile width enhancement, penile lengthening, and full male-to-female gender reassignment.

Partially because of Bangkok's well-publicized sex industry, hundreds of sex-change clinics have seized on Thailand's recent successes in medical travel, and many prey on the vulnerable. Thus, as with any other medical procedure, patients should conduct careful investigations, including thorough reference checks and redoubled research on clinic accreditation and physician experience.

■ TYPICAL TREATMENTS AND COSTS

Cardiovascular:
Coronary Artery Bypass Graft:
$22,000-$24,000
Bypass + Valve Replacement (single):
$25,000-$26,300
Pacemaker (single-chambered):
$3,700-$4,650

Orthopedic:
Birmingham Hip Resurfacing:
$14,300-$14,900
Joint Replacement:
Knee: $11,200-$11,800
Hip: $12,400-$13,000

Cosmetic:
Breast Augmentation: $2,050-$3,040
Breast Lift/Reduction: $4,400
Facelift (higher figure includes neck):
$2,800-$8,000
Liposuction (stomach, hips, and waist):
$2,500-$3,000
Tummy Tuck: $2,900-$4,400

Dental:
Porcelain Veneer: $215-$350
Crown (all porcelain): $465-$620
Crown (porcelain fused to gold): $430
Inlays and Onlays: $215-$250
Implant: $2,150
Root Canal: $100-$230
Full Denture (per jaw): $430-$580
Extraction (surgical, per tooth): $60

Vision:
Glaucoma: $2,300-$2,500

Weight Loss:
LAP-BAND System: $12,400-$14,000

Other:
Gall Bladder Removal: $4,650-$5,260
Prostate Surgery (TURP): $4,100-$4,700

■ HEALTH TRAVEL AGENTS

BridgeHealth International, Inc. (also Medical Tours International)
5299 DTC Boulevard, Suite 800
Greenwood Village, CO 80111
Tel: 1 800 680.1366 (US toll-free); 1 303 457.5745
Fax: 1 303 779.0366
Email: info@bridgehealthintl.com
Web: www.bridgehealthintl.com

For more information on BridgeHealth International, see Costa Rica.

Companion Global Healthcare, Inc.
c/o Blue Cross Blue Shield of South Carolina
I-20 at Alpine Road, AF-324
Columbia, SC 29219
Tel: 1 803 264.3256
Fax: 1 803 264.7063
Email: David.Boucher@BCBSSC.com
Web: www.CompanionGlobalHealthcare.com

Although this new (2007) agency is a wholly owned subsidiary of Blue Cross Blue Shield of South Carolina, anyone in the US can use its services. However, follow-up care upon return from medical travel is provided in South Carolina only. That situation may change, however, as Blue Cross Blue Shield and other insurance carriers expand their activities and support of low-cost, high-quality medical travel.

Companion Global Healthcare started out working with hospitals in Thailand and Ireland, and it has since expanded its reach to include Singapore and Turkey. Its standard package includes case management, medical record transfer, and travel coordination. Depending on a patient's diagnosis and treatment, Blue Cross Blue Shield may pay part of the cost. Uninsured customers and clients of other insurance companies pay overseas providers directly. Representatives of this agency say they bring the Blue Cross Blue Shield reputation for reliability and quality to their global healthcare services.

Healthbase Online, Inc.

287 Auburn Street
Newton, MA 02466
Tel: 1 888 691.4584 (US toll-free); 1 617 418.3436
Fax: 1 800 986.9230 (US toll-free)
Email: info.hb@healthbase.com
Web: www.healthbase.com

For more information on Healthbase Online, see India: Chennai.

International Medical Resources, LLC

9492 Good Lion Road
Columbia, MD 21045
Tel: 1 410 992.3436
Fax: 1 410 992.3437
Email: info@medinfoonline.com
Web: www.medinfoonline.com

This US-based agency sends patients to large, well-established medical centers and specialty hospitals in Bangkok and Singapore. International Medical Resources (IMR) founder James Perry says that the medical

providers he uses provide unique services (for example, intracardiac stem cell therapy and robotic prostate surgery), services typically unavailable in the US (such as Birmingham hip resurfacing), and exceptional quality and personal service. Unlike staff members in some other health travel firms, Perry and his team have significant medical experience. Perry is a PA (physician associate) with over 25 years of surgical and medical experience. While US liability concerns preclude IMR from offering specific medical advice (practicing medicine over the Internet), Perry believes that his medical expertise gives his agency an advantage in communicating with physicians and hospitals and evaluating the quality of services.

Several of this agency's core staff members are Thai, and still more have lived and traveled in Thailand, engaging in a wide variety of sport, leisure, and cultural activities. "We are happy to share our 'local knowledge' with clients who are interested," Perry says.

Med Journeys

2020 Broadway, Suite 4C
New York, NY 10023
Tel: 1 888 633.5769 (US toll-free); 1 212 931.0557
Fax: 1 212 656.1134
Email: sonnyk@medjourneys.com
Web: www.medjourneys.com

For more information on Med Journeys, see India: Delhi.

MedRetreat

2042 Laurel Valley Drive

Vernon Hills, IL 60061

Tel: 1 877 876.3373 (US toll-free)

Fax: 1 847 680.0484

Email: customerservice@medretreat.com

Web: www.medretreat.com

For more information on MedRetreat, see Malaysia.

Planet Hospital

23679 Calabasas Road, Suite 150

Calabasas, CA 91302

Tel: 1 800 243.0172 (US toll-free); 1 818 665.4801

Fax: 1 818 665.4810

Email: rudy@planethospital.com

Web: www.planethospital.com

For more information on Planet Hospital, see Singapore.

The Taj Medical Group, Limited

408 West 57th Street, Suite 9N

New York, NY 10019

Tel: 1 877 799.9797 (US toll-free)

Email: info@tajmedical.com

Web: www.tajmedical.com

For more information on Taj Medical Group, see India: Delhi.

■ HOSPITALS AND CLINICS

BANGKOK

Home to 6 million, Bangkok is Thailand's capital city and administrative center and the economic lifeblood of the kingdom. Bangkok is a large, bustling city of extremes—endless traffic jams, glittering golden temples, huge and sprawling shop-

ping complexes, and of course, its thriving and nefarious sex industry.

Despite its highly visible extremes, Bangkok is embedded in tradition, and international travelers are always struck by the overwhelming politeness of the Thai people. Customs and ritual are taken seriously both in the cities and in the countryside, and learning some cultural dos and don'ts will be appreciated by your newfound friends and associates.

Bangkok Hospital Medical Center

2 Soi Soonvijai 7, New Petchburi Road

Bangkok, THAILAND

Tel: 011 66 2 310.3100

Fax: 011 66 2 310.3367

Email: info@bangkokhospital.com

Web: www.bangkokhospital.com

Owned by the mammoth Dusit Medical Group, Southeast Asia's largest network of private hospitals, Bangkok Hospital Medical Center (BMC) has now grown to 17 hospitals located throughout Bangkok and Thailand.

BMC is one of the most technologically sophisticated hospitals in the world today. It is an expansive, state-of-the-art medical campus providing comprehensive medical care through multidisciplinary teams of highly trained specialists. With its four hospitals and broad range of specialized clinics, BMC is equipped with all of the diagnostic and treatment facilities not generally available at local hospitals. The center has received JCI accreditation and is known throughout the world for delivering world-class, award-winning healthcare.

The flagship of Thailand's largest hospital group, BMC has more than 650 full-time and consulting physicians, 700 nurses, and numerous teams of support technicians and specialists. BMC boasts that many of their internationally trained and certified physicians have returned to their homeland committed to improving the quality of national healthcare through advanced treatments and procedures.

BMC boasts four hospital buildings: **Bangkok International Hospital, Bangkok Heart Hospital, Bangkok Hospital,** and **Wattanasoth Cancer Hospital,** with two supporting buildings for dentistry and rehabilitation. The main three focuses at BMC are cardiology, oncology, and neurology.

Bangkok International Hospital (BIH) was the first Thai medical center to serve international patients. Its **International Medical Center** improved and expanded its services in 2002 and now serves more than 140,000 patients annually from over 60 countries. Sixteen specialized centers, ranging from orthopedics to neurology to cardiology, have brought together internationally trained physicians and state-of-the-art medical technology to attract visitors from all parts of the world.

BMC's team of 60 specialists helps overseas visitors overcome cultural and language barriers, in addition to providing the usual amenities, including visa assistance, liaison services with embassies, airport pickup, around-the-clock contact for medical assessments, advice on treatment options and doctors' appointments, arrangements for special diets, arranging shopping and sightseeing tours, liaison with embassies and international organizations, and insurance claims liaison assistance.

Bangkok Heart Hospital is Thailand's first and only dedicated private heart hospital. It is equipped with the most advanced technology and staffed by dedicated personnel who deal with nearly every heart condition, including diagnostics, interventional cardiology, cardiac surgery, and rehabilitation. It boasts Thailand's only DaVinci robotic system, which is used in the newer minimally invasive surgeries. Procedures include cardiac magnetic resonance imaging (MRI), computed tomography (CT) angiogram, adult stem cell therapies, radiofrequency ablation, pacemaker, and an all-artery cardiac bypass surgery.

Wattanasoth Cancer Hospital (WSH) is the only dedicated private cancer hospital in Thailand. The center is equipped with state-of-the-art technologies, including positron emission tomography (PET) and CT scan for fast and accurate diagnosis, NOVALIS for intensity-modulated radiosurgery and radiotherapy, and Gamma Knife for radiosurgery of the brain.

At the **Bangkok Neuroscience Center,** 12 neurologists and 14 neurosurgeons treat a host of diseases and traumas, including headache, dizziness, and vertigo; stroke and its aftermath; seizures; Parkinson's and related diseases; Alzheimer's; brain and spinal cord injury; tumors of the brain and spinal cord; muscle and nerve diseases; paresthesia of the limbs, trunk, or face; developmental disorders; and genetic anomalies. The center's test and instrumentation inventory includes CT, MRI, cerebral angiogram, electroencephalography (EEG), EEG monitoring, brainstem auditory evoked response, somatosensory evoked response, neurosonology carotid ultrasound, transcranial Doppler, and a spinal cord stimulation drug infusion system. Specialties within the center include clinics for stroke and cardiovascular disorders, pain, headache, epilepsy, movement disorders, neuromuscular diseases, and neurogenetics. Neurosurgeons specialize in head trauma and spinal cord injuries, tumor and skull-base surgery, cerebral hemorrhage, aneurysms, spinal surgery, Parkinson's disease, movement disorders, and epilepsy. The Neuroscience Center deploys the Leskell Gamma Knife, a new radiosurgical device that enables doctors to treat deep-seated brain lesions without the risks of open-skull surgery. Hundreds of precisely targeted beams of cobalt gamma radiation painlessly "cut" through brain tumors, blood vessel malformations, and other abnormalities, allowing neurosurgeons to correct disorders not currently treatable using established procedures. With Gamma Knife treatment, patients experience less discomfort and greatly shortened recovery periods. There are only 180 Gamma Knives in use worldwide as of this writing.

BMC's rooms rival the best hospitals in the US. They include a guest sofa-bed for a companion, personal telephone for international calls, microwave oven, refrigerator, personal safe, free Internet access, free English-language newspaper, and an inpatient library. The BMC campus offers all the amenities from concierge services and luxury accommodations to translation and visa assistance, ensuring that every patient's stay is comfortable.

Bangkok Nursing Home Hospital
9/1 Convent Road
Silom, Bangrak
Bangkok, THAILAND 10500
Tel: 011 66 2 686.2700
Fax: 011 66 2 632.0577
Email: info@bnhhospital.com
Web: www.bnhhospital.com

Don't be fooled by the name—Bangkok Nursing Home Hospital (BNH) is not a nursing home in the American sense of the word. It is a modern, full-service 120-bed hospital that meets international standards. Founded in the nineteenth century, BNH is one of Thailand's oldest healthcare facilities and was the first international hospital in Thailand. More than 300,000 international patients visit BNH annually from 150 different countries.

The hospital has nearly 440 physicians from every medical service area. Specialties include the **Spine Centre, Women's Health Centre,** and the **International Travel Medicine Clinic.** The **Preecha Aesthetic Institute** (see below) is also housed within BNH.

BNH operates a special center for spinal and orthopedic surgery. Since opening in 2005, the Spine Centre has performed over 200 complex surgeries, nearly half of them for international patients. The surgical team has also implanted over 100 disc prostheses, a rate higher than some centers in the US or EU. The center's total artificial disc replacement (TADR) is a minimally invasive surgery; the patient experiences less blood loss and significantly less pain. Early ambulation leads to fewer complications, shorter length of stay, and faster return to work and a normal life.

With typically a 70–80 percent cost saving compared to what patients can negotiate from a US and EU hospital for a similar procedure, the success rate runs an impressive 90 percent, well above international averages of 60–70 percent.

Preecha Aesthetic Institute

7th Floor, BNH Hospital
9/1 Convent Road
Silom, Bangruk
Bangkok, THAILAND 10500
Tel: 011 66 2 632.2540
Fax: 011 66 2 632.2542
Email: consult@pai.co.th
Web: www.pai.co.th

Preecha Aesthetic Institute (PAI) offers a full range of cosmetic and reconstructive plastic surgery at centers situated in various hospitals in the heart of Bangkok. PAI's services include facial contouring, eye therapies, rhinoplasty, cheekbone contouring, hair transplant and laser hair removal, breast surgery, jaw contouring, labiaplasty, vaginoplasty, and various surgeries of the ear, lips, and chin. The institute's 30 physicians specialize in sex reassignment surgery, mammoplasty, rhinoplasty, facial feminization surgery, and body contouring.

The institute is operated by Dr. Preecha Tiewtranon, often called simply Dr. Preecha. In more than 34 years of practice, Dr. Preecha has personally performed more than 30,000 cosmetic and plastic surgeries. He reigns as Bangkok's undisputed leader in gender reassignment. His techniques have become standard practice throughout the world, and he trained most of Thailand's qualified sex reassignment surgeons. From 1980 to 2005, Dr. Preecha personally performed more than 3,500 sex reassignment and facial feminization surgeries.

The Preecha facility at Bangkok Nursing Home Hospital is well supported by medical departments, including cardiology, endocrinology, intensive care, and emergency care.

Bumrungrad International Hospital

33 Sukhumvit 3 (Soi Nana Nua)
Wattana
Bangkok, THAILAND 10110
Tel: 011 66 2 667.1000
Fax: 011 66 2 667.2525
Email: info@bumrungrad.com
Web: www.bumrungrad.com

Established in 1980, Bumrungrad International Hospital is the largest private hospital in Southeast Asia, serving more than 1 million patients per year, including more than 400,000 international patients who visit from 190 countries.

This 554-bed facility provides a full range of tertiary healthcare services, including 19 operating rooms equipped for most general surgery and surgical specialties; some are minimally invasive, including cardiothoracic, orthopedic, urological, ophthalmological, laser, transplant, and otolaryngological (ear, nose, and throat) surgeries.

Bumrungrad International was the first hospital in Asia to obtain JCI accreditation (2002) and the first to be reaccredited. At this writing, it is one of Thailand's three JCI-accredited hospitals, and it was the first Asian hospital to receive JCI disease-specific accreditations for its stroke and heart attack programs.

Of its 900 physicians, surgeons, and consultants, approximately 200 are US board-certified.

Bumrungrad International's 34 clinical specialties include endocrinology (diabetes and metabolism), nephrology (kidneys), neurology, and nutrition. Bumrungrad International's **Heart Center** offers pacemaker implantation, invasive and noninvasive procedures for congenital heart disease, valvoplasty (balloon valve treatment) and valve replacement, and coronary artery bypass graft (CABG). The hospital's **Horizon Regional Cancer Center** employs such advanced techniques as image-guided radiotherapy and HD brachytherapy. Orthopedic procedures, such as hip replacements and resurfacing, are also popular among international patients.

Directed by a US-trained medical director, Bumrungrad International sponsors an active continuing medical education program for its physicians, who also participate in clinical research through the **Bumrungrad International Clinical Research Center.**

The hospital commissions an independent research firm to conduct a customer satisfaction survey each year. In the most recent survey, nine out of ten international patients reported being satisfied with their experience and said they would recommend the hospital.

For patients who wish to recover near the hospital, Bumrungrad International offers two Bumrungrad Residences and Bumrungrad Suites. For rates, room pictures, and further information, visit the hospital's Web site.

Samitivej Sukhumvit Hospital
133 Sukhumvit 49, Klongtan Nua
Vadhana
Bangkok, THAILAND 10110
Tel: 011 66 2 711.8000
Fax: 011 66 2 391.1290
Email: info@samitivej.co.th
Web: www.samitivej.co.th

Samitivej Sukhumvit Hospital is one of four hospitals in Bangkok belonging to the Samitivej group. This one is JCI accredited. Sukhumvit currently has 270 beds, 87 examination suites, 1,200 caregivers, 400 specialists, and a full-service **International Patient Center.** Sukhumvit is one of the few Thai hospitals to have received the Prime Minister's Award for Most Recognized Service (2004). It is accredited by Thailand's Hospital Accreditation Board. Americans will feel at home with a 7-Eleven, Starbucks, and ATMs on the ground level of the hospital.

Specialty centers include

■ **Eye Clinic:** specializes in general ophthalmology, retinal and vitreous conditions, glaucoma, pediatric ophthalmology and strabismus, oculoplastic reconstruction, and ocular oncology.

■ **Hemodialysis Department:** for patients with acute or chronic renal (kidney) failure. The center deploys artificial kidney machines. It has been certified by the Royal College of Physicians of Thailand. Known throughout Thailand for its success rates in kidney transplants, the Hemodialysis Department receives its kidneys from the Thai Red Cross's Organ Donation Center.

■ **Liver and Digestive Institute:** where a team of gastroenterologists treats the full gamut of liver and digestive abnormalities, including cirrhosis, fatty liver disease, pancreatitis, gall bladder infection, and bile duct infection. Specialty surgeries include procedures on the liver, bile ducts, gall bladder, esophagus, stomach, and small and large intestine, as well as liver transplantation.

The other hospitals in the group are

■ **Samitivej Srinakarin:** Samitivej's newest addition in Bangkok. It has 17 stories and

400 beds, located on Bangkok's east side, a few minutes from the newly opened Suvarnabhumi International Airport. The hospital's 21 acres of landscaped gardens and fountains foster an environment of tranquility not commonly found on the grounds of US hospitals. The **Cancer Center** and **Oncology Clinic** focus on prevention, screening, diagnosis, and treatment of out-service patients. A full team of multilingual medical oncologists, radiation oncologists, physicists, technicians, oncology nurses, and intravenous nurses render Bangkok's best in cancer treatment. Seven dental units, three x-ray operating suites, a panoramic x-ray machine, a laser system, and an intraoral camera make Srinakarin's **Dental Center** a state-of-the-art, one-stop shop, with no need for multiple trips to outside labs. The full range of dental services and oral surgeries is offered, including orthodontics, root canals, full and partial dentures, crowns and bridges, implants, extractions, bone graft surgery, and treatment of gum diseases.

■ **Samitivej Sriracha:** A 150-bed hospital located 130 kilometers (about 80 miles) southeast of Bangkok. Since its opening more than ten years ago, Samitivej Sriracha has become a key healthcare provider for corporate and industries in the Eastern seaboard. Sriracha's proximity to the resort towns of Pattaya and Hua Hin also attracts many tourists looking for quality healthcare facilities. The hospital has 15 intensive care units and six operating rooms. Its special services include the **Children's Clinic, Dental Services,** and **Wellness Center.**

■ **Samitivej Srinakarin Children's Hospital:** Thailand's first and only dedicated private hospital for children. The hospital offers a mind-boggling array of pediatric specialties and subspecialties, ranging from pediatric snoring to bone marrow transplant.

Specialty centers include

■ **Allergy Clinic:** diagnoses and treats asthma, hay fever, atopic dermatitis, food allergy, drug allergy, and chronic sinusitis.

■ **Growth, Endocrine, and Diabetes Center for Children:** diagnoses and treats growth hormone deficiency, thyroid disease and abnormalities, precocious and delayed puberty, ambiguous genitalia (including micropenis or undescended testis), adrenal gland disease or disorder, obesity, juvenile diabetes, and other endocrine system disorders.

■ **Pediatric Hearing Center:** provides complete hearing evaluations and diagnostics, sales of analog and digital hearing aids (much less expensive in Thailand than in the US), and cochlear implants.

■ **Pediatric Cardiology Clinic:** offers diagnosis and treatment for congenital heart diseases, abnormal heart rhythm, heart muscle inflammation, pericardial diseases, valve diseases, aortic aneurysm, rheumatic diseases, and Kawasaki disease.

■ **Pediatric Nephrology Clinic:** provides early detection of kidney disease and abnormalities, as well as treatment for childhood nephrotic syndrome.

■ **Pediatric Orthopedic Clinic:** focuses on early detection and treatment of bone and joint diseases, as well as sports injuries, brachial plexus palsy and arm and shoulder paralysis due to difficult deliveries, pediatric spinal disorders (e.g., congenital scoliosis), congenital hip dislocation, and cerebral palsy.

- **Infectious Disease Clinic:** focuses on rare, complicated, or drug-resistant infectious diseases, as well as diagnosis and treatment for all infectious diseases, including bloodstream infections (septicemia), meningitis, pneumonia, and pediatric HIV.

Bangkok Dental Group
Siam Square Street 2
Unit 236/3–236/4 (Level 2–4)
Pratuwan
Bangkok, THAILAND 10330
Tel: 011 66 2 658.4774
Email: contact@bangkokdental.com
Web: www.bangkokdental.com

and

Bangkok Dental Home
1701/12 Phaholyothin Road
Jatujuk
Bangkok, THAILAND 10900
Tel: 011 66 2 930.1144
Email: contact@bangkokdental.com
Web: www.bangkokdental.com

and

Bangkok International Dental Center
157 Ratchadapesik Road
Din Daeng District
Bangkok, THAILAND 10400
Tel: 011 66 2 692.4433
Fax: 011 66 2 248.6196
Email: contact@bangkokdentalcenter.com
Web: www.bangkokdentalcenter.com

Bangkok is peppered with dental clinics. You can probably find three of them for every temple in the town! A few cater specifically to international tourists, and the Bangkok Dental Group (BDG) is one of the most enduring and expansive of them. The group's three locations around Bangkok have treated more than 1,500 foreign visitors since opening their doors in 2003. Together the centers employ 45 full-time dental specialists and surgeons, with a staff of nearly 90 practicing in 20 treatment rooms. Most of BDG's dentists have been trained and certified overseas, and a large and comforting number received their degrees in the US. All practitioners' credentials are posted on the BDG Web site, grouped by area of expertise.

Specialties include aesthetic and cosmetic dentistry, crowns (porcelain and zirconium), root canals, periodontics (gum disease), orthodontics (including braces, retainers, and invisible braces), implantology, and prosthodontics (including full and partial dentures).

PHUKET

Once a brisk trading port, the island of Phuket (pronounced approximately "poo-GET") is now a leading tourist center nestled within a cluster of 40 islands in the Andaman Sea. Known as the "Pearl of the Andaman," Phuket's culturally mixed and multinational setting has fostered a major center of medical travel, with the emphasis on travel.

Where a health traveler to Thailand might favor Bangkok for more invasive treatment, such as orthopedic or cardiovascular surgery, those seeking less physically taxing procedures (such as cosmetic surgery, dental care, and ophthalmological treatments) might well be tempted to head to the resort beaches of this beautiful island.

Although smaller, Phuket's hospitals are as good and the treatment specialties nearly as robust. If you're willing to stay a little farther from the epicenter of Thailand's healthcare, Phuket's beaches, five-star resorts, and relaxed surroundings are alluring. Phuket's medical infrastructure has largely recovered from the devastating effects of the Indian Ocean tsunami of 2004.

Bangkok Hospital Phuket

2/1 Hongyok Utis Road
Muang District
Phuket, THAILAND 83000
Tel: 011 66 76 254.425
Fax: 011 66 76 254.430
Email: info@phukethospital.com
Web: www.phukethospital.com

A sister hospital to Bangkok Hospital Medical Center (see above), Bangkok Hospital Phuket (BPK) belongs to the Bangkok Hospital Group, a network of 15 private hospitals that form the largest healthcare provider in Southeast Asia. Sixty full-time specialists, 40 consulting physicians, and 207 nurses make this 200-bed center Phuket's largest and most prestigious medical facility.

As with its sister hospital in Bangkok, BPK opened its own **International Medical Service Center** in 2005, catering exclusively to medical travelers. Specialties include closed- and open-heart surgery, keyhole surgery, and hip and knee replacement. Its **Aesthetic Center** provides a full range of plastic surgeries (cosmetic and reconstructive). The hospital also boasts a full-service dental clinic.

As with all hospitals within the group, BPK is accredited through Thailand's Institute of Hospital Quality Improvement and Accreditation. The hospital, which was damaged extensively in the 2004 tsunami, is now housed in a new building.

Phuket International Hospital

44 Chalermprakiat Ror 9 Road
Phuket, THAILAND 83000
Tel: 011 66 76 249.400
Fax: 011 66 76 210.936
Email: info@phuket-international-hospital.com
Web: www.phuket-international-hospital.com

Founded in 1982, Phuket International Hospital (PIH) was the first private hospital to open its doors on the island. Extensively remodeled during 2007, a new wing of the hospital contains a new outpatient facility and more patient rooms, which have increased the hospital's occupancy to 150 beds. PIH has many areas of specialization. It is internationally recognized for its plastic surgery. Other areas include orthopedic surgery, dentistry, and general surgery. It treats more than 2,000 patients from the US and Canada annually.

PIH aggressively promotes its medical checkup packages tailored for Western patients. A variety of tests and exam packages are offered at prices well below fees encountered in the US.

For those interested in alternative therapies, the **Traditional Health Center** at PIH offers an array of traditional Chinese medical treatments, including acupuncture, massage, and cupping (the use of suction cups in place of needles at acupuncture points).

Inpatient room rates are attractive (deluxe private rooms for less than $60 per day), and the rooms include bathroom, bedside sofa, separate lounge area, and refrigerator.

■ RECOVERY ACCOMMODATIONS

Although you won't find any medical services in these oases of tranquility, if you are feeling well enough for a brief journey—yet still want to be close to your doctor—you may find just the perfect recuperative environment at one of these retreats. Fisherman's Village is about a two-hour drive from Bangkok. Mukdara Beach is near Phuket.

Fisherman's Village
170 Moo 1
Haad Chao Samran
Phetchaburi, THAILAND 76100
Tel: 011 66 3 244.1370
Fax: 011 66 3 244.1380
Email: info@fishermansvillage.net
Web: www.fishermansvillage.net

Mukdara Beach Villa and Spa Resort
Khao Lak
26/14 Moo 7 Khuk Khak
Takuapa, Phang-Nga, THAILAND 82190
Tel: 011 66 76 429.999
Fax: 011 66 76 486.199
Email: info@mukdarabeach.com
Web: www.mukdarabeach.com

■ HOTELS: DELUXE

BANGKOK

The Emerald Hotel
99/1 Ratchadapisek Road
Din Daeng
Bangkok, THAILAND 10400
Tel: 011 66 2 276.4567
Fax: 011 66 2 276.4555
Email: info@emeraldhotel.com
Web: www.emeraldhotel.com

Imperial Queen's Park Hotel
199 Sukhumvit Soi 22
Bangkok, THAILAND 10110
Tel: 011 66 2 261.9000
Fax: 011 66 2 261.9530
Email: queenspark@imperialhotels.com
Web: www.imperialhotels.com

InterContinental Bangkok (near Bumrungrad International Hospital)
973 Ploenchit Road
Patumwan
Bangkok, THAILAND 10330
Tel: 011 66 2 656.0444
Fax: 011 66 2 656.0555
Email: intercon@ihgbangkok.com
Web: www.bangkok.com/intercontinental

Centre Point Saladaeng Service Apartments (near Bangkok Nursing Home Hospital)
5 Soi Saladaeng 1 Silom Road
Bangkok, THAILAND 10500
Tel: 011 66 0 2267.5500
Fax: 011 66 0 2267.5501
Web: www.centrepoint.com

Novotel Suvarnabhumi (at the airport and near Samitivej Srinakarin Hospital)
999 Suvarnabhumi Airport Hotel
Moo 1 Nongprue Bang Phli Samutprakarn
Bangkok, THAILAND 10540
Tel: 011 66 2 131.1111
Fax: 011 66 2 131.1188
Email: reservation@novotelsuvarnabhumi
.com
Web: www.novotel.com

President Solitaire
Sukhumvit Soi 11
Bangkok, THAILAND 10110
Tel: 011 66 2 255.7200
Fax: 011 66 2 253.2330
Email: enquiry@presidentsolitaire.com
Web: www.presidentsolitaire.com

PHUKET

Le Méridien Phuket Beach Resort
29 Soi Karon Nui, Tambon Karon
Amphur Muang
Phuket, THAILAND 83100
Tel: 1 800 315.2621 (US toll-free); 011 66 76
370.100
Fax: 011 66 76 340.479
Email: reservations.phuketbeach@
lemeridien.com
Web: www.starwoodhotels.com

Phuket Merlin Hotel
158/1 Jawaraj Road
Muang District
Phuket, THAILAND 83000
Tel: 011 66 76 2 128.6670
Fax: 011 66 76 216.429
Web: www.merlinphuket.com

■ HOTELS: MODERATE

BANGKOK

Amari Atrium Hotel (near Bangkok International Hospital)
1880 New Petchburi Road
Bangkok, THAILAND 10310
Tel: 011 66 2 718.2000
Fax: 011 66 2 718.2002
Email: atrium@amari.com
Web: www.amari.com/atrium/ath.htm

Siam Beverly Hotel
188 Ratchadapisek Road
Huaykwang
Bangkok, THAILAND 10320
Tel: 011 66 2 275.4397
Fax: 011 66 2 275.4049
Email: info@siambeverly.com
Web: www.siambeverly.com

Radisson Hotel
92 Soi Saengcham
Rama 9 Road
Huay Kwang
Bangkok, THAILAND 10320
Tel: 1 800 333.3333 (US toll-free); 011 66 2
641.4777
Fax: 011 66 2 641.4884
Email: radisson@radisson.com.th
Web: www.radisson.com/bangkok.th

Swissôtel Le Concorde (near Bangkok Dental Group and Preecha Aesthetic Institute)
204 Ratchadapisek Road
Huay Kwang
Bangkok, THAILAND 10320
Tel: 011 66 2 694.2222
Fax: 011 66 2 694.2223
Email: Bangkok-leconcorde@swissotel.com
Web: www.swissotel.com

Chatra Court
49 Soi Sukhumvit 19
Wattana
Bangkok, THAILAND 10110
Tel: 011 66 2 651.1310
Fax: 011 66 2 253.5830
Email: reservation@chatracourt.com
Web: www.chatracourt.com

Majestic Grande Hotel
12 Sukhumvit Soi 2
Bangkok, THAILAND 10110
Tel: 011 66 02 262.2999
Fax: 011 66 02 262.2900
Email: info@majesticgrande.com
Web: www.majesticgrande.com

Holiday Inn Resort Phuket
52 Thaweewong Road
Patong Beach
Phuket, THAILAND 83150
Tel: 1 800 315.2621 (US toll-free); 011 66 76
340.608
Fax: 011 66 76 340.435
Email: reservations@holidayinn.com
Web: www.holidayinn.com

PHUKET

Burasari Patong Resort Hotel
18/110 Ruamjai Road
Tambon Patong, Amphur Kathu
Phuket, THAILAND 83150
Tel: 011 66 2 678.0101
Fax: 011 66 2 678.0102
Email: contact@burasari.com
Web: www.burasari.com

DESTINATION: **TURKEY**

■ AT A GLANCE

Istanbul, Kocaeli, and Izmir

Language:	Turkish (English widely spoken)
Time Zone:	GMT +2
Country Dialing Code:	90
Electricity:	220V, Plug type B
Currency:	New Turkish lira
Visa Required?	Yes
Recommended Immunizations:	Hepatitis A; Boosters for Typhoid and Polio
Treatment Specialties:	Cardiovascular Surgery, IVF, Organ Transplantation, Cosmetic Surgery, Dental, Oncology
Leading Hospitals and Clinics:	*Istanbul:* Memorial Hospital, Gayrettepe Florence Nightingale Hospital, Acibadem Healthcare Group; *Kocaeli:* Anadolu Medical Center; *Izmir:* Kent Hastanesi Hospital
JCI-Accredited Hospitals:	*Istanbul:* Acibadem Healthcare Group, Alman Hastanesi/Deutsches Krankenhaus, Caglayan Florence Nightingale Hospital, Dünya Eye Hospital, Hisar Intercontinental Hospital, Memorial Hospital, Medline Alarm Saðlýk Hizmetleri A.Þ., Gayrettepe Florence Nightingale Hospital, Vehbi Koc Foundation American Hospital, Yeditepe University Hospital; Ozel Medicana Hospital; *Ankara:* Bayindir Hospital, Hacettepe University Adult Hospital, Mesa Hastanesi, Turkish Red Crescent Society Middle Anatolia Regional Blood Center; *Izmir:* Kent Hastanesi Hospital; *Kocaeli:* Anadolu Medical Center; *Bursa:* Üniversitesi Saglik Kuvuluslan
Standards and Accreditation:	Republic of Turkey Ministry of Health; Turkish Society of Plastic, Reconstructive and Aesthetic Surgery; Turkish Medical Association; JCI

■ TREATMENT BRIEF

Turkey has one foot in Europe and the other in the Near East. It's an enormous country of diverse people and landscapes, ranging from the bustling commercial centers of Istanbul to the quiet agricultural villages of the eastern provinces. As a major player on the world scene both politically and economically, Turkey is poised to play its part in the global healthcare arena. It's now promoting medical travel in a big way, and Turkish medical institutions are serving some 15,000 foreign patients each year.

Few medical travelers realize that Turkey has more JCI-accredited healthcare facilities than any other country combined! The number as of this writing is 20, and more are being added to the list annually. Prices in Turkey compare favorably with even the lowest available in Asia, and the quality of healthcare is consistently outstanding, with many doctors Western-trained and fluent in English. The Turkish government enforces rigorous quality standards in all its institutions, and healthcare is no exception. Technology, facilities, and personnel are consistently top-notch.

Turkey has developed a booming trade in vacation tourism in the last three decades, so extending the traditional Turkish warmth and hospitality to medical travelers is not a stretch. The Turkish Cultural and Tourism Ministry has spent more than $100 million to spread the word that Turkey is welcoming health travelers. The country has much to offer. Turkish cuisine is among the best in the world, and—if you have the time and feel well enough for a vacation—you are sure to enjoy the port cities of Mar-maris and Fethiye, the stone dwellings of Cappadocia, or the hot springs of Pamukkale.

■ TYPICAL TREATMENTS AND COSTS

Cardiovascular:
Coronary Artery Bypass Graft:
$16,500-$18,000
Bypass + Valve Replacement (single):
$18,000
Bypass + Valve Replacement (double):
$27,000

Orthopedic:
Birmingham Hip Resurfacing: $9,700
Joint Replacement:
Knee: $8,200-$12,000
Hip: $9,700-$11,250
Ankle: $9,700
Shoulder: $9,700

Cosmetic:
Breast Augmentation: $3,500-$4,650
Breast Lift/Reduction: $5,000-$6,350
Facelift: $6,000-$6,300
Liposuction (one region): $3,000-$3,200
Tummy Tuck: $4,950-$5,800

Dental:
Porcelain Veneer: $290-$480
Inlays and Onlays: $365-$660
Implant: $1,800
Extraction (surgical, per tooth): $320-$360

Vision:
Glaucoma: $4,200
LASIK (per eye): $950

Other:

Gall Bladder Removal: $7,000

Prostate Surgery (TURP): $6,500

■ HEALTH TRAVEL AGENTS

BridgeHealth International, Inc. (also Medical Tours International)

5299 DTC Boulevard, Suite 800

Greenwood Village, CO 80111

Tel: 1 800 680.1366 (US toll-free); 1 303 457.5745

Fax: 1 303 779.0366

Email: info@bridgehealthintl.com

Web: www.bridgehealthintl.com

For more information on BridgeHealth International, see Costa Rica.

Companion Global Healthcare, Inc.

c/o Blue Cross Blue Shield of South Carolina

I-20 at Alpine Road, AF-324

Columbia, SC 29219

Tel: 1 803 264.3256

Fax: 1 803 264.7063

Email: David.Boucher@BCBSSC.com

Web: www.CompanionGlobalHealthcare.com

For more information on Companion Global Healthcare, see Thailand.

MedRetreat

2042 Laurel Valley Drive

Vernon Hills, IL 60061

Tel: 1 877 876.3373 (US toll-free)

Fax: 1 847 680.0484

Email: customerservice@medretreat.com

Web: www.medretreat.com

For more information on MedRetreat, see Malaysia.

WorldMed Assist

1230 Mountain Side Court

Concord, CA 94521

Tel: 1 866 999.3848 (US toll-free)

Fax: 1 925 905.5898

Email: whoeber@worldmedassist.com

Web: www.worldmedassist.com

For more information on WorldMed Assist, see India: Bangalore.

■ HOSPITALS AND CLINICS

Memorial Health Group
Memorial Hospital

Piyale Paşa Bulvari Okmeydani-Şişli

Istanbul, TURKEY 34385

Tel: 011 90 212 314.6666

Fax: 011 90 212 314.6667

Email: internationalpatients@memorial.com.tr

Web: www.memorial.com.tr

Memorial Hospital was the first JCI-accredited healthcare institution in Turkey. The facility is a member of the American Hospital Association (AHA).

This 200-bed hospital opened in 2000, and now has a staff of 150 physicians, many of them trained in the US or Europe. Most speak fluent English. In the international healthcare arena, Memorial is best known for cardiovascular surgery, in vitro fertilization (IVF), and organ transplantation. In 2004 the Turkish Ministry of Health licensed Memorial as the first private hospital to carry out organ transplantation (kidney and liver). Memorial's **IVF and Genetics Center** generated the first IVF pregnancy via micro-injection in Turkey. It is also the first center in Turkey with an in-house genetics lab capable of performing genetic inspections and resolving genetic issues prior to fertilization. Memorial recently made a large investment in a complete technological renovation of its radiology department.

Memorial's **International Patient Center** services include initial screening and diagnosis, evaluation, and recommendation from Memorial physicians; scheduling of medical appointments; coordination of the admissions process; cost estimates for anticipated treatment; airport pickup/dropoff transportation; English-speaking staff and language interpretation; and lodging and transportation arrangement for patients and family members.

Memorial has its own five-star guesthouse for recovering patients and their families (www.memorial.com.tr). Those who prefer a deluxe hotel may enjoy the nearby Grand Cevahir Hotel (www.gch.com).

Gayrettepe Florence Nightingale Hospital
Cemil Aslan Güder Sokak, No. 8
Gayrettepe, Istanbul, TURKEY
Tel: 011 90 212 288.3400
Web: www.florence.com.tr

The Gayrettepe Florence Nightingale Hospital started operations in 1997 as the third hospital in a group owned by the Turkish Cardiology Foundation. It earned JCI accreditation in 2003. Florence Nightingale's bronchoscopy unit provides radiotherapy from inside the lung. Doctors there claim the unit shortens the treatment period for lung cancer, enhances the effectiveness of treatment, and cuts in half problems stemming from radiotherapy. Florence Nightingale is particularly well known for its in vitro fertilization (IVF) and fertility units. Prospective parents can choose from a wide variety

of methods, such as inoculation, classic test-tube baby, microinjection, testicular sperm aspiration (TESA), testicular sperm extraction (TESE), microsurgical epididymal sperm aspiration (MESA), percutaneous epididymal sperm aspiration (PESA), and implantation of frozen embryos.

Six operating suites are used for a wide variety of procedures, including microlaparoscopy, laser cataract removal, and prostate surgery. Imaging technologies include digital angiography, computer tomography (CT), mammography, x-ray, and ultrasound. In the nuclear medicine and nuclear cardiology units, images are provided by the gamma camera to determine the extent of damage from myocardial infarction.

The **Gayrettepe Oncology Centre** seeks to employ the best cancer treatment practices available. It is the only oncology center in Turkey to model itself after the modern "comprehensive cancer center" found at only 23 sites in the US. In accordance with US standards, its fully equipped diagnosis, medical oncology, and radiation oncology treatment units work in cooperation. The center can connect online with cancer centers in the US via satellite.

Acibadem Healthcare Group
Altunizade Mahallesi Fahrettin Kerim Gökay
Caddesi No. 49 Üsküdar
Istanbul, TURKEY 34662
Tel: 011 90 216 544.3892
Fax: 011 90 216 340.7728
Email: international@asg.com.tr
Web: www.acibadem.com.tr

JCI-accredited Acibadem Healthcare Group operates six hospitals in Turkey, with eight more soon to be added to the club. More than 1,000 physicians and 5,000 staff members provide healthcare services in 20 different locations (including Izmir and Bodrum) through a network of general hospitals, medical centers, outpatient clinics, laboratories, and an ophthalmology center. Acibadem's partners include Istanbul International Hospital and International Etiler Outpatient Clinic. Acibadem signed a partnership agreement with Harvard Medical International in 2003 to provide high-level professional development of the healthcare team, especially nurses. Acibadem's **International Patient Center** provides complete services for patients visiting member hospitals from countries outside Turkey. Staff members assist patients with treatment plans, package pricing, and accommodation arrangements.

Anadolu Medical Center
Anadolu Caddesi No. 1
Cayirova Mevkii Bayramoglu
Cikisi Gebze, Kocaeli, TURKEY 41400
Tel: 011 90 262 678.5513
Fax: 011 90 262 654.0053
Email: asli.akyavas@anadolusaglik.org
Web: www.anadolusaglik.org

Affiliated with Johns Hopkins in Baltimore, this JCI-accredited hospital has 209 beds and has been operating since 2005. Anadolu Medical Center has earned praise for its architecture and location atop a hill bordered by woodlands and olive groves, with a clear view of the ocean. Its 2-million-square-foot campus is home to treatment facilities, medical offices, and health-related retail stores. With nearly 100 physicians in attendance, Anadolu has earned some impressive honors, including a "Designated Center of Integrated Oncology and Pallia-

tive Care" recognition from the European Society for Medical Oncology. The Canada Operational Support Command honored Anadolu for the high-quality healthcare provided to the Canadian Intermediate Staging Team during their stay in Turkey in 2006–2007.

Anadolu treats nearly 700 international patients annually, serving them through its **International Patient Services Department.** The hospital provides transportation free of charge from the airport to local hotels and to medical appointments and treatment facilities. For those who are well enough, Anadolu offers international patients a free tour of Istanbul with a private driver and car.

Kent Hastanesi Hospital
8229 Sokak No. 30, Çiğli
Izmir, TURKEY 35580
Tel: 011 90 232 386.7070
Fax: 011 90 232 386.7071
Web: www.kenthospital.com

With 121 beds, eight surgery suits, and 21 intensive care units, Kent Hastanesi Hospital received its JCI accreditation in 2006. Its specialty centers include the **Sleep Disorders Center, Plastic Surgery Center, IVF Center, Diabetes Center,** and **Urology Center.** Kent physicians employ state-of-the-art diagnostic and treatment technology. Kent often turns to the Mayo Clinic for training and consultation. Diagnostic images from radiology, coronary angiography, nuclear medicine, and bone densitometry are achieved digitally and made available for use within the hospital, as well as to local and international medical practitioners in a fashion that maintains patient confidentiality. Kent's laboratory is certified for testing all biochemical, hematological, microbiological, and hormonal parameters. Kent's **Cardiology Diagnostic Unit** is equipped with electrocardiogram (EKG), Holter monitor, echocardiography, and stress EKG equipment. The unit provides coronary angiography, angioplasty, stenting, and pacemaker placement. Kent offers the full range of minimally invasive and endoscopic surgical procedures.

■ HOTELS: DELUXE

Note: The major commercial centers and tourist destinations of Turkey abound with family-owned and -operated *pensiones*, small hotels, and modest guesthouses that are clean, quiet, and inexpensive. If you prefer local color to large, luxury accommodations (and your recuperative needs are moderate), you may wish to consider arranging such housing. We list here only a few of the larger hotels recommended by the Istanbul hospitals described above.

Hotel Hegsagone
Balyanos Koyu Kaptan Sokak No. 13
Bayramoğlu Gebze
Kocaeli, TURKEY
Tel: 011 90 262 653.5959
Fax: 011 90 262 653.8549
Email: hotel@hegsagone.com
Web: www.hegsagone.com

The Marmara Pendik
Sahil Yolu, Ankara Caddesi No. 239
Alt Kaynarca, Pendik
Istanbul, TURKEY 34890
Tel: 011 90 216 362.1010
Fax: 011 90 216 362.8375

Email: residence-info@themarmarahotels.com
Web: www.themarmarahotels.com

Sisus Hotel
Dalyanköy Yat Limani Çeşme
Izmir, TURKEY
Tel: 011 90 232 724.0330
Fax: 011 90 232 724.9656
Email: info@sisushotel.com
Web: www.sisushotel.com

■ HOTELS: MODERATE

Bayramoğlu Resort Hotel
Bayramoğlu Caddesi No. 229
Bayramoğlu-Darica-İzmit-Kocaeli
TURKEY
Tel: 011 90 262 653.4030
Fax: 011 90 262 653.4033
Email: info@bayramogluresort.com
Web: www.bayramogluresort.com

Zeus Hotel
Bayramoğlu Grup Sokak No. 10
Bayramoğlu, Istanbul, TURKEY
Tel: 011 90 262 653.3036
Fax: 011 90 262 653.7254
Web: www.otelzeus.com

Izmir Palas Hotel
Atatürk Bulvari
Izmir, TURKEY 35210
Tel: 011 90 232 465.0030
Fax: 011 90 232 422.6870
Email: info@izmirpalas.com.tr
Web: www.izmirpalas.com.tr

UNITED ARAB EMIRATES (UAE)

■ AT A GLANCE

Dubai and Abu Dhabi

Language:	Arabic, Persian (English widely spoken)
Time Zone:	GMT +4
Country Dialing Code:	971
Electricity:	240V, Plug type G
Currency:	UAE dirham
Visa Required?	Yes
Recommended Immunizations:	Hepatitis A; Typhoid Booster
Treatment Specialties:	Cardiovascular, Dermatology, Oncology, Orthopedic
Leading Hospitals and Clinics:	American Hospital Dubai, Tawam Hospital, Skin Laser Dubai, Oasis Hospital
JCI-Accredited Hospitals:	*Abu Dhabi:* Al Rahba Hospital; Al Corniche Hospital; *Al Ain (in Abu Dhabi state):* Oasis Hospital, Tawam Hospital; *Dubai:* Al Wasl Maternity and Paediatric Hospital, Thalassemia Center (of Al Wasl Maternity and Paediatric Hospital), American Hospital Dubai, Dubai Hospital, Rashid Hospital, International Modern Hospital; *Sharjah:* Zulekha Hospital
Standards and Accreditation:	College of American Pathologists (CAP), German-Arab Medical Society, International Pan Arab Critical Care Medicine Society (IPACCMS), Society of International Radiology, JCI

■ TREATMENT BRIEF

While many Americans shy away from traveling to an Arab country for healthcare, much less for a vacation, the United Arab Emirates (UAE) is surprisingly safe and welcoming. On the healthcare front, the UAE already claims five JCI-accredited hospitals and a number of specialty clinics.

Slightly smaller than the state of Maine, the UAE is a federation of seven emirates or states. Bordered by Oman and Saudi Arabia, the UAE was once considered a desert wasteland. Now it is an international blend of Eastern values and Western technologies—without the Western crime rates.

The city of Abu Dhabi is the capital of the UAE and also the center of government for the state of the same name. Two JCI-accredited hospitals are located in Al Ain in the state of Abu Dhabi, with another in the city itself.

The state of Dubai, the second largest emirate, is situated on the Persian Gulf. The city of the same name is one of the Middle East's most popular beach resorts. Dubai has two JCI-accredited hospitals.

For the past decade, Arab nationals have traveled to Thailand, Singapore, India, and other Asian hospitals for healthcare. After a purse tally, the Dubai government decided it was time to reclaim its regional base of patients. More than $100 million has been raised to realize this vision, which will include facilities for medical care and wellness, research, and education.

Harvard University has shown an interest in the region and has undertaken several initiatives. The **Harvard Medical School Dubai Center (HMSDC)** Institute for Postgraduate Education and Research promotes cross-national collaboration on key education and research projects. The **Dubai Harvard Foundation for Medical Research (DHFMR)** seeks to support a regional community of leaders in medicine and the life sciences.

If you're interested in learning more about healthcare in the Middle East, you may want to familiarize yourself with ArabMedicare Medical Tourism Center of North Carolina. Although not a health travel agent, the clearinghouse has been promoting hospitals and clinics in the Middle East since 1999. For more information, go to www.arabmedicare.com.

Note: Unfortunately, politics remain an issue in the UAE, and travelers with an Israeli passport or with Israeli stamps in their passports will be denied entry into the country.

■ TYPICAL TREATMENTS AND COSTS

Cardiovascular:
Coronary Artery Bypass Graft:
  $37,000-$40,900
Bypass + Valve Replacement (single):
  $50,600
Bypass and Valve Replacement (double):
  $57,500

Orthopedic:
Joint Replacement:
  Knee: $40,250
  Hip: $46,000
  Ankle: $43,700
  Shoulder: $46,200

Dental:

Crown (all porcelain): $575

Porcelain Veneer: $575

Inlays and Onlays: $345

Implant: $2,070

Extraction (surgical, per tooth): $200-$260

■ HEALTH TRAVEL AGENTS

Planet Hospital

23679 Calabasas Road, Suite 150

Calabasas, CA 91302

Tel: 1 800 243.0172 (US toll-free); 1 818

665.4801

Fax: 1 818 665.4810

Email: rudy@planethospital.com

Web: www.planethospital.com

For more information on Planet Hospital, see Singapore.

■ HOSPITALS AND CLINICS

American Hospital Dubai

19th Street, Old Metha Area

P.O. Box 5566

Dubai, UNITED ARAB EMIRATES

Tel: 011 971 4336.7777

Fax: 011 971 4336.5176

Email: info@ahdubai.com

Web: www.ahdubai.com

Opened in 1996, American Hospital Dubai (AHD) is an acute-care hospital devoted to providing American standards of healthcare in the Middle East. In 2000 the hospital was the first facility in the Middle East to be certified by JCI; JCI accreditation was renewed in 2003 and again in 2006.

AHD is located in the Bur Dubai dis-

trict, which is near the city center and the beaches. AHD currently has 143 beds and is expanding to 360 by 2009. The 60 full-time hospital physicians are US board-certified or are equivalent physician specialists. By the end of the expansion, the hospital will have 110 physicians.

AHD is a multicultural organization with a staff representing 35 nationalities. English is the main language spoken, although other common languages include Arabic, French, and German.

AHD offers general surgery, including laparoscopic and neuralgic, in addition to gastrointestinal endoscopies.

Centers of excellence include

■ The **Cancer Care Unit** offers quiet, relaxing suites and state-of-the-art treatment.

■ The **Diabetes Center** treats all diabetic needs, including diagnosis, medical care and supervision, information and education, and family support.

■ The **Endocrinology and Digestive Disease Center** offers diagnosis and management of digestive and liver diseases. Services include upper and lower gastrointestinal (GI) endoscopy and enteroscopy (lower intestine).

■ The **Heart Center** comprises two areas of treatment: interventional cardiology and cardiothoracic surgery. The center frequently performs angiograms and angioplasties and specializes in minimally invasive cardiac surgery and beating-heart bypass surgery, both relatively new techniques. In addition, the center is committed to introducing advanced techniques, such as endoscopic and robotic procedures, as they become available.

■ The **Total Joint Replacement Center** is the first of its kind in the Middle East. The center's director has performed more than 4,000 joint replacements, and more than 550 joint replacements are performed yearly, making it the largest knee center in the Middle East. Although knee joint replacement is a specialty, the center offers an extensive range of full or partial artificial joints using minimally invasive surgical intervention techniques.

■ The **Dialysis Unit** has private rooms, and separate clinics treat all ages: children, adolescents, adults, and the elderly.

■ AHD's **International Patient Center** offers the usual amenities, including assistance with appointments and consultation, interpreters for non-Arabic speaking patients, Internet connections in rooms, fax, photocopy, courier, and laundry service. Arrangements can be made for ambulance pickup (with a mobile intensive care unit and trained paramedics) at the airport, which is less than a 15-minute ride from AHD. Once a health traveler checks in, an international patient coordinator assists in making appointments and coordinating referrals to the outpatient clinic, laboratory, pathology, medical imaging, and inpatient surgical procedures.

Dubai Hospital
Al-Braha Area
Dubai, UNITED ARAB EMIRATES
Tel: 011 971 4 219.5000; 011 971 4 271.4444
Fax: 011 971 4 219.5613
Email: DHWeb@dohms.gov.ae
Web: http://web.dohms.gov.ae/dh/

Established in 1983, this 630-bed hospital received JCI accreditation in 2007. Dubai Hospital comprises numerous specialized departments and clinics, including ophthalmology, orthopedics, pediatrics, physiotherapy, obstetrics, urology, radiology, nuclear medicine, endocrinology, nephrology, rheumatology, oncology, and otolaryngology. It has 22 executive-style suites for VIP patients, with a choice of sea or city views. Suite prices start at about $400 per night. Services for health travelers include express check-in and check-out, a 24-hour medical team, special food and beverages, and wireless Internet connection. Treatment prices are listed on the hospital's Web site.

International Modern Hospital
P.O. Box 121735
Dubai, UNITED ARAB EMIRATES
Tel.: 011 971 4 398.8888
Fax: 011 971 4 398.4444
Email: info@imh.ae
Web: www.imh.ae

JCI-accredited in 2007, International Modern Hospital is located in the heart of Dubai, convenient to New Dubai and Dubai Internet City. This privately operated facility is organized around the full range of departments and clinics, including otolaryngology, neurology, general surgery, orthopedics, pediatrics, cardiology, dermatology, plastic surgery, and internal medicine. It is affiliated with more than 20 insurance companies; a list of them is provided on its Web site.

Skin Laser Dubai

Al Ghurair City, 641-B, Office Tower 4
P.O. Box 14477
Dubai, UNITED ARAB EMIRATES
Tel: 011 971 4222.2663
Fax: 011 971 4221.9292
Email: drmmehta@emirates.net.ae
Web: www.skinlaserdubai.com

Founded in 1990, Skin Laser Dubai employs seven full-time staff members who speak English, Arabic, and Hindi-Urdu. Each year the clinic sees approximately 5,000 patients from more than 100 countries, including the US and European nations.

This clinic was one of the first in the Middle East and Asia to offer laser technology for skin treatments. The center now treats cellulite, psoriasis, vitiligo, pigmented lesions (including tattoo removals), unwanted hair, and spider veins with various laser procedures. In addition, the center offers skin filler injections, including Botox, Restylane, and Perlane. Dr. Mahaveer Mehta has performed more than 5,000 laser hair reductions and 5,000 laser skin surgeries.

Oasis Hospital

P.O. Box 1016
Al Ain, Abu Dhabi, UNITED ARAB EMIRATES
Tel: 011 971 3722.1251
Fax: 011 971 3722.2007
Email: hr2@oasishospital.org
Web: www.oasishospital.org

Oasis Hospital is located in Al Ain, the second largest city in the state of Abu Dhabi. Al Ain has been a vital link between the Indian Ocean and the Arabian Gulf for thousands of years due to its strategic position and good water supply.

The hospital started in the 1960s as nothing more than huts constructed from mud and palm branches. No traces of those humble origins remain today. The present hospital building opened in 1990, and a new outpatient clinic was added in 1995. In 2006 a government grant allowed Oasis to plan future construction of new inpatient and outpatient facilities. In 2007 Oasis became the first private hospital in the emirate of Abu Dhabi to receive JCI accreditation.

The hospital delivers about 1,900 babies and treats over 50,000 outpatients annually. Its medical services are especially strong in the area of obstetrics and pediatrics. Oasis also runs outpatient clinics for diabetes, pain management, urology, and minimally invasive surgery.

Tawam Hospital

P.O. Box 15258
Al Ain, UNITED ARAB EMIRATES
Tel: 011 971 3767.7444
Fax: 011 971 3767.7634
Email: webmaster@tawam-hosp.gov.ae
Web: www.tawam-hosp.gov.ae

Tawam Hospital is located 100 miles from the cities of Abu Dhabi and Dubai. The 477-bed center meets the standards of European and North American hospitals, and its nursing care meets or exceeds international standards. The hospital's nursing team is a culturally diverse staff of 900 representing 33 different nationalities. Johns Hopkins International manages Tawam, which earned its JCI accreditation in 2006.

Tawam is a full-service hospital with several specialties (excluding cardiovascular surgery).

The **Department of Oncology** is the cancer referral center for the UAE and other

Gulf States. Established in 2004, the 46-bed department includes hematology, radiology, and palliative care. Nearly half of the rooms are high-efficiency particulate-air (HEPA) filtered. Diagnostic workup is provided for both benign and malignant disorders, including all types of solid tumors and hematological disorders. The medical staff includes more than a dozen oncology specialists.

The **Dental Centre** is a freestanding dental hospital 15 minutes from the main hospital. The center was one of the first dental facilities in the Gulf region to provide a complete implant dentistry service, specializing in one- and two-stage dental implant replacements. Two clinics perform oral and facial surgery. The center employs a total of 120 people, including 16 general dentists and 14 consultants or specialists, representing every clinical dental specialty. The majority of its dentists have Western qualifications or experience. Some have held appointments at American, Canadian, or European universities.

The **Department of Surgery** is the newest medical department at Tawam. It covers all subspecialties except for cardiovascular surgery. The department has six fully equipped operating rooms, and more than 4,000 inpatient and outpatient surgeries are performed each year. Its most common surgical procedures include arthroscopic surgery for knee and hip replacements; ear, nose, and throat (ENT) surgery using endoscopes; prostatic surgery; neurosurgery; and reconstructive surgery, especially to treat burn cases.

Tawam's **Clinical Nutrition Department** offers a unique service in the management of inherited metabolic diseases, such as disorders of amino acid metabolism and fatty acid oxidation.

Zulekha Hospital
P.O. Box 457
Sharjah, UNITED ARAB EMIRATES
Tel: 011 971 6 565.8866
Fax: 011 971 6 565.6699
Email: info@zulekhahospitals.com
Web: www.zulekhahospitals.com

The Zulekha Hospital in Sharjah is one of five healthcare facilities operating under Zulekha management; the others are in Dubai. In business since 1992, this 75-bed hospital is home to 35 doctors and surgeons and boasts a 1:1 nurse-to-patient ratio. More than 400,000 patients have been treated at the Zulekha-Sharjah facility, and 5,000 surgeries have been performed. Specialty units include cardiac care, intensive care, burn treatment, and intensive care for newborns. Each department is headed by a minimum of two specialist physicians. The hospital offers discounted health checkup and corporate packages. Insurance companies can be billed directly, and patients can elect to stay in private or semi-private rooms or VIP suites. Zulekha-Sharjah received JCI accreditation in 2007.

■ RECOVERY ACCOMMODATIONS

Although recovery accommodations are not available in Dubai or Abu Dhabi, the UAE has a number of deluxe and moderately priced hotels.

■ HOTELS: DELUXE

Deluxe hotels in the UAE can be expensive, so make sure to include lodging in your budget plan. Note that the Möevenpick Hotel is directly across the street from American Hospital Dubai.

Möevenpick Hotel Bur Dubai
19th Street, Old Metha Area
P.O. Box 32733
Dubai, UNITED ARAB EMIRATES
Tel: 011 971 4336.6000
Fax: 011 971 4336.6626
Email: hotel.burdubai@moevenpick.com
Web: www.moevenpick-hotels.com

JW Marriott Hotel Dubai
Abu Baker Al Siddique Road
Dubai, UNITED ARAB EMIRATES 16590
Tel: 1 800 228.9290 (US toll-free); 011 971
    4262.4444
Fax: 011 971 4262.6264
Email: marriott@emirates.net.ae
Web: www.marriott.com

Renaissance Dubai Hotel
Salah Al Din Road, Deira
P.O. Box 8668
Dubai, UNITED ARAB EMIRATES
Tel: 1 800 HOTELS.1 (US toll-free); 011 971
    4262.5555
Fax: 011 971 4269.7358
Email: rendubai@emirates.net.ae
Web: www.renaissancehotels.com

Mercure Grand Jebel Hafeet Al Ain
Jebel Hafeet
P.O. Box 244760
Al Ain, UNITED ARAB EMIRATES
Tel: 011 971 3783.8888
Fax: 011 971 3783.9000
Email: resa@mercure-alain.ae
Web: www.mercure.com

Le Méridien Abu Dhabi
Tourist Club Area
Abu Dhabi, UNITED ARAB EMIRATES 46066
Tel: 011 971 2644.6666
Fax: 011 971 2644.0348
Email: lemeridien.abudhabi@lemeridien.com
Web: www.starwoodhotels.com

■ HOTELS: MODERATE

Khalidia Hotel Apartments
Al Maktoum Street
P.O. Box 63890
Dubai, UNITED ARAB EMIRATES
Tel: 011 971 4228.2280
Fax: 011 971 4221.1222
Email: khappt@emirates.net.ae
Web: www.khalidiahotelapartments.ae

Avari Hotel
Deira
P.O. Box 50400
Dubai, UNITED ARAB EMIRATES
Tel: 011 971 4295.6666
Fax: 011 971 4295.9459
Email: info@avari-dubai.co.ae
Web: www.avari.com/avaridubai.htm

Al Massa Hotel
P.O. Box 19483
Al Ain, UNITED ARAB EMIRATES
Tel: 011 971 3762.8884
Fax: 011 971 3762.7500
Email: maasarht@emirates.net.ae

Khalidia Palace Hotel
P.O. Box 4010
Abu Dhabi, UNITED ARAB EMIRATES
Tel: 011 971 2666.2470
Fax: 011 971 2666.0411
Email: kphauh@emirates.net.ae
Web: www.khalidiapalacehotel.ae/home.htm#

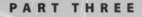

PART THREE

Resources
and References

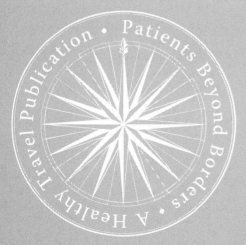

ADDITIONAL RESOURCES

Other Editions of *Patients Beyond Borders*

Each year, Healthy Travel Media publishes new, specialized editions of *Patients Beyond Borders*. Want to know more about Singapore? See the *Patients Beyond Borders: Singapore Edition*. Country-specific volumes are also underway for India, Korea, Malaysia, and Taiwan. A treatment-specific series is coming soon as well, beginning with the *Patients Beyond Borders: Orthopedic Edition*. Visit www.patients beyondborders.com to check on special editions for your destination or treatment.

World, Country, and City Information

The World Factbook. Cataloged by country, *The World Factbook*—compiled by the US Central Intelligence Agency (CIA)—is an excellent source of general, up-to-date information about the geography, economy, and history of countries around the world. Go to www.cia.gov; in the left column, find "Library and Reference," then click on "The World Factbook."

Lonely Planet. This feisty travel book publisher has compiled a collection of useful online snippets (mostly as teasers to get you to buy their books), along with useful links. Go to www.lonelyplanet.com and search for your country of interest to find information on transport, events, and more.

World Travel Guide. The publishers of the *Columbus World Travel Guide* sponsor the Web site www.worldtravelguide .net. The site offers good information on countries and major metropolitan areas throughout the world. Go to the Web site's "Choose Guide" search to find information on airports, tours, attractions, cruises, and more.

World Atlas

Google Earth. If you've not downloaded Google Earth, go there and do so. It's truly one of the wonders of the online world. After you download it, you can zoom to your home's rooftop or "fly" to any continent, country, or city on the planet just by typing in the appropriate keywords. Legends include city names, roads, terrain, populated places, borders, 3-D buildings, and more. Go to http:// earth.google.com/ and follow the download instructions.

Encarta Atlas. Encarta, Microsoft's easy-to-use, free atlas allows you to quickly click your way around the planet, and then obtain information on your country of interest. Go to www.encarta.com and click on the "World Atlas" tab.

Passports and Visas

Travisa. Dozens of online agencies offer visa services. We've found Travisa, at www.travisa.com, to be reliable and accessible by telephone as well. The agency offers good customer service and follow-up. Travisa's Web site also carries information links to immunization requirements, travel warnings, current weather, and more.

Currency Converter

www.xe.com. To learn quickly how much your dollar is worth in your country of interest, go to the www.xe.com homepage and click on "Quick Currency Converter."

International Hospital Accreditation

Joint Commission International. Mentioned frequently throughout this book, the Joint Commission International (JCI) remains the only game in town for international hospital accreditation. For a current list of accredited hospitals by country, go to www.jointcommission international.org/23218/iortiz.

Medical Dictionary

Merriam-Webster's Medical Dictionary. If a multisyllabic medical term stumps you, don't run out and purchase an unabridged brick of a medical dictionary. Several free online medical glossaries provide more than you probably want to know on most health topics. *Merriam-Webster's Medical Dictionary* is provided on a number of sites, including Medline-Plus (http://medlineplus.gov) and InteliHealth (www.intelihealth.com). The simplest access is through http://dictionary.reference.com. Just type in a medical word or phrase and voila! For a richer exploration of a given medical term, sources such as MedicineNet (www.medicinenet.com) offer articles, services, and a thicket of sponsored links.

Medical Information

MedlinePlus is a US-government sponsored medical site that brings together a wealth of information from sources such as the National Library of Medicine (the world's largest medical library), the National Institutes of Health, *Merriam-Webster's Medical Dictionary,* and the *United States Pharmacopeia.* Go to http://medlineplus.gov and click any of the various choices in the left column. The online tour at www.nlm.nih.gov/medlineplus/tour/medlineplustour.html helps you navigate this massive site.

Medical Travel Resources

Medical Tourism Insight is a monthly, online newsletter written for the medical travel industry as well as employers, benefits managers, government officials, and prospective patients. Coverage includes objective and timely information on overseas medical care and related issues, such as health insurance and employee health benefits. The Web site is www.medical tourisminsight.com.

The ***International Medical Travel Journal*** (IMTJ) is the world's leading journal for the medical travel industry. While geared more toward industry professionals than consumers, it does provide a free online guide for potential patients at www.imtjonline.com. There's a free email newsletter, too, and a paid subscription service for those who are serious about industry news.

International Society of Travel Medicine. If you are looking for information about immunizations, infectious diseases, or other aspects of medical travel, check out the Web site of the International Society of Travel Medicine (ISTM) at www.istm.org. This organization maintains offices in Georgia and in Munich, Germany, to promote safe and healthy travel and to facilitate education, service, and research activities in the field of travel medicine. Most useful to the health traveler is the society's searchable database of health travel practitioners.

International Medical Travel Association. Based in Singapore, the International Medical Travel Association (IMTA) and its small but growing membership advocate international patients' rights, quality assurance standards for international hospitals, excellence in continuity of care, and other patient-provider issues. For more information, visit www.intlmta.org.

Beauty from Afar. If you're seeking more specialized information on cosmetic or aesthetic surgery or dental care, author and medical traveler Jeff Schult can fill you in on the main destinations, leading clinics and facilities, and third-party agents. Published in July 2006 (Stewart, Tabori & Chang), this 224-page paperback is written in an anecdotal style, providing numerous first-hand accounts that give prospective patients a thorough perspective on the health travel experience.

Medical Tourism in Developing Countries, by Milica Z. Bookman and Karla R. Bookman (Palgrave Macmillan, 2007), explores the international marketplace for medical services and its dollars-and-cents potential for developing countries. While it's more an academic work than a consumer guide, physicians, administrators, and healthcare officials will find this book's economic perspective and vast bank of data on the industry instructive.

1 888 STAR.012. Star Hospitals (www.starhospitals.net), a North American healthcare service, operates this toll-free call center staffed entirely by medical professionals. Staff members provide potential clients with information and guidance on member hospitals in India, Singapore, and Thailand.

A couple of magazine articles are worth a trip to your local library or an online search to dig up. If you are considering in vitro fertilization, you need to read "How Far Would You Go to Have a Baby?" by Brian Alexander, which appeared in the May 2005 issue of *Glamour.* On broader topics, Jennifer Wolff's "Passport to Cheaper Health Care?" assesses the pros and cons of medical travel. You'll find it in the October 2007 issue of *Good Housekeeping* or online.

Web Resources

Medical Nomad. A group of medical professionals, technology geeks, and consultants established www.medicalnomad.com in 2004 to bring together an impressive body of information, including specific data on treatments, clinics, physicians, accreditation, and other topics of interest to the health traveler. Medical Nomad's extensive database allows readers to search by procedure, provider, and destination, with clinic and country summaries as well as lay summaries of common treatments.

The Google Guide. While you may not wish to become a wild-eyed expert on the nuances of search engines, a little additional knowledge can greatly enhance your efficiency in narrowing your health travel choices. Consultant and Internet search guru Nancy Blachman (co-author of the book *How to Do Everything with Google*) has posted a useful online tutorial entitled "The Google Guide." Go to www.googleguide.com, click on "Novice," and you'll find a wealth of information on conducting Internet searches that will greatly improve your online health travel quests. Most of this information applies to other search engines as well, including Yahoo, MSN, and AOL.

RevaHealth.com is an Internet-based searchable database of healthcare providers. Its unique directory system and powerful search engine allow patients to find detailed information easily. The platform at www.RevaHealth.com also lets patients select providers and talk to them directly for a consultation.

Personal Memoirs

State of the Heart, by Maggi Ann Grace (New Harbinger, 2007), is a nonfiction narrative that describes the odyssey Maggi Grace and Howard Staab undertook when Howard's heart valve suddenly malfunctioned. The local hospital in Durham, North Carolina, estimated $200,000 to fix it, and Howard had no health insurance. Part travelogue, part critique of the US healthcare system, and part medical drama, this memoir describes the couple's frantic search for alternatives to mortgaging the rest of their lives in exchange for Howard's treatment. It covers their trip to the Escorts Heart Institute and Research Center in New Delhi, India, the surgery, and its aftermath. It is also the story of how a woman, alone and consumed with worry, navigated Third World streets clogged with cattle to find such basic necessities as chocolate, pencils, and friendship.

MEDICAL GLOSSARY

Many medical terms are used in this book. The following is a list of the most commonly used terms. For further information, plase consult your doctor.

Acute-care. Providing emergency services and general medical and surgical treatment for sudden severe disorders (as compared with long-term care for chronic illness).

Addiction. Occurs when a person has no control over the use of a substance, such as drugs or alcohol. Also includes addictions to food, gambling, and sex.

Aesthetics. A general term for medical treatments and surgical procedures undertaken to improve appearance. Such procedures include (but are not limited to) facelifts, tummy tucks, laser resurfacing of skin, Botox injection, cosmetic dentistry, and others.

Alzheimer's disease. A degenerative disorder of neurons in the brain that disrupts thought, perception, and behavior.

Anesthesia. Loss of physical sensation produced by sedation. Anesthesia may be given as (1) general, which affects the entire body and is accompanied by loss of consciousness; (2) regional, affecting an entire area of the body; and (3) local, which affects a limited part of the body (usually superficial).

Angiography. An x-ray procedure that uses dye injected into the coronary arteries to study circulation in the heart.

Angioplasty. A procedure that uses a tiny balloon on the end of a catheter to widen blocked or constricted arteries in the heart.

Arthroscopy or arthroscopic surgery. The use of a tubelike instrument utilizing fiber optics to examine, treat, or perform surgery on a joint.

Bariatric. Pertaining to the control and treatment of obesity and allied diseases.

Birmingham hip resurfacing (BHR). A metal-on-metal hip replacement system, surgically implanted to replace a hip joint. The BHR is called a resurfacing prosthesis because only the surface of the femoral head (ball) is removed to implant the femoral head-resurfacing component.

Bone densitometry. A method of measuring bone strength, used to diagnose osteoporosis.

Botox. A nonsurgical, physician-administered injection treatment to temporarily reduce moderate to severe wrinkles on the face.

Cardiac. Pertaining to the heart.

Cardiac catheterization. The insertion of a catheter into the arteries of the heart to diagnose heart disease. See also **angiography.**

Cardiothoracic. Of or relating to the heart and the chest.

Cardiovascular. Pertaining to the heart and blood vessels that comprise the circulatory system. See also **vascular surgery.**

Cataract. Cloudiness of the lens in the eye, which affects vision. Cataracts, which often occur in older people, can be corrected with surgery to replace the damaged lens with an artificial plastic lens known as an intraocular lens (IOL).

Colonoscopy. An examination of the interior of the colon, using a thin, lighted tube (called a colonoscope) inserted into the rectum.

Computed tomography (CT). Sometimes known as CAT scan. A noninvasive diagnostic tool that uses x-rays to provide cross-sectional images of the body. Used to detect cancer, determine heart function, and provide images of body organs. May be used in conjunction with **positron emission tomography (PET).**

Coronary artery bypass graft (CABG). Surgical procedure to create alternative paths for blood to flow around obstructions in the coronary arteries, most often using arteries or veins from other parts of the body.

Cosmetic surgery. Plastic surgery undertaken to improve appearance. See also **plastic surgery.**

Craniofacial. Relating to the head and face.

CyberKnife. A tool for radiosurgery that delivers precise high-dose radiation to a tumor. Can be used for tumors of the pancreas, liver, and lungs.

Diabetes. A chronic disease characterized by abnormally high levels of sugar in the blood.

Discectomy. Removal of all or part of an intervertebral disc (a soft structure that acts as a shock absorber between two bones in the back).

Electrocardiogram (EKG or ECG). A diagnostic test that measures the heart's electrical activity.

Endocrinology. The branch of medicine that studies hormonal systems and treats disorders that arise when hormones are out of balance.

Endoscope. A slender, tubular optical instrument used as a viewing system for examining an inner part of the body and, with an attached instrument, for performing surgery or detecting tumors.

Extracorporeal shock wave therapy (ESWT). A noninvasive treatment that involves delivery of shock waves to a painful area.

Gamma Knife. A form of radiation therapy that focuses low-dose gamma radiation on a precise target, such as a tumor of the brain or breast.

Gastroenterology. The branch of medicine that studies and treats disorders of the digestive system.

Genetics. The study of inheritance.

Gynecology. The branch of medicine that studies and treats females, especially as related to their reproductive system.

Hematology. The study of the nature, function, and diseases of the blood and of blood-forming organs.

Hemopoietic or hematopoietic. Pertaining to the formation of blood.

Hepatitis. Inflammation of the liver caused by a virus or toxin. There are different forms of viral hepatitis. Vaccines are available for hepatitis A and B. There is no vaccine for hepatitis C.

Hepatobiliary. Relating to the bile ducts.

Hepatology. The branch of medicine that studies and treats disorders of the liver.

Holter monitor. A wearable electronic device used to obtain a continuous recording of the heart's electrical activity. See **electrocardiogram.**

Immunization. Inoculation with a vaccine to render a person resistant to a disease.

Immunology. The branch of medicine that studies and treats disorders of the body's mechanisms for fighting disease, especially infectious diseases.

Implant. *In dentistry:* a small metal pin placed inside the jawbone to mimic the root of a tooth. Dental implants can be used to help anchor a false tooth, a crown, or a bridge. *In fertility treatment:* to place an embryo in the uterus.

Intensive Care Unit (ICU). The ward in a hospital where 24-hour specialized nursing and monitoring are provided for patients who are critically ill or have undergone major surgical procedures.

International Organization for Standardization (ISO). An organization based in Geneva, Switzerland, that approves and accredits the facilities and administrations of hospitals and clinics, but not their practices, procedures, or methods.

Intracytoplasmic sperm injection (ICSI). A type of fertility treatment in which a single sperm cell is inserted into an egg using special micromanipulation equipment.

Intrauterine insemination (IUI). Introduction of prepared sperm (either the male partner's or a donor's) into the uterus to improve chances of pregnancy.

In vitro fertilization (IVF). Known as the test-tube baby technique. Eggs are fertilized outside the body, and then embryos are introduced back into the woman's uterus.

Joint Commission International (JCI). The international affiliate accreditation agency of the Joint Commission, which inspects and accredits healthcare providers worldwide using US-based standards.

Laparoscope. A thin, lighted tube used to examine and treat tissues and organs inside the abdomen.

LAP-BAND System. An adjustable silicone band inserted laparoscopically around the upper part of the stomach, thereby reducing the food storage area of the stomach and promoting weight loss.

LASIK (laser-assisted *in situ* keratomileusis). A laser procedure to reduce dependency on eyeglasses or contact lenses by permanently changing the shape of the cornea, the clear covering of the front of the eye.

Liposuction. The surgical withdrawal of fat from under the skin, using a small incision and vacuum suctioning.

Lithotripsy. A procedure that breaks up kidney stones or gallstones using sound waves. Also called extracorporeal shock wave lithotripsy (ESWL).

Magnetic resonance imaging (MRI). A noninvasive diagnostic tool that produces clear images of the human body without the use of x-rays. MRI, which uses a large magnet, radio waves, and a computer, is used to diagnose spine and joint problems, heart disease, and cancer.

Mammography. X-ray imaging of the breast for detection of cancer.

Maxillofacial. Of or pertaining to the jaws and face.

Microsurgical epididymal sperm aspiration (MESA). Obtaining immature sperm cells from the epididymis (which joins the testicle to the vas deferens), in cases where obstruction in the genital tract leads to absence of sperm in the ejaculate. The recovered sperm can be used for intracytoplasmic sperm injection (ICSI).

Minimally invasive surgery. Any of a variety of approaches used to reduce the trauma of surgery and to speed recovery. These approaches include "keyhole" surgery, endoscopy, arthroscopy, laparoscopy, or the use of small incisions.

Myocardial infarction. Heart attack.

Neonatology. The branch of medicine specializing in the care and treatment of newborns.

Nephrology. The medical specialty that deals with the kidneys.

Neurology. The branch of medicine that studies and treats disorders of the nervous system, including the brain.

Neuro-oncology. The branch of medicine that studies and treats cancers of the nervous system.

Neuro-ophthalmology. The branch of medicine that studies and treats disorders of the nerves in the eye.

Neurosurgery. Surgery on the brain or other parts of the nervous system.

Obstetrics. The branch of medicine focusing on pregnancy and childbirth.

Oncology. The branch of medicine that studies and treats cancer.

Ophthalmology. The branch of medicine that studies and treats disorders of the eye.

Orthodontics. The branch of dentistry dealing with the prevention and correction of irregular tooth positioning, as by means of braces.

Orthopedics. The branch of medicine that studies and treats diseases and injuries of the bones and joints.

Osteoporosis. Thinning of the bones and reduction in bone mass, which increases the risk of fractures and decreases mobility, especially in the elderly.

Otolaryngology. The branch of medicine that studies and treats ear, nose, and throat disorders.

Pacemaker. An electronic device surgically implanted into a patient's chest to regulate the heartbeat.

Parkinson's disease. A movement disorder most common among the elderly.

Pathology. The branch of medicine that focuses on the laboratory-based study of disease in cells and tissues, as opposed to clinical examination of symptoms.

Pediatric. Of or pertaining to children.

Periodontics. The branch of dentistry dealing with the study and treatment of diseases of the bones, connective tissues, and gums surrounding and supporting the teeth.

Physiotherapy or physical therapy. The treatment or management of physical disability, malfunction, or pain by exercise, massage, hydrotherapy, and other techniques without the use of drugs, surgery, or radiation.

Plastic surgery. The branch of medicine focusing on corrective operations to the face, head, and body to restore function and (sometimes) to improve appearance (also called cosmetic surgery).

Polio (poliomyelitis). A paralyzing disease caused by a virus and characterized by inflammation of the motor neurons of the brain stem and spinal cord.

Positron emission tomography (PET). Also known as PET imaging or PET scan. A diagnostic tool that captures images of the human body by detecting positrons or tiny particles from radioactive material. Used to detect cancer and determine heart function; used most recently as an early clue to Alzheimer's. May be used in conjunction with **computed tomography (CT)**.

Prosthodontics. The branch of dentistry that deals with replacing of missing teeth and other oral structures with artificial devices.

Psychiatry. The branch of medicine that studies and treats mental disorders.

Radiofrequency ablation. The use of electrodes to generate heat and destroy abnormal tissue.

Radiology. The branch of medicine dealing with capturing and interpreting images, such as x-rays, CT scans, and MRI scans.

Radiosurgery. The use of ionizing radiation, either from an external source (such as an x-ray machine) or an implant, to destroy cancerous or diseased tissue.

Radiotherapy. Treatment of disease with radiation, especially by selective irradiation with x-rays or other ionizing radiation or by ingestion or implantation of radioisotopes.

Reconstructive surgery. The branch of surgery dealing with the repair or replacement of malformed, injured, or lost organs or tissues of the body, chiefly by the transplant of living tissues.

Rehabilitation. The process of restoring health and improving functioning.

Renal. Relating to the kidneys.

Rheumatology. The branch of medicine that studies and treats disorders characterized by pain and stiffness afflicting the extremities or back.

Stem cell. An unspecialized or undifferentiated cell that can become specialized to perform the functions of diverse tissues in the body.

Stent. A tube inserted into a blood vessel or duct to keep it open. Stents are sometimes inserted into narrowed coronary arteries to help keep them open after balloon angioplasty.

Tertiary care. Care of a highly specialized nature.

Testicular epididymal sperm aspiration (TESA). A surgical procedure to obtain sperm from within the testicular tissue.

Transplant. *Organ transplant:* the surgical insertion of an organ from a donor (living or deceased) into a patient to replace an organ that is diseased or malfunctioning; transplants are available for heart, liver, lungs, pancreas, kidney, cornea, and some other organs. *Stem cell transplant:* a procedure in which stem cells are collected from the blood of the patient (autologous) or a matched donor (allergenic) and then reinserted into the patient to rebuild the immune system. *Bone marrow transplant:* a procedure that places healthy bone marrow from the patient (autograft) or a donor (allograft) into a patient whose bone marrow is damaged or malfunctioning.

Typhoid. An infectious, potentially fatal intestinal disease caused by bacteria and usually transmitted in food or water.

Ultrasound. The use of high-frequency sound waves in therapy or diagnostics, as in the deep-heat treatment of a joint or in the imaging of internal structures.

Urology. The branch of medicine that studies and treats urinary tract infections (UTIs) and other disorders of the urinary system.

Vascular surgery. The branch of medicine focusing on the diagnosis and surgical treatment of disorders of the blood vessels, excluding the heart, lungs, and brain.

Wellness. An area of preventive medicine that promotes health and well-being though various means, such as diet, exercise, yoga, tai chi, social support, and more.

X-rays. A form of electromagnetic radiation, similar to light but of shorter wavelength, which can penetrate solids; used for imaging solid structures inside the body.

INDEX

Specific treatments are in *italics*. Hospital names are in **bold**. The main discussion of each health travel agency is listed first with the page number in **bold**. Main treatment categories are indexed; specific treatments may be found in the text.

A

accommodations. *See* hotels; recovery accommodations
accreditation, hospital, 23–24, 61, 63–64, 170, 191–192, 391
Acibadem Healthcare Group, 373–374
addiction recovery, Antigua and Barbados, 202
Aesthetic Plastic Surgery Institute, 296
aftercare protocol. *See* post-treatment care
agents. *See* health travel agents; health travel planners
air travel
  airport transportation, 85
  arrival challenges, 168
  booking ahead, 38–39
  budgeting for, 76–77, 83
  and deep vein thrombosis, 142–143, 161–162
  health travel planner's help with, 51, 76–77
  wheelchair assistance, 77
Albert Einstein Jewish Hospital, 211
alcohol, 162
Al-Essra Hospital, 280
Alexandra Hospital, 326
all-in-one package deals, 107–108
American Hospital Dubai, 378–379
Anadolu Medical Center, 374

Angel's Touch Dental Clinic, 300–301
anticoagulants, 161
Antigua and Barbados, 201–205
Apollo Dental Centre, 258
Apollo Hospital/Chennai, 258
arbitration, 159
Artemis Health Institute, 245–246
Ascot Hospital, 306–307
Asian Heart Institute and Research Center, 265
Asian Hospital and Medical Center, 316
Assaf Harofeh Medical Center, 273
Assuta Hospital I.V.F. Center, 276
ATM cards/machines, 123, 180
Australian Council of Healthcare Standards, 64

B

Bair's Eye Clinic, 349–350
Baja Oral Center, 296
Bangkok Dental Group, 365
Bangkok Hospital Medical Center, 359–361
Bangkok Hotel Phuket, 366
Bangkok International Dental Center, 365
Bangkok Nursing Home Hospital, 361
banking, 122–124, 180
Barbados. *See* Antigua and Barbados
Barbados Fertility Centre, 204
bariatric surgery. See weight loss surgery
Bay View Private Hospital, 336–337
Beauty in Prague, **226–227**
BestMed Journeys, **263**
birth control pills, 161
blood clots, 142–143, 161–162
blues, home again, 147–148
booking air travel and accommodations, 76–77
Brazil, 206–213
BridgeHealth International, **216**, 357, 372
brokers. *See* health travel planners
Budget Planner form, 90–93

New Titles in the *Patients Beyond Borders* Series

Patients Beyond Borders

For the most current information on books in the *Patients Beyond Borders* Series, please visit www.patientsbeyondborders.com.

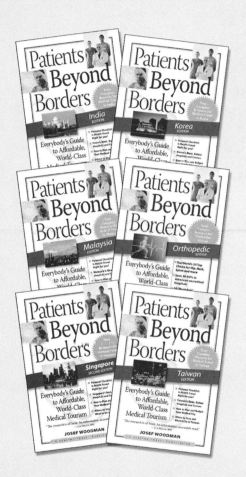

ABOUT THE AUTHOR

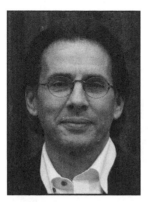

As President of Healthy Travel Media, **Josef Woodman** has spent more than three years touring 100 medical facilities in 14 countries, researching contemporary medical tourism. As co-founder of MyDailyHealth and Ventana Communications, Woodman's pioneering background in health, wellness, and Web technology has allowed him to compile a wealth of information about global health travel, telemedicine, and new developments in consumer and institutional medical care. Woodman has lectured at the UCLA School of Public Health and Harvard Medical School, and has conducted seminars and workshops in a dozen countries. He serves on the Advisory Board of the Global Healthcare Summit and as Program Co-Chairman of the Global Healthcare Congress. Woodman has emerged as an outspoken advocate of global consumer healthcare and medical travel.